Color Atlas and Text of

NEUROPATHOLOGY

David I. Graham

MBBCH PHD FRCPATH FRCPSG FRSE

Professor, Department of Neuropathology
Institute of Neurological Sciences
Southern General Hospital
Glasgow, UK

Jeanne E. Bell

MBCHB MD MRCPATH

Consultant Neuropathologist
Neuropathology Laboratory
University of Edinburgh
Western General Hospital
Edinburgh, UK

James W. Ironside

BMSC (HONS) MBCHB MRCPATH

Consultant Neuropathologist
Neuropathology Laboratory
University of Edinburgh
Western General Hospital
Edinburgh, UK

Mosby-Wolfe

London Baltimore Barcelona Bogotá Boston Buenos Aires Caracas Carlsbad, CA Chicago Madrid Mexico City Milan Naples, FL New York
Philadelphia St. Louis Seoul Singapore Sydney Taipei Tokyo Toronto Wiesbaden

Published in 1995 by Mosby-Wolfe, an imprint of Times Mirror International Publishers Limited.

Printed and bound by Grafos S. A. Arte Sobre Papel, Barcelona, Spain.

ISBN 0 7234 1954-X

For full details of all Times Mirror International Publishers Limited titles, please write to Times Mirror International Publishers Limited, Lynton House, 7–12 Tavistock Square, London WC1H 9LB, England.

A CIP catalogue record for this book is available from the British Library.

Library of Congress Cataloging-in-Publication Data Applied for.

Project Manager: Alison Taylor

Layout Artist: Lindy van den Berghe

Cover Design: Pete Wilder

Illustration: Richard Prime

Production: Jane Tozer

Index: Nina Boyd

Publisher: Fiona Foley

Contents

Foreword

The subject of neuropathology is well endowed with reference textbooks that cover the subject matter of neurological disease in a comprehensive and systematic fashion. Many of these texts, however, are too detailed for non-specialists who require a more conceptual understanding of the various disease processes afflicting the nervous system. It is difficult also for standard textbooks to remain entirely up-to-date given the rapid explosion of knowledge in recent years as a result of developments in cellular and molecular biology and the new imaging technologies.

The authors of this Atlas have set themselves the rather formidable task of bridging the gap between the standard reference textbook in neuropathology and the more pragmatic requirements of physicians engaged in training in pathology and their contemporaries in the cognate clinical specialities. Whenever possible, the authors have embraced the new developments in neurobiology and imaging techniques, although they have taken the positive decision to limit this to those most relevant to clinical practice. The end-product is a treatise that is easy to read, highly informative and extremely well illustrated. It combines an account of the anatomical basis and general principles of neurological disease with a more systematic but concise description of the specific disease entities affecting the nervous system. The *Color Atlas and Text of Neuropathology* provides a most useful adjunct to standard textbooks and will be of considerable value to those working and training in clinical neurosciences. The authors are to be congratulated on such a successful outcome to a most difficult task.

Colin C Bird
MBChB PhD FRCPath FRCPE FRSE
Professor of Pathology
University of Edinburgh
Edinburgh, UK

Preface

Originally conceived as a second edition of the *Colour Atlas of Neuropathology,* written by Dr C. S. Treip, it soon became apparent that the requirements of the principal readers of this Atlas had changed considerably since 1978 when the first edition was published. Discussion with pathologists in training and with neurologists, neurosurgeons and psychiatrists, who have rather specialised requirements, had indicated the need for a concise but comprehensive text of neuropathology that was well illustrated and which covered most of the conditions commonly encountered in the clinical neurosciences.

This Atlas is not intended either as a practical manual of diagnostic neuropathology or a comprehensive account of the many diseases that afflict the brain and spinal cord. Rather, the book provides basic information about many of the more important of these disorders. Many of the figures are recently acquired from our own material but we also searched the neuropathology archives in Edinburgh and Glasgow in order to find the best and most appropriate illustrations. Fortunately this task has not been too difficult because of the meticulous care taken by our predecessors Drs A. Gordon, J. F. Maloney and Professor J. H. Adams, respectively, to establish a comprehensive photographic collection in their departments. Because of the changed circumstances in which neuropathology is practiced today, many of the illustrations are quite unique and record a range of material which is simply not immediately available. Therefore, it is with great pleasure that we dedicate this Atlas and Text to our mentors without whom this work would not have been possible.

It is not possible to achieve a true understanding of neuropathology without having some knowledge of the anatomy and normal histology of the nervous system and the way in which the brain and spinal cord react to various disease processes. This information, together with guidance on the way in which neuropathology is practiced, is contained within chapters 1 and 2. The remaining chapters are devoted to the main features of specific diseases and disorders, many of which are illustrated comprehensively. Because each chapter provides only essential information, this Atlas and Text is intended to complement the many excellent reference books that exist on neuropathology. A guide towards further reading is given at the end of each chapter.

Although much of the material used in this Atlas and Text has been taken from the current and archival collection in our departments, there are certain disorders for which suitable illustrative material has been difficult to obtain. Therefore, we are particularly grateful to friends and colleagues who have provided material for inclusion in this book. Particular thanks go to Professor H. Goebel (Figures 8.17, 8.20, 8.22, 8.28, 8.39), Drs P. Piltz (Figure 5.23), Dr A. J. Franks, Dr J. M. MacKenzie, Dr Christine M. L Smith, Professor S. Lucas, Dr W. R. Timperley and Mr C. Turner for their contributions and to Dr Jean Keeling for some of the illustrations in the chapter on congenital and perinatal disorders. Figure 6.12 is reproduced from *General and Systematic Pathology* by kind permission of Professor J. C. E. Underwood (editor) and Churchill Livingstone. We are also very pleased to acknowledge the technical expertise of Mr W. M. Shade and Mr F. Donnelly (Edinburgh) and Mr L. Miller (Glasgow) and their staff for having prepared suitable material for photography.

Particular thanks are given to Mrs Helen Boyd, Mrs Sheena Graham and Mr Roddy Melrose for their untiring secretarial assistance.

Finally, and by no means least, at times when the task of completing this Atlas and Text seemed almost beyond reach, our thanks go to Fiona Foley and Alison Taylor from Mosby-Wolfe Publishing for their constant encouragement and support.

David I. Graham
Jeanne E. Bell
James W. Ironside

1. Anatomical Basis of Clinical Signs and Symptoms and Autopsy Techniques

Neuropathology is a specialised branch of histopathology, concerned with the diagnosis and understanding of disease processes in the brain, spinal cord, peripheral nerve and muscle. It is closely allied to the cognate disciplines of clinical neurology and neurosurgery, as well as to psychiatry. There are also very close links with paediatric and forensic medicine, with neuropathology being a bridge between these clinical disciplines and the basic neurosciences.

To understand the pathology of the central nervous system (CNS), it is important to have basic knowledge of the normal structure, function and metabolism of the CNS and of the basic signs and symptoms of disease. It is also important to be able to integrate the information derived from specialised investigations, such as in neuroradiology and neurophysiology.

In recent years, the localisation and characterisation of lesions *in vivo* has been greatly improved by the advent of high-resolution computed tomographic (CT) scanning, magnetic resonance imaging (MRI) and spectroscopy (MRS), single photon emission computed tomography (SPECT) and proton emission tomography (PET). These advances have been paralleled by the application of modern laboratory methods, such as neurochemistry, molecular genetics and molecular biological techniques. Nevertheless, accurate clinicopathological correlation still relies on traditional methods, such as the examination of cerebrospinal fluid (CSF), microscopy of biopsy specimens, and autopsies. These methods remain the cornerstone of clinical neuropathology.

ANATOMICAL BASIS OF CLINICAL SIGNS AND SYMPTOMS

Until recently, the precise anatomical localisation of symptoms and signs was based on clinicopathological correlations. However, with the development of functional and structural imaging, it has been found that the concepts of localisation are not always correct, and that some tasks have such a complex functional integration that precise clinical localisation is not possible. The following account provides a summary of the present understanding of the principal functional correlations of the cerebral cortex, thalamus, hypothalamus and pituitary gland, basal ganglia, brainstem, cerebellum and spinal cord.

CEREBRAL CORTEX

The two cerebral hemispheres can each be divided into the frontal, parietal, temporal and occipital lobes. According to studies of patients with lateralised hemisphere disease, one of the cerebral hemispheres is the major or dominant hemisphere. This is usually the left hemisphere, which is dominant in all right-handed and approximately 95% of left handed persons. Verbal linguistic, calculating and analytical functions reside in the dominant hemisphere, while visual, spatial and perceptual skills are located in the non-dominant hemisphere. The degree of disability and the symptomatology occurring in cortical disease varies, being influenced by the nature of the disease and its speed of progression, and the plasticity of the cerebral hemisphere.

Frontal lobe disease

The principal symptoms are listed in **1.1**. The motor cortex lies immediately in front of the central sulcus. This is the point at which the areas subservient to movement in the face, arm and trunk are represented on the lateral surface of the hemisphere, and to move-

Symptoms and signs of frontal lobe disease	
Contralateral hemiplegia	Expressive dysphasia when Broca's area is diseased in a dominant hemisphere
Frontal incontinence	Behavioural disturbances due to involvement of prefrontal areas (apathy, akinetic mutism, emotional lability)
Primitive reflexes (snout, grasp)	
Apraxia of gait	Due to damage to corpus callosum

1.1 Symptoms and signs of frontal lobe disease.

ment in the leg on the medial surface. Certain functions, such as hand or lip movements, have the greatest area of representation, in contrast to the movement of a large joint which is only represented by a small amount of cortical area.

If damage is maximal on the medial surface of the frontal lobe, e.g. following occlusion of an anterior cerebral artery, there will be paralysis of the leg, but sparing of the trunk, upper limb and face. In contrast, if mainly the lateral surface of a frontal lobe is affected, e.g. following occlusion of the middle cerebral artery, the reverse will be true. The face or trunk will show paralysis, while the leg will be relatively spared.

Unilateral disease is usually caused by cerebrovascular disease or tumours, while bilateral disease is usually due to a large midline tumour, hydrocephalus, neurodegenerative disease, or complications of a saccular aneurysm on the anterior communicating artery.

Parietal lobe disease

The principal symptoms and signs are listed in **1.2**. The main sensory cortex lies behind the central sulcus and has a similar topography and representation to the motor cortex. Unilateral disease is usually due to cerebrovascular disease, tumour, or abscess. Bilateral disease is less common and usually caused by an infarction in the arterial boundary zones.

Temporal lobe disease

The principal symptoms and signs are listed in **1.3**. The temporal lobe is made up of a lateral cortex, buried insular cortex and the deep limbic lobe, which includes part of the rhinencephalon, hippocampus and associated structures. Unilateral disease may be due to cerebrovascular disease, tumour, or an abscess from middle-ear disease, while bilateral disease may be caused by herpes simplex virus encephalitis, vascular disease, metabolic disease such as in Wernicke's encephalopathy, or Alzheimer's disease.

Symptoms and signs of parietal lobe disease
Contralateral loss of discriminatory sensation
Receptive dysphasia due to involvement of dominant hemisphere
Impaired calculation
Impaired handwriting
Impaired ability to read
Loss of body image and spatial orientation due to involvement of non-dominant hemisphere
Visual disturbances if optic radiation is affected

1.2 Symptoms and signs of parietal lobe disease.

Symptoms and signs of temporal lobe disease
Receptive dysphasia if dominant hemisphere affected
Cortical deafness (rare)
Limbic system disease may result in memory loss and aggressive or antisocial behaviour
Upper homonymous quadrantanopia if optic radiation is damaged
Epilepsy with memory disturbance, déja vu or jamais vu, transient hallucinations of smell and taste and formed visual hallucinations

1.3 Symptoms and signs of temporal lobe disease.

Symptoms and signs of occipital lobe disease
Unilateral cortical lesion produces loss of vision in homonymous fields
Cortical blindness occurs with extensive bilateral lesions of striate cortex
Visual hallucinations
Visual agnosia

1.4 Symptoms and signs of occipital lobe disease.

Occipital lobe disease

The principal symptoms and signs are listed in **1.4**. The occipital lobe is concerned with the perception of vision (the visual cortex) and its interpretation (the parastriate cortex).

Signs and symptoms often develop as a result of cerebrovascular disease within the distribution of the vertebrobasilar arteries and their principal branches, the posterior cerebral arteries.

Thalamic disease

The principal symptoms and signs are listed in **1.5**. The thalami are a pair of masses of grey matter, which lie in the upper part of the lateral wall of the third ventricle.

Each thalamus has four regions: anterior, posterior, medial and lateral. The efferent connections project to the frontal lobes, hypothalamus, cingulate gyrus, medial parietal cortex, and subfrontal cortex. The afferent connections are received from the mamillary bodies, hippocampus, frontal lobes, amygdala, hypothalamus, basal ganglia and sensory afferent pathways.

Thalamic syndromes are often due to cerebrovascular disease and rarely to fatal familial insomnia—a type of prion disease (*see Chapter 7*).

DISEASE OF THE HYPOTHALAMUS AND PITUITARY GLAND

The hypothalamus lies in the lateral wall of the third ventricle, and is connected to the reticular formation of the midbrain (alertness), the limbic system (behaviour and memory), and the autonomic nuclei of the brainstem and spinal cord. The precise localisation of function to specific areas of the hypothalamus is uncertain, but to a large extent the hypothalamus controls the release of hormones from the anterior pituitary gland, body temperature, fluid balance, circadian rhythm and reproductive function. Broadly speaking, involvement of the hypothalamus results in one of four syndromes (**1.6**). Damage may result from trauma, vascular disease or tumour. The symptoms and signs of anterior pituitary gland lesions are often due to either decreased or increased production of hormones (**1.7**). In most instances, an adenoma is the usual cause of hormonal hypersecretion (*see Chapter 10*). However, some adenomas act simply as space-occupying masses, and the first signs of their presence are related to the effects of their mass. These include a raised intracranial pressure or visual field defects, particularly bitemporal hemianopia, caused by pressure upon the optic chiasm.

Symptoms and signs of thalamic disease	
Anterior thalamic region	If in dominant hemisphere, may cause dysphasia, inattention and memory impairment May cause a movement disorder of contralateral limbs (hemiballismus)
Dorsomedial thalamic region	Recent memory loss Apathy and agitation Impaired attention Sleep abnormalities, particularly insomnia
Ventrolateral thalamic region	Contralateral sensory loss
Posterior thalamic region	Hemianaesthesia or contralateral sensory loss Visual field loss Pain (anaesthesia dolorosa)

1.5 Symptoms and signs of thalamic disease.

Symptoms and signs of disease of the hypothalamus and pituitary gland	
Anterior hypothalamus	Cachexia Diabetes insipidus Hypothermia
Posterior hypothalamus	Hypothermia Apathy Coma
Medial hypothalamus	Excessive water intake Inappropriate antidiuretic hormone secretion Obesity Memory impairment Aggression
Lateral hypothalamus	Reduced water intake Dehydration Emaciation Apathy

1.6 Symptoms and signs of disease of the hypothalamus and pituitary gland.

DISEASE OF THE BASAL GANGLIA

The main symptoms and signs are given in **1.8**. These periventricular masses of grey matter lie anterior to the thalami and include the corpus striatum (putamen and caudate nucleus), substantia nigra, globus pallidus, and subthalamic nuclei. The basal ganglia are responsible for the control and modulation of movements and the maintenance of posture.

DISEASE OF THE BRAINSTEM

This is classically divided into the midbrain, pons and medulla. Each region contains cranial nerve nuclei and ascending and descending pathways. The principal structures in the midbrain include the colliculi, cerebral peduncles, third and fourth cranial nerve nuclei and the medial longitudinal fasciculus. As well as the principal symptoms and signs of contralateral spastic hemiplegia, diplopia and impairment of vertical eye movements, and convergence, there are three distinctive midbrain syndromes (**1.9**). The pons is linked to the cerebellum by the anterior and middle cerebellar peduncles, and contains the VIIth and VIIIth cranial nerve nuclei, and the medial longitudinal fasciculus. There are four principal pontine syndromes (**1.10**). In the lower part of the brainstem, there is the medulla oblongata, which contains part of the fourth ventricle. As well as the sensory and

Symptoms and signs of increased pituitary gland activity	
Growth hormone	Gigantism in children Acromegaly in adults
Prolactin	Delayed puberty in children Amenorrhoea, galactorrhoea and infertility in adult women Impotence and infertility in adult men
Thyrotrophin	Hyperthyroidism
Luteinising and follicle-stimulating hormones	Precocious puberty in children Infertility, hypogonadism and polycystic ovary syndrome in adults

1.7 Symptoms and signs of increased pituitary activity.

Types of movement disorder associated with basal ganglia disorders	
Chorea	Brief involuntary jerk-like movements or fidgeting Classically seen in Huntington's disease but may also occur in metabolic and drug-induced disorders Usually due to disease of the caudate nucleus or putamen
Athetosis	Slow writhing movements Seen in Wilson's disease and perinatal hypoxia Due to disease in cortex, globus pallidus or substantia nigra
Dystonia	Sustained muscle contractions with a twisting and repetitive nature Disease of contralateral basal ganglia
Hemiballismus	Violent flinging or flailing movements Due to lesions in the contralateral subthalamic nucleus
Tremor	In Parkinson's disease, tremor occurs at rest, is coarse and associated with rigidity and paucity of movement

1.8 Types of movement disorder associated with disorders of the basal ganglia.

Midbrain syndromes	
Weber's syndrome	Ipsilateral IIIrd nerve palsy and contralateral hemiplegia
Benedikt's syndrome	Tremor, ipsilateral IIIrd nerve palsy and contralateral cerebellar signs
Parinaud's syndrome	Impairment of upward gaze and convergence

1.9 Midbrain syndromes.

motor long tracts, it also contains the 11th and 12th cranial nerve nuclei, and the vital centres involved in respiration and control of the heart. Several syndromes have been recognised (**1.11**).

As well as vascular disease, other pathologies in the posterior cranial fossa may affect the brainstem, e.g. tumours arising in the posterior fossa or the cerebellopontine angle.

DISEASE OF THE CEREBELLUM

Connected to the pons and medulla by the paired cerebellar peduncles, the cerebellum consists of two large hemispheres and a small unpaired medial portion called the vermis. The function of the cerebellum is to modulate motor activity, controlling and coordinating movements and maintaining stance, posture and gait. The main symptom of cerebellar disease is ataxia, which is characterised by:

- difficulty in performing rapid tasks with the limbs;
- unsteadiness of the feet while walking;
- walking and turning with the feet placed widely apart

Slurring of speech (dysarthria) and tremor and nystagmus may also occur. A variety of specific syndromes are recognised (**1.12**), and may occur as part of a developmental abnormality, vascular disease, tumour, multiple sclerosis, degenerative disorders or a non-metastatic manifestation of an occult tumour.

DISEASE OF THE SPINAL CORD

The spinal cord extends from the base of the skull, where it is continuous with the medulla, to the first lumbar vertebra, below which it is connected to the sacrococcygeal region by the filum terminale. The major ascending tracts carry sensation to the cerebellum, thalamus and cerebral cortex. Some of the fibres terminate in the dorsal horn, before crossing over to form the lateral and anterior spinothalamic

Pontine syndromes	
Dorsolateral	Ipsilateral Horner's syndrome is associated with contralateral loss of pain and temperature from limbs and body, as well as ipsilateral cerebellar ataxia, impaired lateral ocular gaze, deafness and nystagmus
Paramedian	VIth and VIIth cranial nerve palsies, and loss of touch and contralateral proprioception
Basilar	If unilateral, this results in contralateral hemiplegia and VIth and VIIth nerve palsies
Bilateral disease	Will result in quadriplegia

1.10 Pontine syndromes.

Medulla oblongata syndromes	
Dorsolateral	Also known as Wallenberg's syndrome or lateral medullary syndrome Ipsilateral Horner's syndrome with contralateral loss of pain and temperature perception; ipsilateral loss of facial sensation; vertigo and vomiting; ipsilateral ataxia and palsies of XIth and XIIth cranial nerves
Paramedian	If bilateral, the result is the 'locked-in' syndrome in which the patient is quadriplegic and unable to communicate, though fully conscious

1.11 Medulla oblongata syndromes.

Cerebellar syndromes	
Anterior	Patient walks with a broadened gait but with coordinated limbs, and without speech disturbance or abnormal ocular movements
Posterior	The gait is profoundly disturbed, with an inability to stand without swaying
Hemispheric	Unilateral disease results in a lack of coordination of ipsilateral limbs, unsteadiness of gait, slurring of speech or dysarthria, and nystagmus
Pancerebellar	Marked disturbance of gait and balance, ataxia in all limbs, altered ocular movements and dysarthria

1.12 Cerebellar syndromes.

tracts, which carry the sensations of pain, temperature and light touch. Other fibres in the dorsal roots pass into the dorsal horns, and then ascend in the posterior column to end in the nucleus gracilis and nucleus cuneatus. They decussate within the medulla to form the medial lemnisci which then pass to the thalamus and on to the primary sensory cortex. These fibres carry the sensations of vibration, weight, proprioception and pressure.

The major descending pathway is the corticospinal tract, which arises predominantly from the primary motor cortex, and passes down through the internal capsule into the cerebral peduncle of the midbrain, and thence into the basis of the pons, with projections to the motor cranial nerves. It then descends to the pyramidal decussation in the lower part of the medulla, and then passes on to the ventral horn cells of the spinal cord.

Spinal cord disease tends to result in a combination of motor, sensory, and autonomic dysfunction. Localisation to a specific level requires knowledge of the segmental innervation of limb reflexes, the level of decussation of the spinothalamic fibres, and the assessment of motor and sensory levels. The history and clinical examination may help to distinguish extrinsic extramedullary lesions from intrinsic or intramedullary ones. A complete transection of the spinal cord in the cervical region results in quadriplegia, and in the thoracic region in paraplegia. Below the level of transection, there is a loss of all sensory function to pain and temperature. Bladder and bowel function are lost and there may be autonomic disturbances in blood pressure and temperature control.

The symptoms and signs of spinal cord syndromes are listed in **1.13**. Although trauma is often the cause, there are many other causes of spinal cord disease, such as degenerative disease, tumour, nutritional and metabolic disorders, and inflammatory processes. Demyelination, as seen in multiple sclerosis, is common.

Spinal cord syndromes	
Complete transection	Loss of power below level of transection Loss of all sensory function to pain and temperature and loss of discriminatory sensation below the level of transection Loss of bladder and bowel function Disturbances in autonomic function
Hemicord or Brown–Séquard syndrome	Loss of discriminatory sensation on the same side of the body as the lesion Ipsilateral limb paralysis Loss of temperature and pain perception on the contralateral side
Central syndrome	Results in dissociated sensation with loss of pain and temperature and retention of discriminatory sensation With progression there is ventral horn cell involvement Further extension results in loss of discriminatory sensation and both upper and lower motor neuron tract signs
Selective involvement of ascending and descending pathways	Involvement of dorsal root entry zones and posterior columns Involvement of posterior and lateral columns Involvement of ventral horns Involvement of combined ventral horn cells and corticospinal tracts

1.13 Spinal cord syndromes.

AUTOPSY TECHNIQUES

It is essential for the pathologist to have sufficient clinical information to determine the type of neurological illness. In unusual or atypical cases, it is particularly important to discuss the case with the clinicians involved before the autopsy is done. This is to identify the appropriate tissues for sampling for microbiological or neurochemical study, and to decide whether the spinal dorsal root ganglia, peripheral nerve and muscle should be removed, in addition to the brain and spinal cord.

Prior discussion or access to the records will also alert the pathologist to potential hazards, such as Creutzfeldt–Jakob disease or an infection with hepatitis B or C viruses or human immunodeficiency virus (HIV).

REMOVAL OF THE BRAIN AND SPINAL CORD

The brain

After reflecting the scalp, a saw-cut is made through the calvaria immediately above the supraorbital ridge and continued horizontally around the skull to the occiput. The skull cap is then prised loose by twisting a T-shaped chisel along the saw-cut. If this is done carefully, the dura mater will not be breached, though this may be difficult to prevent when the dura is tightly adherent to the skull, as is common in the elderly. If the dura and skull are tightly adherent, they can be separated by a malleable retractor.

The tenseness of the dura should be established, and the patency of the superior sagittal sinus determined by running a fingertip along it or by opening it. The dura is then incised along the line of the saw-cut, the falx is freed from the cribiform plate, and the dura retracted to allow inspection of the bridging veins draining into the sagittal sinus.

The frontal lobe is then retracted gently from the floor of the anterior cranial fossa, taking care not to damage the olfactory bulbs. The optic nerves, internal carotid arteries, pituitary stalk and upper cranial nerves are then cut as they come into view. Further retraction exposes the attachment of the tentorium cerebelli to the base of the skull, which is incised to expose the structures in the posterior fossa. The remaining cranial nerves and the vertebral arteries are cut and the upper end of the spinal cord is transected: the brain is gently removed from the skull taking care not to cause damage.

If the abnormality is in the posterior fossa or upper part of the spinal canal, a central wedge of occipital bone should be removed along with the spines and laminae of the upper cervical vertebrae, so that the brain and upper segments of the spinal cord can be removed in one block.

The spinal cord

The spinal cord may be removed either by an anterior or posterior approach. The anterior approach has the advantage of enabling the autopsy to be carried out through a single midline ventral incision, and permits the dorsal root ganglia and the vertebral arteries in the transverse processes of the cervical vertebrae to be more easily identified.

After the cord has been fully exposed, it should be removed within its dural sheath, avoiding any angulation to minimise distortion of the intrinsic architecture. In some circumstances, it may be necessary to remove the vertebral column *en bloc* and to fix the cord *in situ*.

Abnormalities in the base of the skull

After removing the brain, the dura should be stripped from the bone to identify any abnormalities in the base of the skull. This allows an examination of the various air and venous sinuses, middle ears, orbits, and contents of the pituitary fossa, and identification of any fractures.

Extracranial cerebral arteries in the neck

In cerebrovascular disease, it is necessary to examine the major extracranial cerebral arteries in the neck. Easy access can be achieved through a 'Y'- or 'U'-shaped incision in the neck. This allows identification and block dissection of the arch of the aorta. The dissection includes the internal carotid arteries up to the base of the skull, and the proximal part of the vertebral arteries up to the point where they enter the foramina of the sixth cervical vertebrae.

Neonatal procedures

The procedure for removing and handling the neonatal brain requires separate comment because of the nature of the disease processes presenting in the neonatal period, as well as the physical characteristics of the brain and skull. Briefly, the calvaria is opened with scissors along the sutures so that the flaps of the skull and dura can be sprung out, petal-like. The brain may then be removed as described for adults, after dividing and freeing the falx, but great care is required as the neonatal brain is soft. Very macerated brains may be taken out in an intact dural sac. Removal of the brain under saline has been advocated.

As suspension by the basilar artery (*see below*) is inappropriate for neonatal brains, several flotation methods have been devised. These include fixation in 10% formalin using a mattress of cotton wool, and floating in 20% formalin or in 10% formalin to which glacial acetic acid has been added.

Preliminary inspection

It is rarely necessary to section the brain before fixation. Samples of unfixed brain may be removed for virological or genetic studies, neurochemical analysis or electron microscopy. However, external inspection often reveals preliminary evidence of trauma, cerebrovascular disease or the sequelae of raised intracranial pressure. In cases of proven or suspected meningitis or encephalitis, samples of CSF should be retained for microbiology. In cases of massive subarachnoid haemorrhage, it is advisable to dissect the arteries at the base of the brain prior to fixation and to wash away the blood clot with normal saline.

Fixation and freezing of specimens

There are many diseases of the CNS in which unfixed tissue specimens are needed for enzyme or neurochemical studies. If the disease process is thought to be symmetrical, then after a mid-sagittal cut, half the brain is available for slow freezing. A preferred method is to flash-freeze small samples of the brain taken from predetermined areas of brain, cut either in the coronal, sagittal or horizontal planes.

The usual procedure for fixation is to suspend the brain in a nine-litre (two-gallon) polythene bucket containing neutral 4% formaldehyde in normal saline (10% formalin) for at least two, but preferably three, weeks. The brain is suspended by passing a hook, loop, or a piece of string between the pons and the basilar artery. The brain will then hang freely, with care being taken to ensure that none of its surfaces come into contact with the bottom or sides of the bucket. The fixative should be changed after three days and then at weekly intervals.

The spinal cord, still within the dura, is best fixed vertically in a large measuring cylinder with a weight attached to the caudal dura to prevent distortion. Sometimes, the whole vertebral column needs to be examined.

To ensure adequate fixation, the specimen can either be cut into multiple transverse blocks, or, after laminectomy with the cord *in situ,* the dura can be opened to expose the underlying arachnoid and cord before immersion in a large tank of fixative.

FURTHER READING

Adams JH and Murray MF. *Atlas of Post-Mortem Techniques in Neuropathology*. Cambridge, Cambridge University Press, 1982.

England, MA and Wakely J. *Color Atlas of the Brain and Spinal Cord.* London, Mosby-Year Book, 1991.

Lindsay K, Bone I and Callender R. *Neurology and Neurosurgery Illustrated.* 2nd edn. Edinburgh, Churchill–Livingstone, 1991.

Parsons MA *Color Atlas of Clinical Neurology*. 2nd edn. London, Wolfe Publishing, 1993.

Rowland LP (ed). *Merritt's Textbook of Neurology*. 8th edn. Philadelphia, Lea and Febiger, 1989.

2. Brain Dissection, Normal Microscopy and Reactions of the Nervous System to Disease

The brain should be fixed by suspension in formalin for three to four weeks, and for not less than 10 days. It should then be washed in running water for at least two hours (and preferably left soaking overnight) before dissection. Even after such thorough washing, the brain should be cut in a well-ventilated room, or preferably on an exhaust-ventilated dissecting bench. The pathologist should be suitably gowned and wearing gloves. Before proceeding, the specimen's identity should be confirmed and the appropriate instruments assembled. These should include:

- a set of metal or plastic dissecting angles;
- a brain knife – long blade for adults and shorter for babies;
- a scalpel;
- a pair of forceps;
- sharp scissors.

It is helpful to cut the specimen on a cork board and to display the slices on a suitably sized tray. Any superficial abnormalities, such as infarction, atrophy (either localised or general), or internal herniation, should be noted. If necessary, they should also be photographed. The condition of the leptomeninges (**2.1, 2.2**), cranial nerves and circle of Willis (**2.3**) should be noted and the weight of the fixed brain recorded.

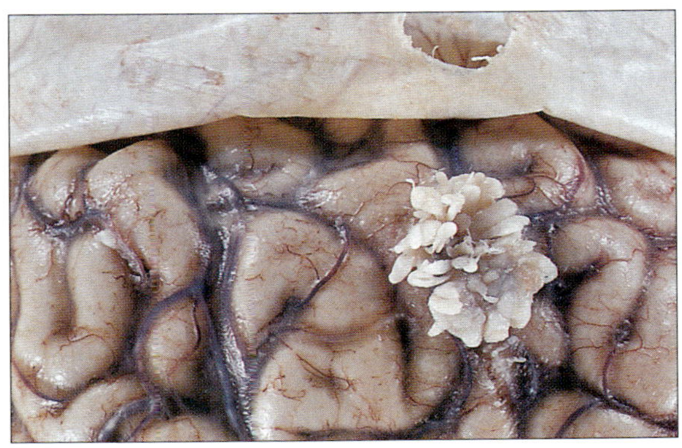

2.1 The meninges. The dura mater has been reflected to reveal transparent meninges within which are blood vessels. Note the normal arachnoid villi in the parasagittal region.

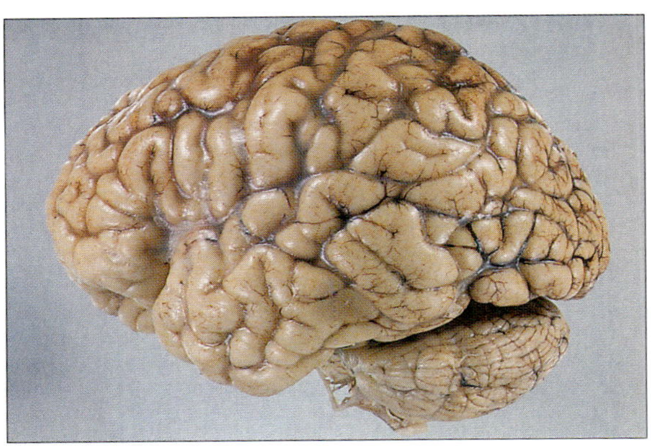

2.2 The meninges. Lateral view of brain to reveal normal lobulation and gyral pattern of a middle-aged subject. The meninges are transparent.

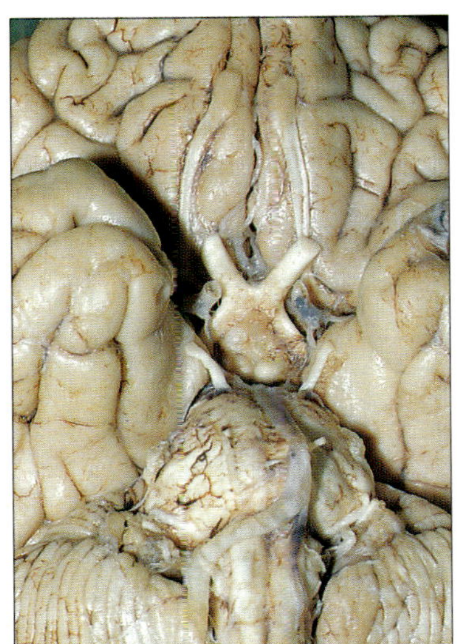

2.3 Base of normal brain. With minimal dissection of the meninges, it is possible to identify the cranial nerves, hypothalamic structures, and blood vessels comprising the circle of Willis (*see also* **2.12**).

DISSECTION AND BRAIN CUTTING

Dissection is carried out in the plane that will result in the best correlation of the morbid anatomy with the neuroradiological findings. The most commonly used planes for slicing are coronal and horizontal.

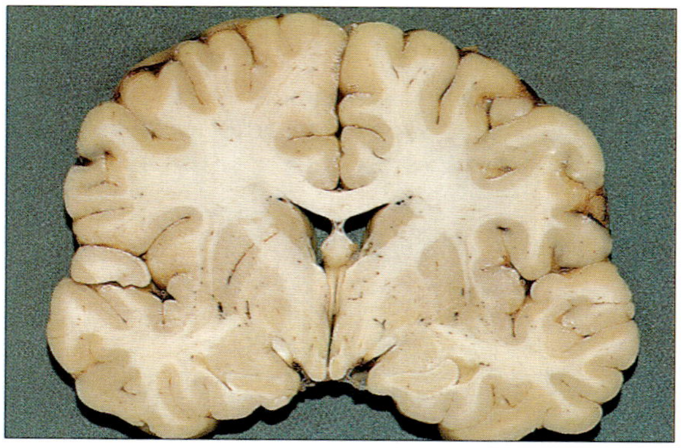

2.4 Coronal slice of normal brain at the level of the mamillary bodies.

The initial procedure is to detach the hindbrain from the cerebrum by a horizontal cut through the upper pons. In adults with degenerative disease, the hindbrain should be weighed and the ratio between it and the weight of the whole fixed brain determined. The normal ratio is 1:8–10; a deviation from this represents disease of either the hindbrain or the cerebral hemispheres. A further transverse cut is made through the cerebral peduncles to obtain a block of the midbrain which includes the aqueduct, substantia nigra and the origin of the IIIrd cranial nerves. The first coronal cut is made through the cerebral hemispheres at the level of the mamillary bodies (**2.4**), and then the hemispheres are cut into slices 1.0cm thick with the aid of two half rectangular dissecting angles. The slices are laid out sequentially, and right and left sides are identified. They are numbered as follows:

- those in front of the initial cut at the level of the mamillary bodies are A1, A2, A3, etc., progressing forward (**2.5, 2.6**);
- those behind it are P1, P2, P3, etc., progressing backwards (**2.7, 2.8**).

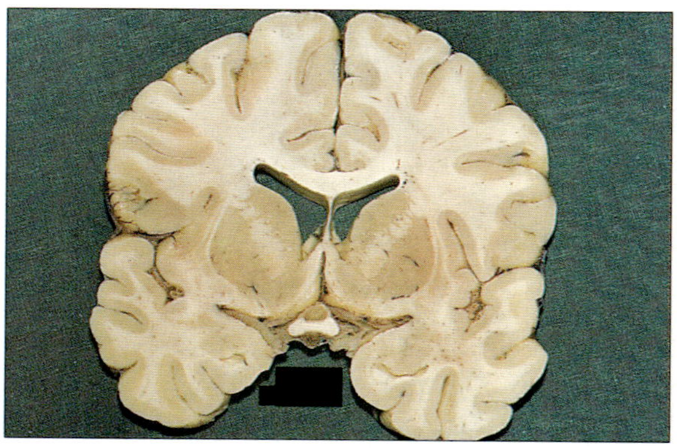

2.5 A1 coronal slice of normal brain at the level of the basal ganglia.

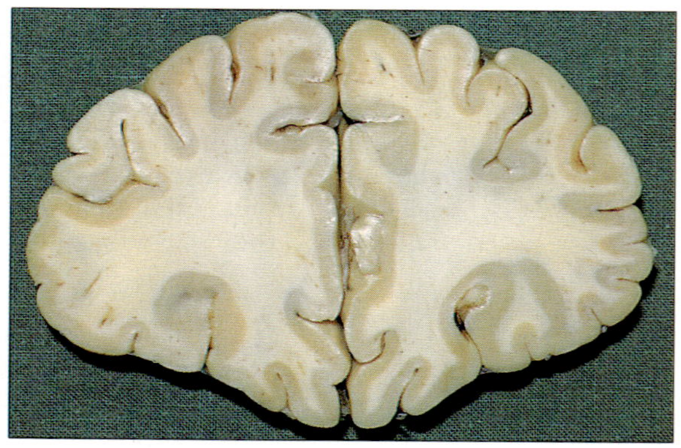

2.6 A4 coronal slice of normal brain at the level of the frontal lobes.

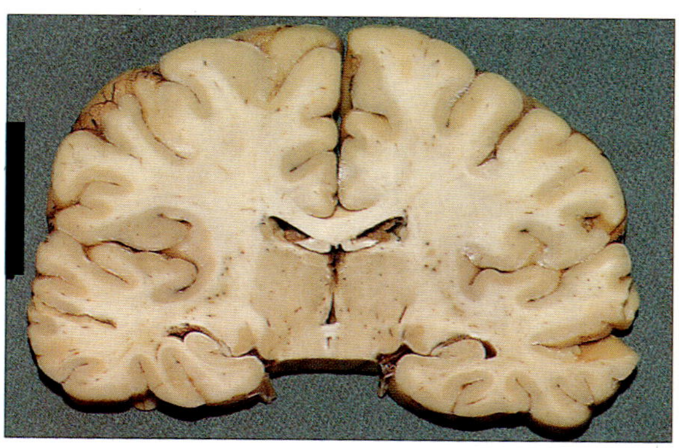

2.7 P1 coronal slice of normal brain at the level of the lateral geniculate bodies.

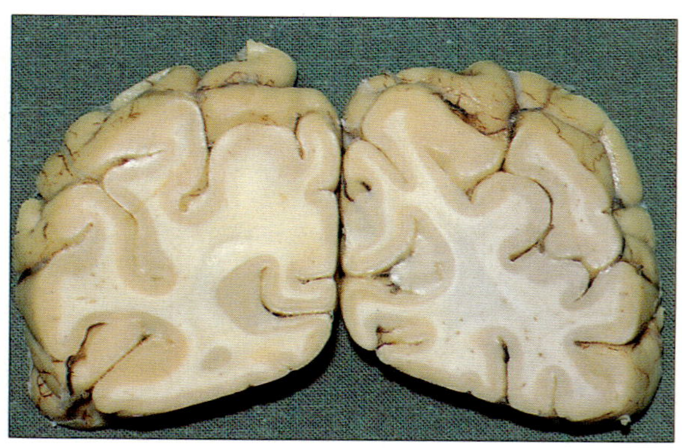

2.8 P6 coronal slice of normal brain at the level of the occipital lobes.

With experience, it is relatively easy to lay out a brain correctly, given some knowledge of the correct positioning of structures and the general shape of the brain at different levels. Alternatively, the brain may be cut in the horizontal plane from a point about 2.0cm above the frontal pole to one about 3.0cm above the occipital pole. As with coronal sectioning, the slices are then laid out upper surface upward with the righthand side on the right (**2.9**).

DISPLAY OF STRUCTURES AND DETECTION OF LESIONS

The structures are normally displayed in coronal and horizontal slices, respectively (**2.4–2.9**). Sometimes, a cerebellar lesion is best displayed by a transverse cut, but it is usually better to separate the cerebellum from the brainstem by cutting through the cerebellar peduncles on each side. The hemispheres can then be cut at right angles to the folia and slightly nearer the vermis than the lateral border. A further cut is then made through the midline of the hemispheres (**2.10**). A series of transverse cuts is made through the brainstem (**2.11**). In order to examine the spinal cord, the dura is opened in the midline along its dorsal and ventral aspects, abnormalities are noted, and a series of transverse cuts is made through the full thickness of the cord. The ventral surface of the cord is easily identified by the single midline anterior spinal artery. Even if the cord has been damaged post mortem, it is usually possible to identify the segments approximately by locating the lowest large ventral nerve root of the cervical plexus. This is usually C8.

Lesions in the brain and spinal cord may be more or less obvious, depending on their nature and size, and the time for which they have been present. The slices should be scanned in a methodical manner and the presence of any asymmetry noted. Palpation may be a sensitive method of locating subtle abnormalities.

HISTOLOGY

The sampling and number of blocks selected for histological examination will be determined by the clinical features, the results of various clinical investigations and the appearances at the time of the brain cut. If the pathology is focal, e.g. tumour or infarct, then one or two blocks may suffice, but if it is diffuse, e.g. cardiac arrest, then it will be necessary to take representative samples of the cortex and basal ganglia, including the thalami, hippocampus, cerebellum and brainstem. The specimen should be stored moist in 10% formol saline, either in a plastic or glass container or in a sealed plastic bag. Prolonged storage (beyond about 12–15 months) causes deterioration of the staining qualities of the tissue, though antigen retrieval is possible using microwave techniques.

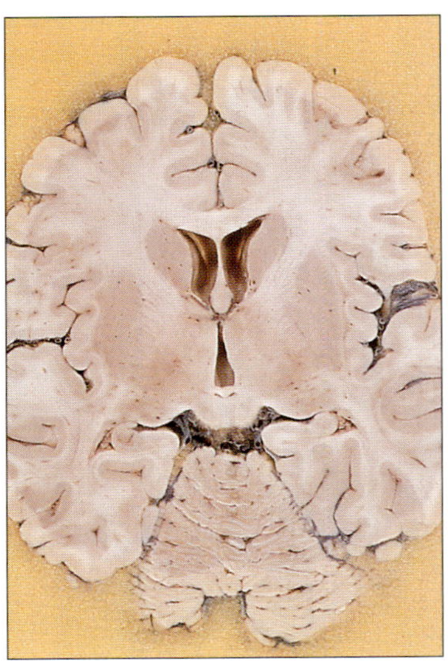

2.9 Horizontal slice of normal brain. This approach allows good correlation with various types of neuroimaging (e.g. MRI, SPECT).

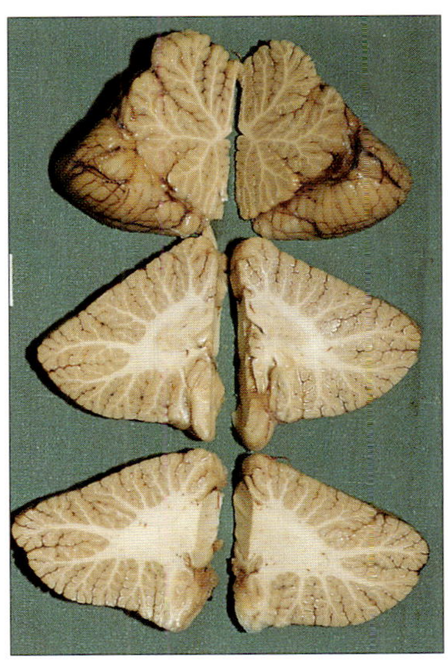

2.10 Normal cerebellum. After bisection the hemispheres have been cut at right angles to the folial pattern on the upper surface of the specimen.

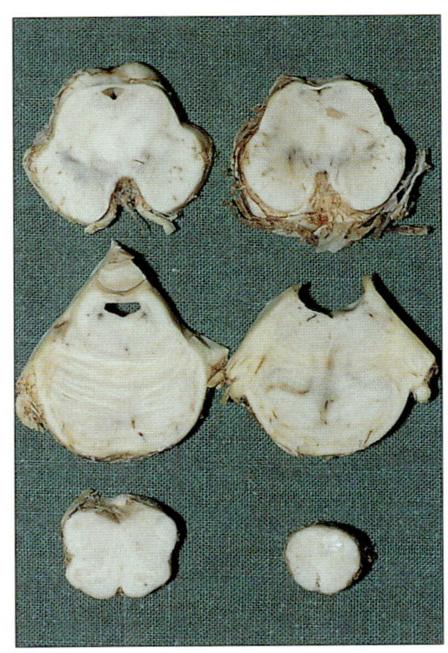

2.11 Normal brainstem. Horizontal slices have been cut at the levels of the midbrain, pons and medulla oblongata.

BLOOD SUPPLY OF THE BRAIN

ARTERIES

The distribution of the arterial supply to the brain is of major importance in determining the position of vascular lesions and their neurological sequelae. The arterial circle of Willis at the base of the brain is derived from the paired internal carotid arteries and the basilar artery. The anterior communicating artery of the circle ensures that there is a cross circulation between the two sides of the brain, though the pontine branches of the basilar artery on the two sides do not anastomose in the brainstem. There is some anastomotic flow between the territories of the carotid and vertebrobasilar arteries through the posterior communicating arteries. Considerable variations in size and symmetry of the circle may occur. The main structures supplied by the principal branches of the circle of Willis are shown in **2.12–2.14**.

The anterior cerebral artery supplies the medial surface of the hemisphere as far back as the parieto-occipital sulcus, plus a strip of the parasagittal cortex on the lateral surface of the cerebral hemispheres not supplied by the middle cerebral artery (**2.13, 2.14**). Deep branches of this blood vessel supply the anterior hypothalamus, and the head of the caudate nucleus.

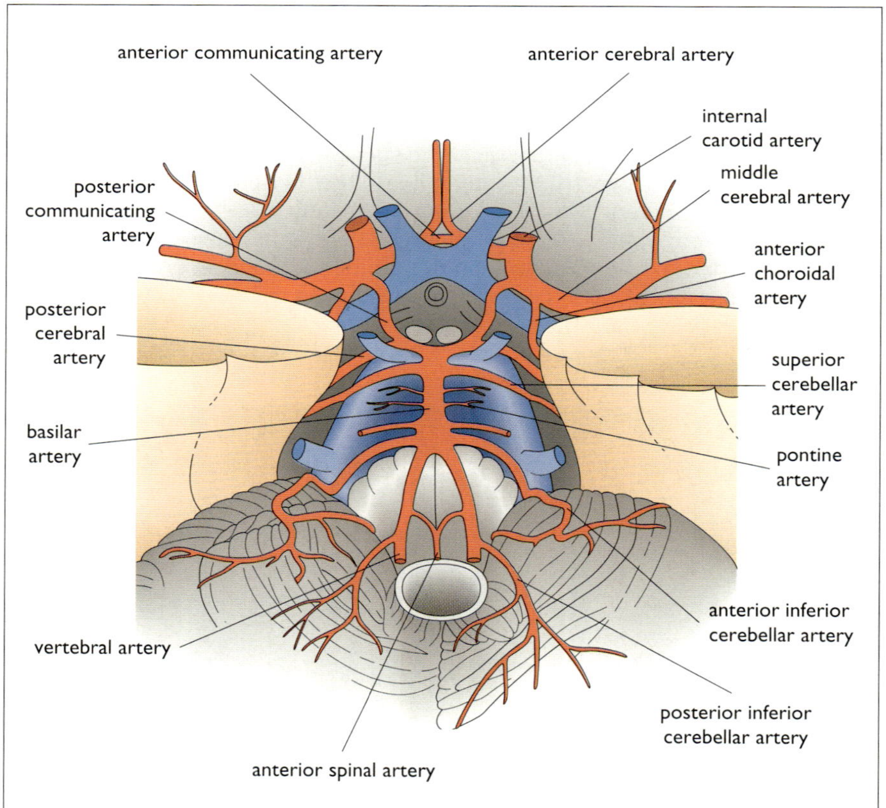

2.12 Circle of Willis. The anterior part of the circle is derived from the internal carotid arteries which divide into the proximal portions of the paired middle and anterior cerebral arteries, and the posterior part of the circle is derived from the vertebrobasilar system which gives origin to the paired posterior cerebral arteries. The circle is completed anteriorly by the anterior communicating artery, which joins the anterior cerebral arteries, and posteriorly by the posterior communicating arteries, which join the posterior cerebral and internal carotid arteries.

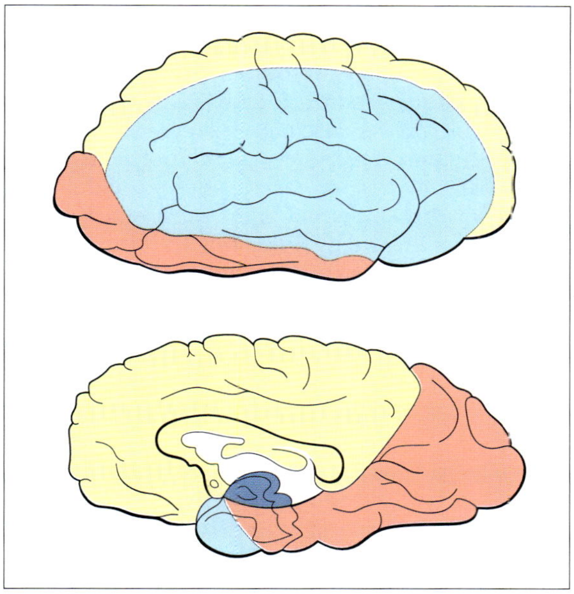

2.13 Arterial blood supply of cerebral hemispheres. Lateral and parasagittal views.

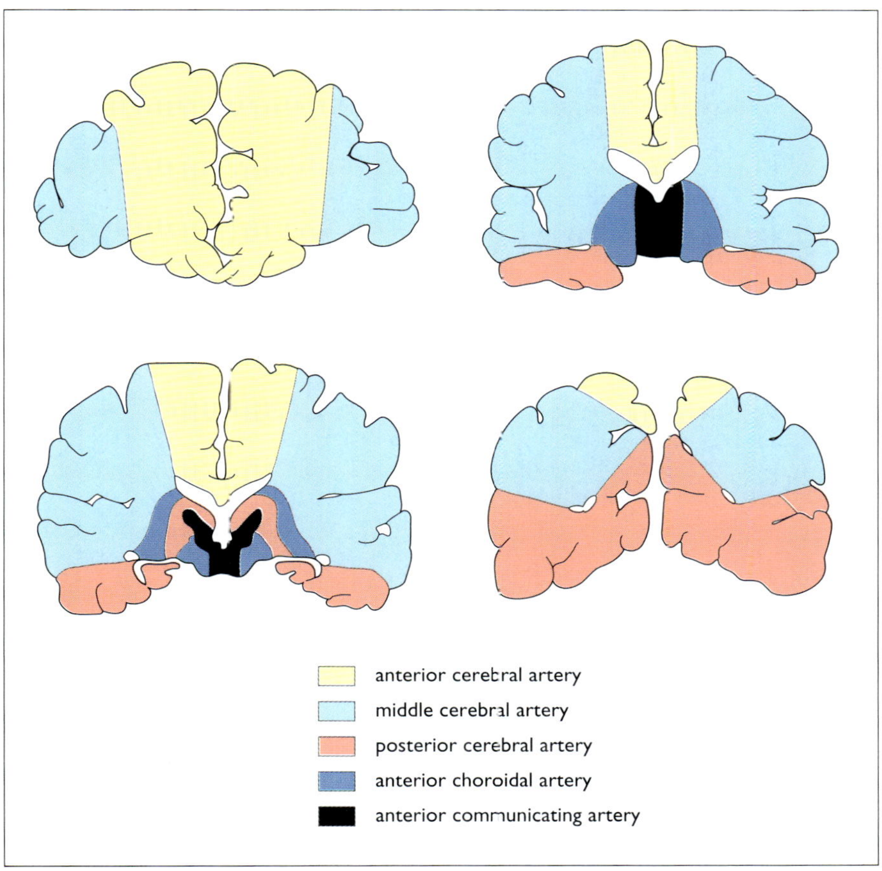

2.14 Arterial blood supply of cerebral hemispheres. Coronal slices. The distributions of the anterior, middle and posterior cerebral arteries are shown.

The middle cerebral artery divides some 2–3cm from its origin and supplies the lateral surface of the cerebral hemisphere, except for strips along the upper border, which are supplied by the anterior cerebral artery, and along the lower border, which are supplied by the posterior cerebral artery (**2.13**). Its lenticulostriate branches supply the basal ganglia, internal capsule, and thalamus. The anterior choroidal artery is a branch of the middle cerebral artery that supplies the anterior basal ganglia, lateral geniculate body, posterior part of the internal capsule and cerebral peduncle. The posterior cerebral artery supplies the cortex of the occipital lobes, including the visual cortex, and the medial and inferior surfaces of the temporal lobes, excluding the temporal poles (**2.13**). Deep branches supply the cerebral peduncles, posterior thalamus, mamillary bodies, midbrain, geniculate bodies and the choroid plexus. The basilar artery supplies the pons, and part of the cerebellum through its anterior, inferior and superior cerebellar arteries (**2.15**). The vertebral artery supplies the lateral part of the medulla oblongata, and the cerebellum through its posterior inferior cerebellar branch.

VEINS

There are three main groups of external cerebral veins which drain the surfaces of the cerebral hemispheres. These are the superior cerebral veins, which drain via the bridging veins into the superior sagittal sinus; the superior middle cerebral vein, which runs forwards in the Sylvian fissure and drains into the cavernous sinus; and the inferior veins, which drain into the nearest venous sinus. Deeper structures are drained by the paired internal cerebral veins, which form when the thalamostriate and choroidal veins run backwards in the roof of the third ventricle. The internal cerebral veins then unite to form the great cerebral vein of Galen which empties into the straight sinus.

BLOOD SUPPLY OF THE SPINAL CORD

The spinal cord is supplied by blood from the anterior and posterior spinal arteries. The single anterior spinal artery lies close to the anteromedial fissure (**2.16, 2.17**). It arises superiorly from the junction of the spinal branches of the vertebral artery and is fed along the cord by branches of the segmental radicular and medullary arteries. The areas supplied include the ventral horns and the white matter of the anterior two-thirds of the cord. The posterior spinal arteries are paired and lie next to the posterior nerve roots. They often originate from the posterior inferior cerebellar arteries. The spinal veins form a plexiform arrangement on the dorsal aspect of the cord and the area of drainage includes the posterior horns, posterior columns and white columns of the posterior third of the cord.

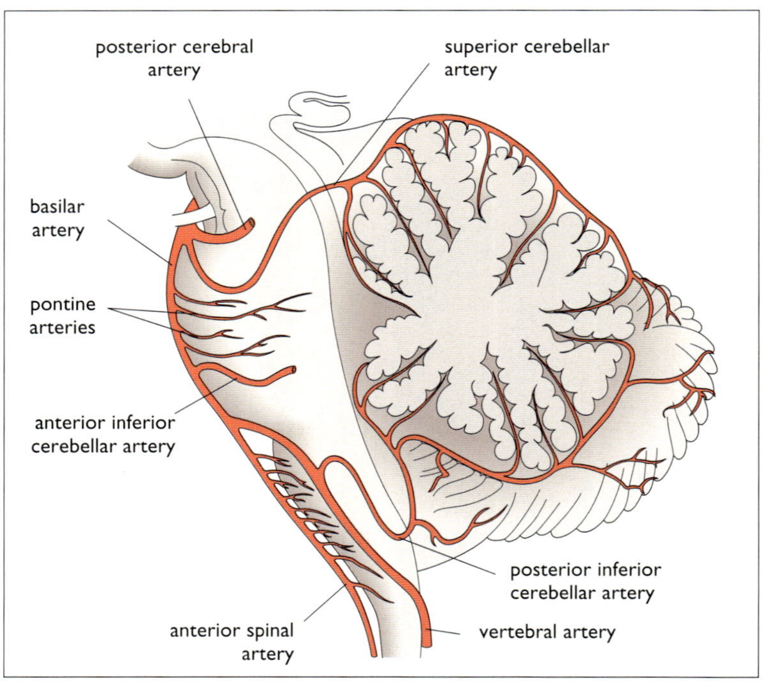

2.15 Arterial blood supply to the hindbrain.

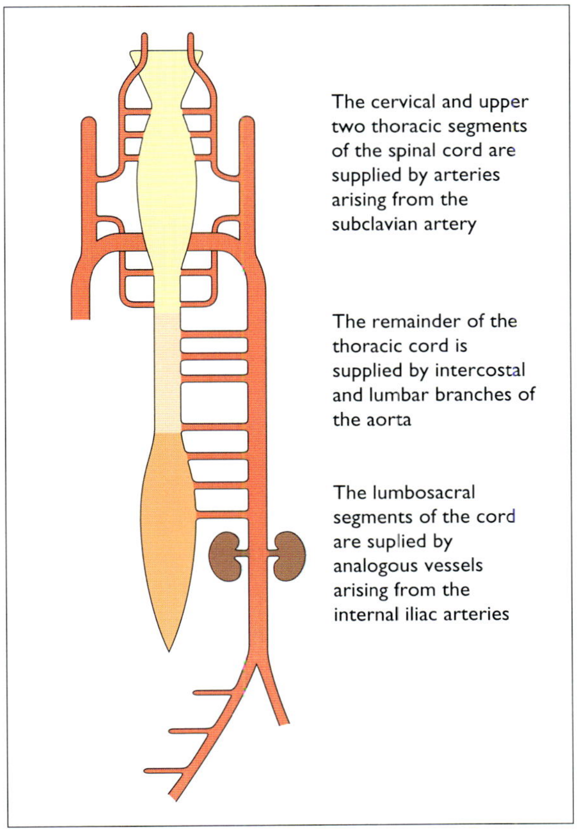

2.16 Arterial blood supply to the spinal cord. The cervical and upper two thoracic segments of the spinal cord are supplied by arteries arising from the subclavian artery. The remainder of the thoracic cord is supplied by intercostal and lumbar branches of the aorta. The lumbosacral segments of the cord are supplied by analogous vessels arising from the internal iliac arteries.

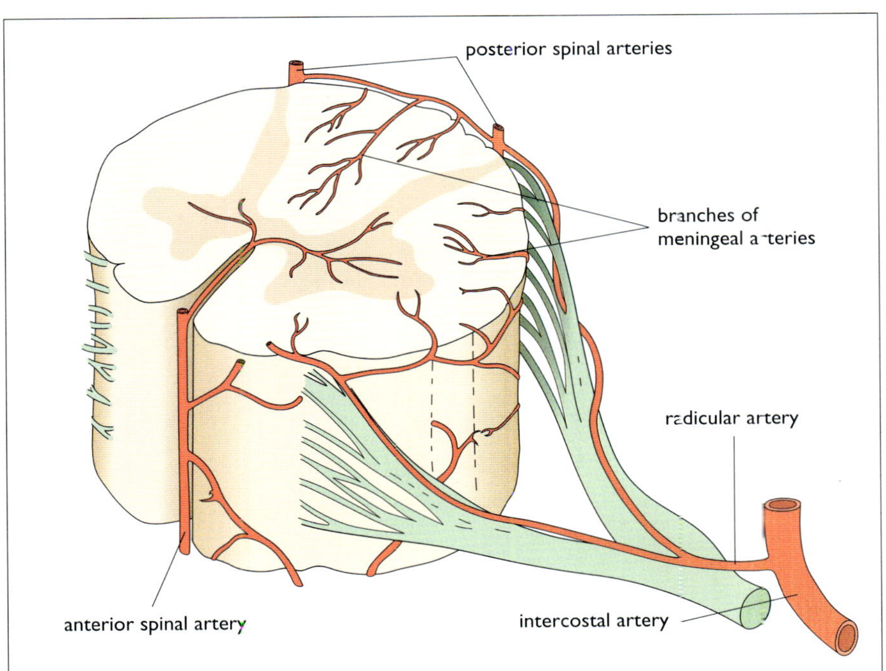

2.17 Arterial blood supply to a segment of the spinal cord.

HISTOLOGICAL TECHNIQUES

Considerable information can be gained about the cellular composition of the tissue from paraffin and frozen-section techniques, the main ones of which are among those listed in **2.18**. From **2.18** it can be seen that a great deal of information can be gained from a limited number of techniques, which are used routinely in neuropathology departments.

PARAFFIN SECTIONS

Many abnormalities of neurons and myelin can be identified in sections stained with haematoxylin and eosin (H & E), provided fairly thick sections (7–8μm) are examined, or cresyl violet (**2.19, 2.20**). By this method, it is easy to recognise the difference between grey and white matter and to gain an overall impression of the architectural arrangements of the

Histological techniques in neuropathology

Preparation	Application	Stain
Paraffin	General purpose	Haematoxylin and eosin Van Gieson
	Neurons, axons and synapses	Cresyl violet may be used with Luxol fast blue or silver impregnation (e.g. Palmgren, Bodian, Holmes) Immunocytochemistry (ICC) for neurofilaments, synaptophysin, neurotransmitters and related enzymes
	Neural crest cells and Schwann cells	ICC for S100 proteins
	Oligodendroglia and myelin	Luxol fast blue (usually combined with cresyl violet) Loyez ICC for carbonic anhydrase C, galactocerebroside, myelin basic protein, anti-Leu 7
	Astrocytes	Phosphotungstic acid haematoxylin (PTAH) Holzer ICC for glial fibrillary acidic protein (GFAP) and glutamine synthetase
	Ependyma	ICC for GFAP
	Choroid plexus	ICC for carbonic anhydrase 2 and transthyretin
	Microglia and macrophages	ICC for CD68 and class II MHC antigen Ricin agglutinin
	Endothelium	ICC for factor VIII-related antigen and angiotensin-converting enzyme Ulex europus lectin
	Meninges	ICC for vimentin
	Pituitary gland	ICC for various hormones
	Pineal gland	ICC for protein gene product (PGP) 9.5
Frozen/Paraffin	Age-related changes of neuritic plaques and neurofibrillary tangles	Silver impregnation, e.g. Von Braunmühl King's amyloid ICC for Aß or ßA4 protein Tau and neurofilaments
	Degenerating myelin	Osmium (Marchi) and cholesterol esters (Sudan)

2.18 Histological techniques in neuropathology.

cerebral cortex, basal ganglia, hippocampus, cerebellum and brainstem. However, immunocytochemistry (ICC)has virtually replaced many of the classic staining methods for cell identification in the CNS. A summary of the various methods is provided here; the reader should refer to the various technical manuals available for further details.

Neurons and axons

A useful stain is the cresyl violet (Nissl) method which stains nuclei and nucleoli and Nissl substance – ribosomes. When combined with a Luxol fast blue stain, myelin stains a rich blue colour, and when combined with a silver stain axons appear black. A commonly used marker for neurons is an antibody raised against neuron-specific enolase (**2.21**) – the gamma homodimer of the enolase enzyme. Most neurons and neuroendocrine cells stain for gamma-enolase while glial cells – particularly astrocytes – stain strongly with antibodies raised to the alpha-enolase homodimer. Antibodies raised to neurofilament proteins are also useful, particularly the 68kD subunit, and antiserum raised to synaptophysin is used as a marker of synaptic density in normal neurons (**2.22**) and of neuronal differentiation in tumours (*see Chapter 10*). Various techniques use

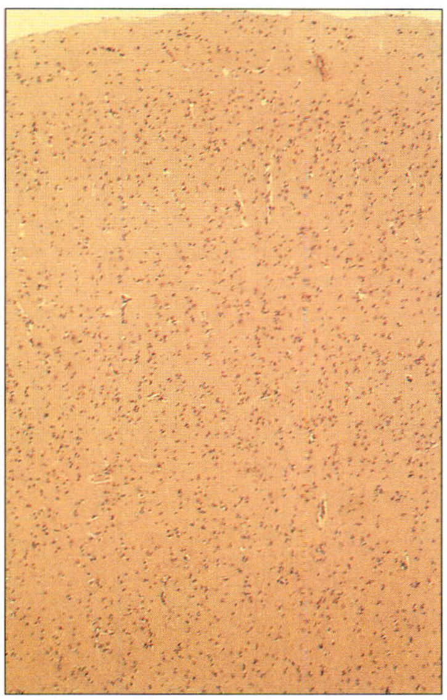

2.19 Cells from the cerebral cortex. With few exceptions, the histological appearances of the cortex are similar throughout the cerebral hemispheres. Beneath the meninges, the cortex has a horizontally disposed laminated appearance reflecting the density and the size of neurons. (H&E)

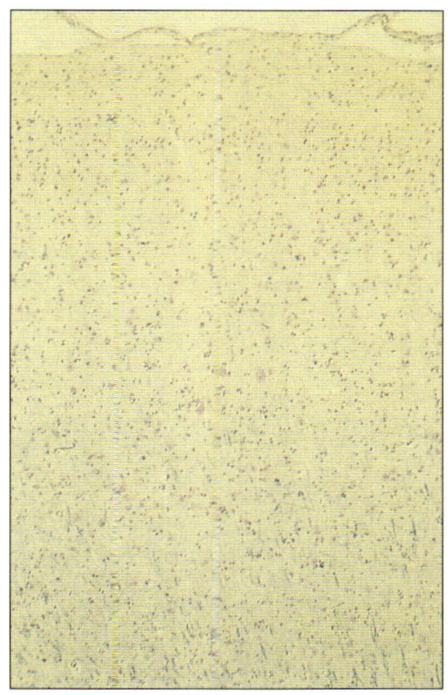

2.20 Cells from the cerebral cortex. (Cresyl violet)

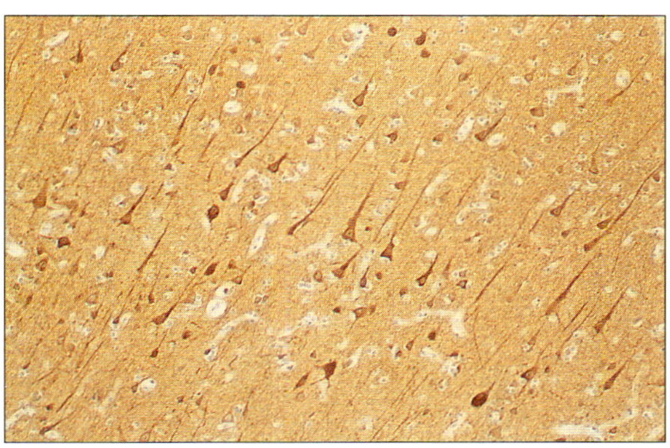

2.21 The cerebral cortex. It is now possible to identify various cell types and particular neuronal populations using a range of antibodies. (ICC for gamma enolase)

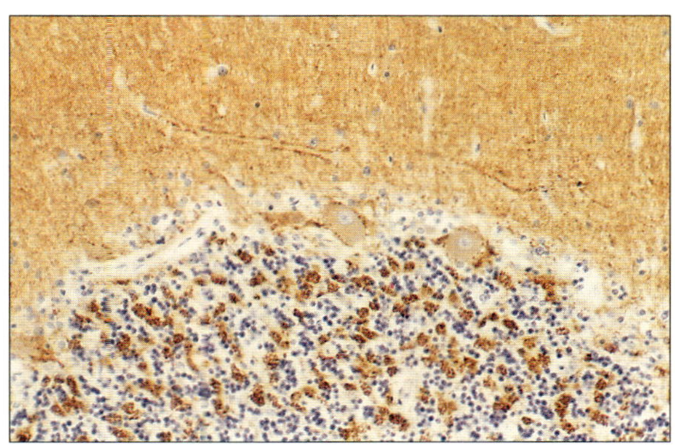

2.22 The cerebellar cortex. The overall amount of synaptic density can be assessed by immunocytochemistry. (ICC for synaptophysin in this example).

silver impregnation for the staining of both neurons (**2.23, 2.24**) and axons (**2.25**). Silver impregnation can be combined with cresyl violet or myelin stains.

Myelin

Definition is poor in H & E-stained sections (**2.26**). One of the traditional methods for myelin is Loyez stain, but a more commonly used technique combines cresyl violet and Luxol fast blue (Klüver–Barrera) stain (**2.27**). These stains are particularly useful in defining anatomical landmarks and in identifying those areas of the CNS where myelin has been lost (*see Chapter 6*).

Oligodendrocytes react with antibodies to galactocerebroside, myelin basic protein, Leu-7, and carbonic anhydrase C.

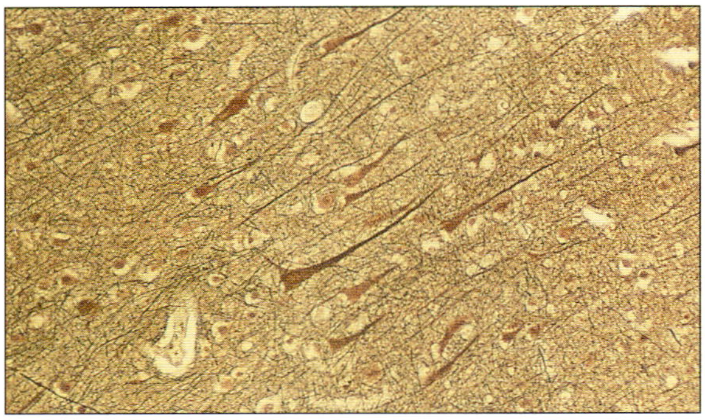

2.23 Neurons in cerebral cortex. It is not possible to determine the full extent of dendritic arborisations and axons in H & E-stained preparations. More detail can be obtained by silver impregnation which reveals the variation in size and shape of the neuronal population. (Palmgren silver)

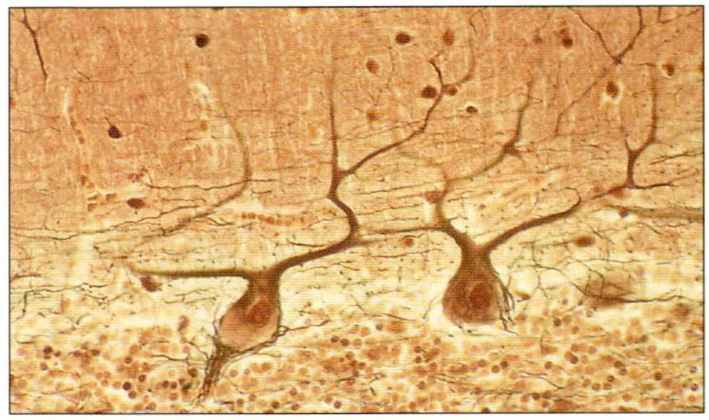

2.24 Purkinje cells in the cortex of the cerebellum. Silver impregnation reveals the extensive dendritic arborisation of the large-bodied Purkinje cells. (Palmgren silver)

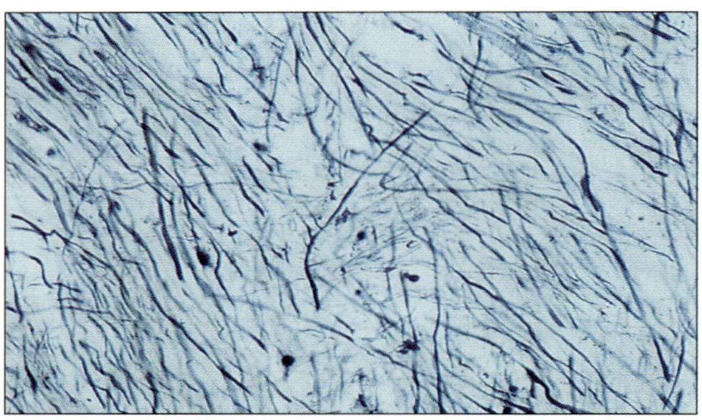

2.25 Axons. These are difficult to identify in H & E-stained sections, but the number, size and shape of axons can be readily seen after silver impregnation. (Holmes silver)

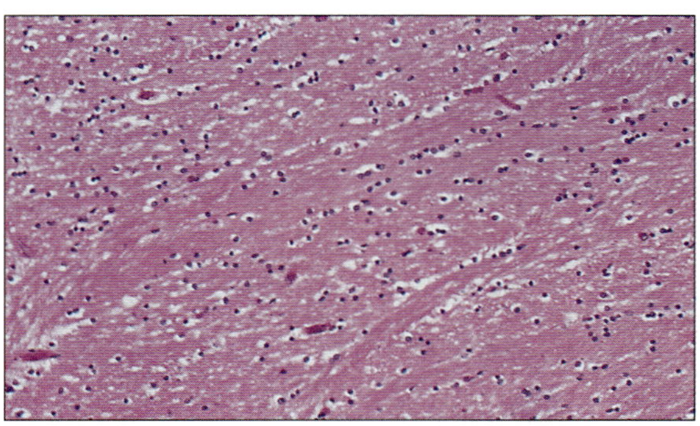

2.26 Myelin. White matter of the brain is made up of large numbers of axons and their myelinated sheaths. (H & E)

2.27 Myelin. (Cresyl violet and Luxol fast blue)

Astrocytes

Although their presence can be identified in H & E-stained sections, positive evidence of glial fibre formation requires use of several specialised techniques. Classically, astrocyte stains have included the Cajal (**2.28**), Holzer and phosphotungstic acid haematoxylin (PTAH) methods, but immunocytochemical techniques to identify glial fibrillary acidic protein (GFAP) are now more commonly used.

Ependymal cells and microglia

Ependymal cells can be seen by immunocytochemistry for GFAP, and their blepharoplasts by PTAH. For microglia, various metallic impregnations have been used in the past (**2.29**), but these have all been superseded by immunocytochemistry, e.g. by the use of antibodies to the CD68 epitope.

Other comments

Cells and tissue originating from the mesoderm can be readily identified in normal CNS by routine H & E staining. However, difficulties may arise in distinguishing between brain tissue and acellular collagen in disease stains. Under these circumstances, the Van Gieson method is particularly useful, and if combined with stains for elastic tissue will reveal the histological structure of blood vessels. As with other aspects of neurohistology, immunocytochemistry is making a significant contribution with its ability to mark:

- endothelium with antibodies to factor VIII-related antigen and angiotensin-converting enzymes;
- muscle with myosin and desmin;
- fibroblasts with vimentin.

If pigment is present, Perls' stain is particularly useful for showing haemosiderin deposits and the Masson–Fontana method identifies melanin. Formalin must be removed from the section by prior treatment with hydrogen peroxide before other pigments can be positively identified. Other pigments that can be identified include lipofuscin and haematoidin.

FROZEN SECTIONS

These are commonly used for rapid intraoperative diagnosis, various metabolic disorders, and myelin abnormalities. Sections cut from formalin-fixed tissue are commonly used to identify age-related changes and those of Alzeimer's disease. Loss of myelin can also be determined by identifying the breakdown products of myelin, which can be stained positively by the Sudan dyes and by the Marchi technique. These lipid end-products are taken up by macrophages, the amount and distribution of which give some indication of chronicity. In the Marchi technique, the degenerate myelin is stained black with osmium tetroxide while normal myelin is left unstained. The material that has been impregnated by the Marchi method can be embedded in paraffin. In general, the Marchi stain identifies demyelinating lesions earlier than do the Sudan dyes.

MICROSCOPY OF THE NORMAL NERVOUS SYSTEM

The cortical ribbon of the cerebral hemispheres has a fairly constant structure with neurons arranged in various layers (**2.19, 2.20**). Beneath the pia mater, it may be easy to identify six layers, the first of which consists of the sparsely cellular molecular layer,

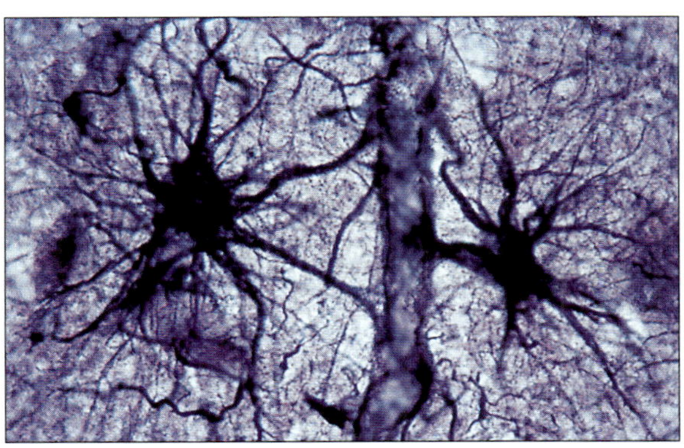

2.28 Astrocytes. These have many processes which help to define the boundaries of the brain at its various surfaces. Part of the anatomical basis of the blood–brain barrier is the envelopment of capillaries by foot processes. (Cajal technique)

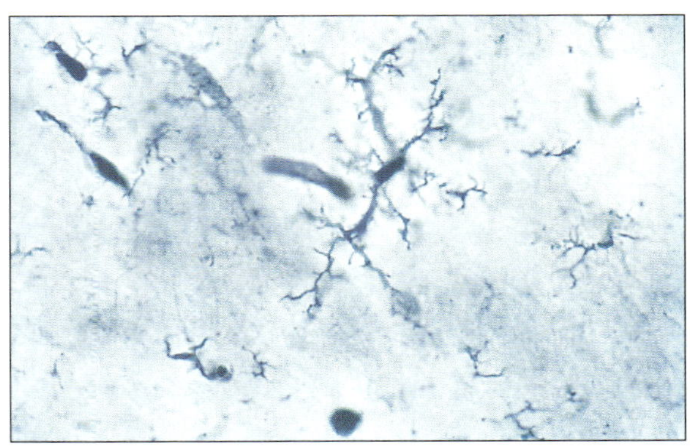

2.29 Microglia. These cells are difficult to see in H & E-stained sections, but can be shown to have short branching processes after silver impregnation. (Hortega silver carbonate)

largely composed of astrocytes. In contrast, layers two and four consist of small darkly staining neurons and layers three, five and six are made up of pyramidal nerve cells.

The neuroanatomy of the hippocampus has a distinctive arrangement in contrast to the cerebral cortex (**2.30, 4.41**). It is essentially comma-shaped, the head of which is enveloped by a band of dark-staining neurons, comprising the dentate fascia that encloses the CA4 sector (endplate) of the hippocampus. The neck is designated CA3 and CA2 – the so-called resistant sector – separates CA3 from CA1. From this endplate region, the cells form an arch; the medial part of this arch merges into a four-layered cortex (the palaeocortex) before it in turn merges with the six-layered neocortex in the collateral sulcus. Another part of the CNS that has an easily recognisable architecture is the cortex of the cerebellum (**2.31, 2.32**). Beneath the pial surface, there is a large pale-staining outer molecular layer, which merges fairly abruptly into the granular cell layer, at the junction of which are large Purkinje cells. A further distinctive part of the nervous system is that of neurons in the Vth cranial nerve and autonomic

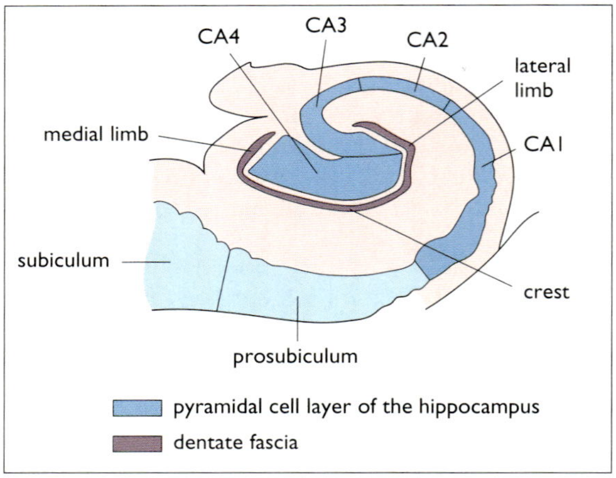

2.30 Hippocampus. Line diagram to show the various subfields. (CA, cornu ammonis and dentate fascia)

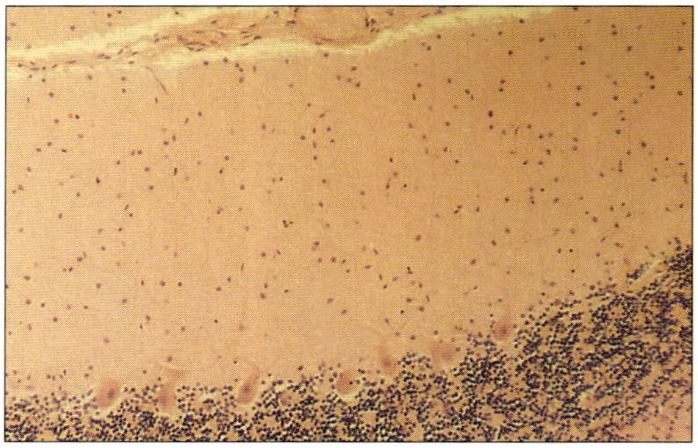

2.31 The cerebellar cortex. The surface of the cerebellar cortex is greatly increased by the folia, each of which has a characteristic pattern. Beneath the meninges, there is a broad pale-staining molecular layer that merges abruptly with the small darkly stained granule-cell layer. Large Purkinje-cell neurons form a single layer between the granule cells and the molecular layer, while between the Purkinje cells is a layer of astrocytes called the Bergmann glia. The extent of the dendritic arborisations from the Purkinje cells can be seen after silver impregnation (*see* **2.24**). (H & E)

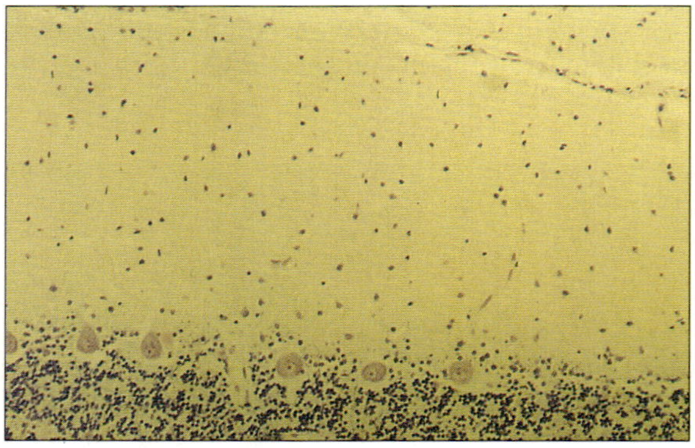

2.32 The cerebellar cortex. (Cresyl violet)

ganglia (**2.33**). In the dorsal root ganglia, the neurons are unipolar spherical-shaped cells, the largest of which measure between 50μm and 100μm in diameter. Each has a peripheral axon, and a central axon that extends into the spinal cord.

NEURONS

Neurons in the CNS vary in size and shape from the small granular cells of the cerebellum, measuring about 5μm in diameter, to the large pyramidal (Betz's) cells of the motor cortex, Purkinje cells of the cerebellum (**2.31, 2.32**), ventral horn cells of the spinal cord (**2.34**) and the specialised nuclei of the hypothalamus (**2.35**), which may measure up to 125μm in diameter. There may be up to 80 dendrites attached to any given neuron, but each neuron gives origin to only a single axon that varies considerably in length ranging from a few millimetres up to 90cm long. Differentiated neurons are post-mitotic cells.

Large neurons are characterised by centrally placed vesicular nuclei with prominent nucleoli within coarsely granular cytoplasm. This granularity is readily seen with light microscopy and is stainable with haematoxylin (**2.35**) and basic aniline dyes, such as cresyl violet. It is composed of RNA-rich stacks of rough endoplasmic reticulum and associated groups of polyribosomes – the Nissl substance (**2.34**). Electron microscopy reveals numerous mitochondria,

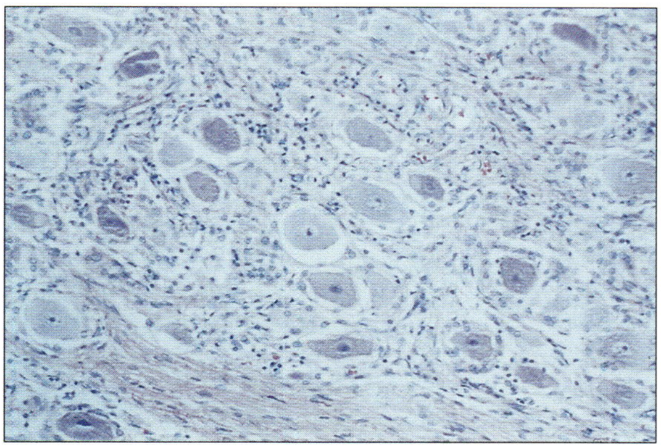

2.33 Sensory neurons in trigeminal nerve ganglion. These large round neurons have a centrally placed nucleus and prominent nucleoli. Each neuron has an afferent (peripheral) and an efferent (central) axon and can measure 30–50μm in diameter. Satellite or capsule cells surround each ganglion cell. Bundles of nerve fibres pass through the ganglion. (H & E)

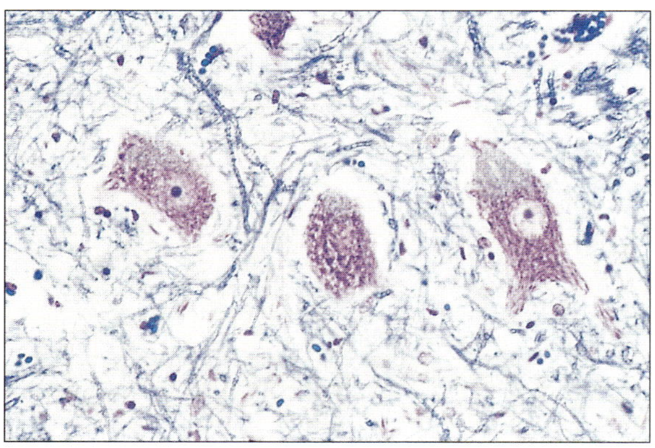

2.34 Ventral horn neurons. The nuclei of these large spinal neurons are slightly eccentric. Nissl substance extends into the dendrites except at the axon hillock. (Luxol fast blue and cresyl violet)

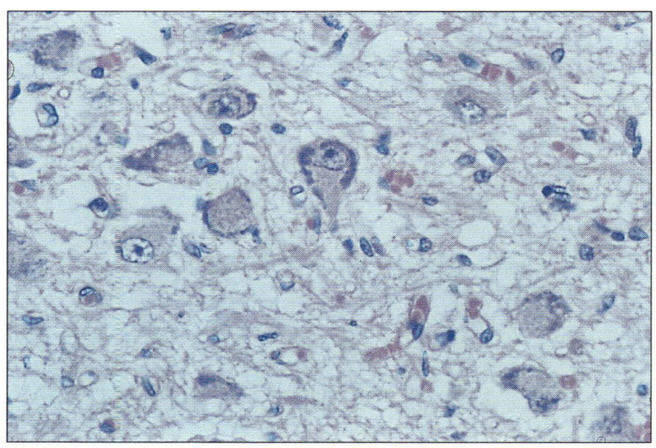

2.35 Large neurons in hypothalamus. The neurons are often circular or slightly triangular in shape, have large vesicular nuclei and prominent nucleoli, and granular basophilic cytoplasm (Nissl substance). Glial cells are of two types: astrocytes with round pale nuclei and oligodendroglia with small darkly staining (lymphocyte-like) nuclei. Small blood vessels are lined by elongated endothelium. The neuropil (background substance) is made up of dendrites, axons, synapses and the processes of astrocytes. (H & E)

a highly developed Golgi apparatus, smooth endoplasmic reticulum and various types of vesicles. In addition, neurofibrils are present. These comprise two main types, namely 20–30nm microtubules and 6–10nm neurofilaments. Since neuronal processes and perikarya are rich in neurofilaments, the overall morphology and extent of neurons can be determined in either paraffin or frozen sections stained by a variety of methods that include silver impregnation and immunocytochemistry. Neurofibrils are also present in axons and dendrites and are concerned with the transport of materials, both away from (anterograde, which has fast and slow components), and towards (retrograde) the cell body of the neuron. Fast anterograde flow transports mitochondria and neurosecretory vesicles at a rate of up to 1000mm/day: in contrast the slow component conveys elements of the cytoskeleton at a rate of up to 5mm/day. Retrograde flow at a rate of about 200mm/day transports lysosomes and various small vesicles back to the perikaryon, where they are either disposed of or recycled. The neurosecretory vesicles are transported to the boutons terminaux, which form synapses on the dendrites and cell body of other neurons. The neurotransmitter is stored in the synaptic vesicle, which may be either dense or clear depending on its function. Some of the vesicles are large. In the hypothalamus, the vesicles take the form of neurosecretory granules which are associated with the peptide hormones, oxytocin and vasopressin, and their carrier proteins.

There are two additional constituents of neurons, which are only found in neurons at particular sites. The first is lipofuscin, which consists of PAS-positive, non-metabolisable substances, stainable by Sudan dyes and generally found in aggregates measuring 1μm in diameter. Although abundant even at an early age in some sites, such as the lateral geniculate nucleus (**2.36**) and anterior horn cells of the spinal cord, it is sparse in other neuronal populations such as the Purkinje cells. In general, there is an accumulation of lipofuscin with age, which has led to its alternative name of 'wear and tear' pigment. The second constituent is neuromelanin, which is present in considerable amounts, normally in the cells of the substantia nigra (**2.37**) and locus ceruleus. Neuromelanin is not found before the age of five years (*see Chapter 9*).

NEUROGLIA

Astrocytes

These are multipolar cells. Many of them possess end-feet that make contact with the basal laminae of both the blood vessels of the blood–brain barrier (**2.28**) and the pia contributing to the glia limitans of the CSF–brain barrier. Astrocytic processes also ensheath the neuronal dendritic and somatic membranes, except at synapses. It has long been recognised that there are two morphologically distinct types of astrocytes – the protoplasmic and fibrous types, which predominate in grey and white matter, respectively. Light microscopy shows rather pale nuclei with granular chromatin and inconspicuous nucleoli. In electron micrographs, astrocytes are characterised by pale nuclei that have heterochromatin, with a relatively loose cytoplasm containing lysosomes, glycogen and large amounts of intermediate filaments composed of GFAP. During development, astrocytes differentiate from the neuroectoderm as GFAP-positive primary radial glia (*see Chapter 9*). Corpora amylacea are rounded laminate bodies of 10–15μm diameter (**2.38**), which are often present in

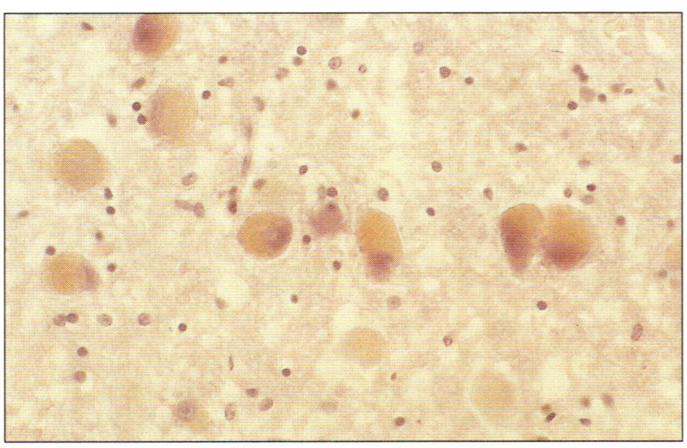

2.36 Lipofuscin. This normal, brown, cytoplasmic constituent accumulates with age. As it increases in amount, it displaces Nissl substance. Staining for acid phosphatase identifies its secondary lysosomal nature. (H & E)

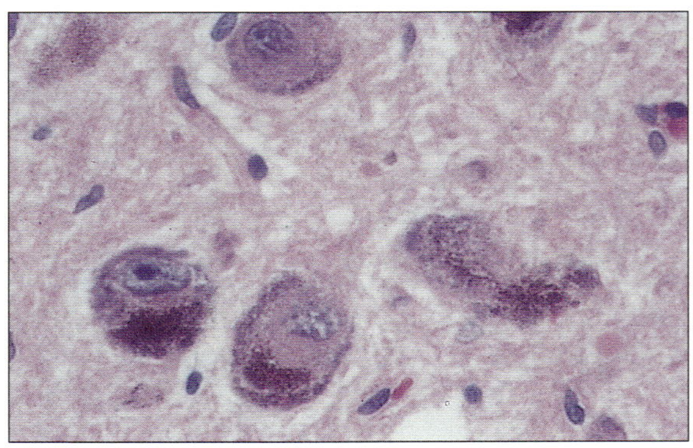

2.37 Neuromelanin. This is a prominent feature of the normal substantia nigra, locus ceruleus and the dorsal nucleus of the vagus. (H & E)

the periventricular and subpial white matter, and in the spinal cord. They are probably derived from astrocytes. They stain greyish-blue in H & E-stained sections and are PAS-positive.

Oligodendrocytes

Oligodendrocytes are responsible for forming and maintaining the myelin in the CNS. Myelin consists of compacted oligodendrocyte cell membrane. This results in a laminated structure of many successive layers of protein and lipid, wrapped around the axon, and producing a characteristic ultrastructural appearance of major and minor dense lines.

Mature oligodendrocytes are galactocerebroside-positive process-bearing cells; their cell bodies are relatively small, and the cytoplasm is rather scanty, but rich in granular endoplasmic reticulum, ribosomes, and mitochondria. Each oligodendrocyte myelinates a single internode of up to 10–15 axons. In the mature CNS, large numbers of oligodendrocytes are disposed in rows as interfascicular cells in white matter tracts. Many oligodendrocytes in grey matter are closely associated with neuronal perikarya as perineuronal satellite cells.

Oligodendrocytes are first recognised in the developing brain during the premyelination phase. Soon after, they engage axons which they immediately begin to myelinate. Myelin acts as an insulating material and prevents excitation of the axolemma, other than at the nodes of Ranvier. At the nodes, the myelin sheaths at either side form end-loops of cytoplasm and attachment zones between the sheath and axon. Conduction of a nerve impulse is mediated through polarization and repolarization at the node in a saltatory fashion.

Ependymal cells

The ventricular system is lined by cuboidal or columnar-shaped ependymal cells, the ventricular surfaces of which are ciliated (**2.39**). The cilia project into the ventricles and their basal bodies (blepharoplasts) stain blue on H & E-stained sections. Gaps in the ependymal covering are common, especially in the occipital horns where small ependymal rosettes are also commonly seen. The blood–CSF barrier is maintained in the choroidal epithelium by tight junctions and desmosomes. A primary function of the choroid plexus cells is secretion of the CSF (**2.40**).

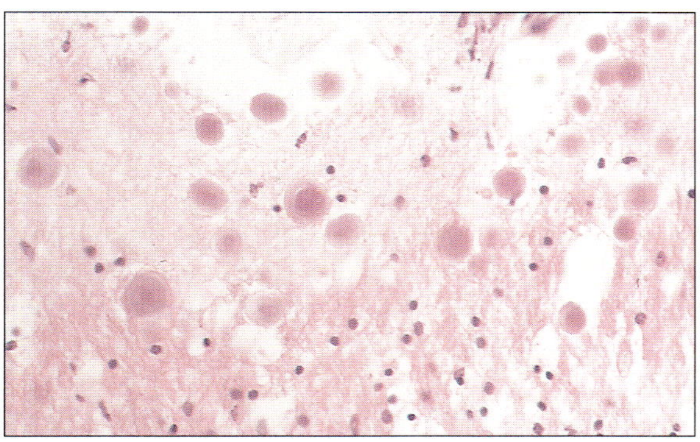

2.38 Corpora amylacea. These spherical basophilic bodies increase in number with age: they show concentric lamellation. (H & E)

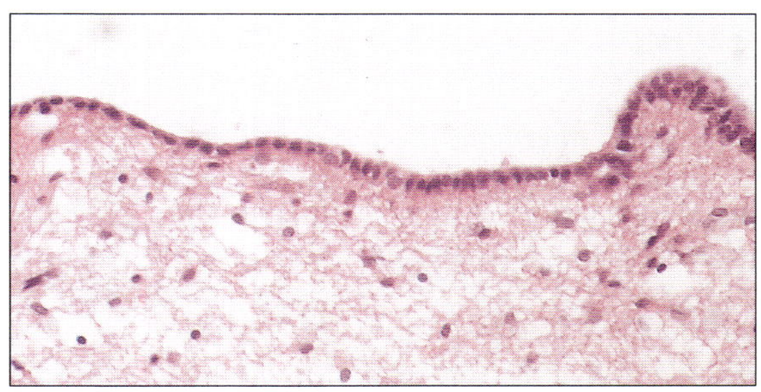

2.39 Ependyma. These ciliated, cuboidal or columnar cells line the ventricular system. (H & E)

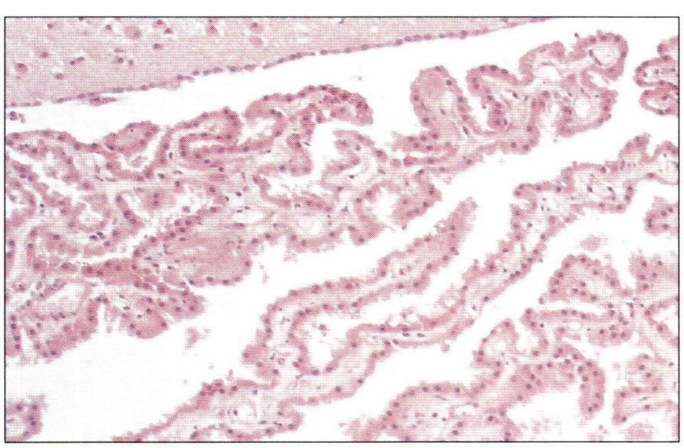

2.40 Choroid plexus. This papillary structure is found in the lateral, third and fourth ventricles. It consists of a core of vascular connective tissue, which is covered by a non-ciliated cuboidal epithelium. With increasing age, it may become calcified and undergo granulomatous degeneration. (H & E)

The subependymal layer is a collection of mitotically active cells scattered along the margins of the ventricles and spinal canal. It appears to comprise a mixture of astrocyte- and oligodendrocyte-progenitor cells, which may give rise to both types of cell after birth.

MICROGLIA

These comprise some 10–20% of the total population of glia in the CNS. They are uniformly distributed with equal numbers in grey and white matter and are made up of small elongated cells with two or three branches. They can be identified ultrastructurally or by the classic technique of silver carbonate of Hortega (**2.29**). Immunocytochemical stains are also available (*see page 2.18*): activated microglia can be identified by demonstrating upregulation of the major histocompatibility complexes I and II; various plant lectins can also be used, e.g. ricinus agglutinin, but they also stain endothelium.

It is generally thought that microglia form a network of antigen-presenting cells in the CNS, with a primary function in immune surveillance. The microglia are thought to arise either from bone-marrow-derived monocytes or from their fetal precursors, and to enter the brain at preferential sites. After migration and mitosis, the cells differentiate into mature microglia.

Experimental evidence suggests that new microglia are supplied from the population already established in the brain, and that monocytes entering the brain after the fetal period become macrophages rather than microglia.

NEUROPIL

This term is used to describe the intercellular matrix in the CNS which in H & E-stained sections appears as 'ground substance' (**2.19**). Under electron microscopy, ground substance consists of a dense complex of glial and neuronal processes, together with some myelin. Between the membranes of adjacent cells, there is a potential extracellular space.

MENINGES AND BLOOD VESSELS

The meninges comprise the dura mater, arachnoid mater and pia mater. The dura mater is made up of two layers, of which the external one forms the inner periostium of the skull and spinal canal. Histologically, it consists of dense collagenous tissue in which there are few blood vessels.

The arachnoid mater is separated from the dura by a potential subdural space and it consists of a thin layer of connective tissue. Attached to its inner surface are cap or arachnoidal cells (**2.41**). The arachnoidal cells aggregate to form arachnoidal granulations (**2.1, 2.42**) and are the means by which CSF is reabsorbed into the venous sinuses that lie between the two layers of the dura.

The pia mater is a thin collagenous membrane that covers the surface of the brain and spinal cord. Between the arachnoid and pia is the subarachnoid space which contains CSF and the blood vessels branching from the circle of Willis to enter the brain.

Histologically, the largest arteries at the base of the brain lack the external elastic lamina found in arteries of equivalent size in other body organs. This

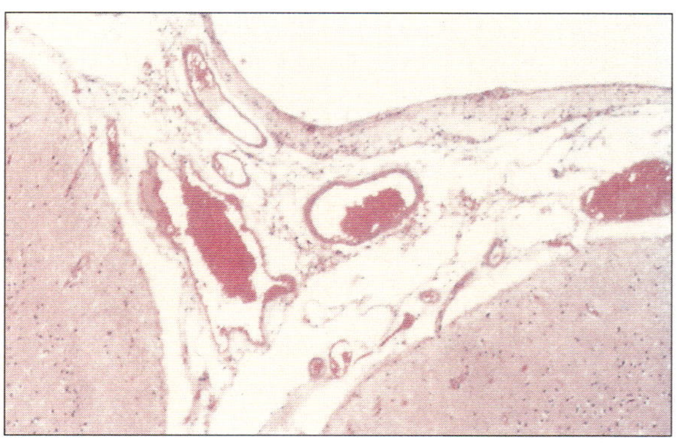

2.41 The meninges. Low-power photomicrograph to show the anatomical features of the arachnoid mater, the subarachnoid space and the pia mater over the surface of the brain. (H & E)

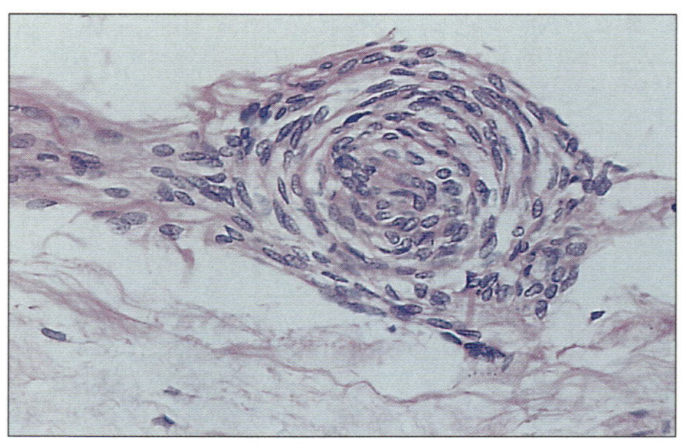

2.42 The meninges. High-power photomicrograph of an arachnoid granulation. (H & E)

is thought to be a factor in the formation of saccular aneurysms (*see Chapter 4*). As part of the normal ageing process, the walls of small blood vessels, especially in the basal ganglia, become encrusted with calcium salts and iron (**2.43**).

Capillaries in the brain, unlike those in other organs of the body, have circumferential tight junctions (zonula occludens) between the endothelial cells. These prevent or retard the passage of large and small molecules from the blood to the intraventricular space (blood–CSF barrier) or the interstitial space (blood–brain barrier). These barriers are characterised by selective permeability to a variety of substances, such as glucose. This permeability is a consequence of metabolic factors, active transport mechanisms, and physical barriers imposed by the anatomy of the endothelium, the basement membrane of the capillary and the foot processes of astrocytes. Experimental studies suggest that astrocytes are responsible for the induction of the blood–brain barrier and probably its maintenance.

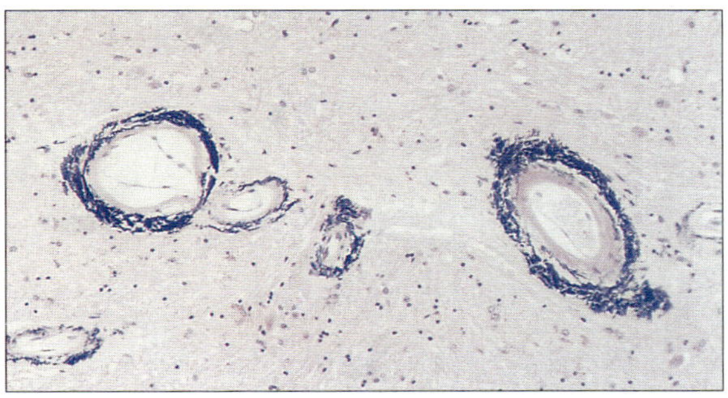

2.43 Siderosis of small blood vessels. There is calcification of small blood vessels in deep grey matter. (H & E)

ARTEFACTS

Various artefacts may arise in the brain and spinal cord as a result of post-mortem changes or difficulties with fixation. These include a band of incomplete fixation at the periphery of a brain, the centre of which is soft and incompletely fixed with pink haloes around small blood vessels.

BRAIN ARTEFACTS

Provided refrigeration has been adequate, post-mortem autolysis is not usually sufficiently advanced to preclude reasonable light microscopy, even several days after death. An exception to this is when the patient has been maintained on a life-support system following the clinical onset of brainstem death. Under these circumstances, the brain undergoes *in vivo* autolysis. At post mortem, this is recognised as the so-called 'respirator brain', which may be increased in weight, semifluid in consistency, and hardens either poorly or not at all in formalin. The tissue is usually discoloured and there is a loss of definition between grey and white matter, with disintegration of midline structures (**2.44**). It is also possible to find fragments of the cerebellar tonsils in the spinal subarachnoid space in cases with advanced changes.

Histologically, neurons have large pale nuclei with indistinct nucleoli and their cytoplasm often appears vacuolated (hydropic cell change). These changes are particularly severe in the granule cells of the cerebellum and appear as the so-called 'grey line' (**2.45**). Another artefact is 'Swiss cheese' change, when smooth-walled cysts occur in the white matter

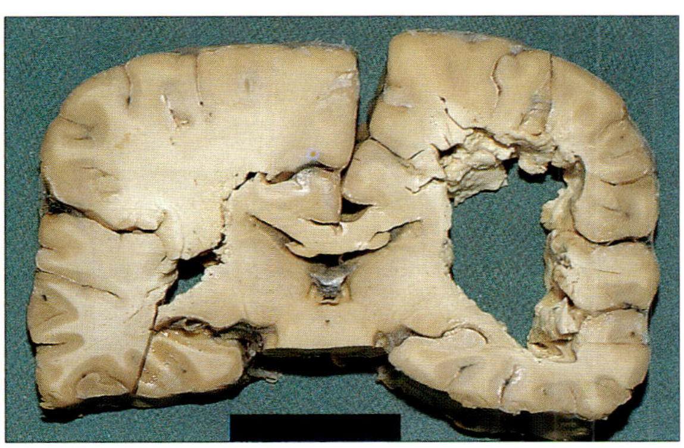

2.44 Post-mortem autolysis. There is loss of anatomical definition and disintegration of tissue.

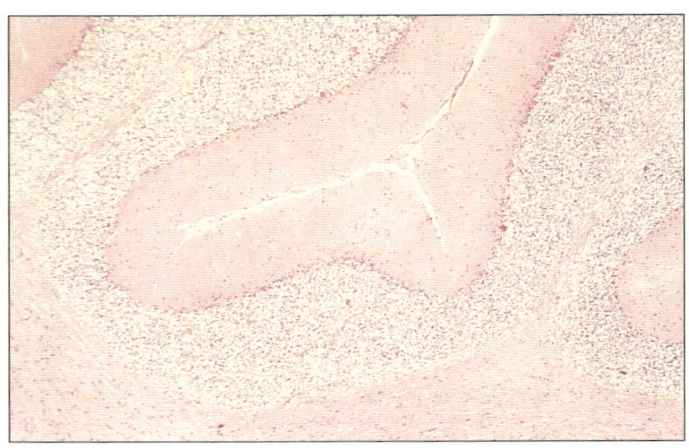

2.45 Post-mortem autolysis. The 'grey-line' is caused by extensive autolysis of the granule-cell layer of the cerebellum. (H & E)

of the brain (**2.46**). These cysts are formed by gas-producing organisms in the absence of any inflammatory reaction.

HISTOLOGICAL ARTEFACT

Histological artefact is seen in many specimens as a result of handling and delayed fixation. The neurons near the surface are shrunken. Nuclei stain deeply with basic dyes and their axons and dendrites are twisted in a corkscrew fashion. This is referred to as 'dark cell change', which can easily be confused with the ischaemic cell process and is particularly common in biopsy material (**2.47**). Other common artefacts include perineuronal and perivascular spaces that are probably due to shrinkage occurring during tissue processing (**2.48**).

Spinal cord artefacts

The spinal cord is particularly prone to artefactual damage following less than perfect removal and excessive handling before fixation. The most characteristic change is the 'toothpaste effect' in which white matter of the dorsal columns is squeezed into adjacent segments.

REACTIONS OF THE NERVOUS SYSTEM TO DISEASE

NEURONS

Neurons are particularly susceptible to hypoxia because they have an obligative aerobic glycolytic metabolism. The structural sequence of events termed the ischaemic cell process is the neuropathological common denominator in all types of hypoxia (*see Chapter 4*). A variety of microscopical changes occur within neurons, some of which are characteristic of specific diseases. These are detailed in the following chapters and include Alzheimer's neurofibrillary degeneration, granulovacuolar degeneration, Hirano

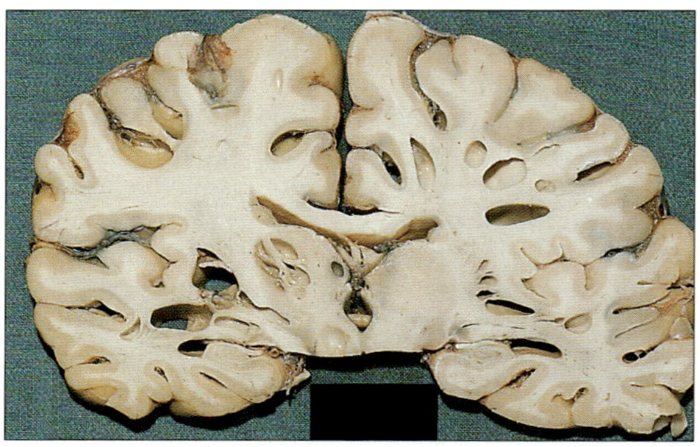

2.46 Post-mortem autolysis. Multiple smooth-walled cysts produce the 'Swiss cheese' change.

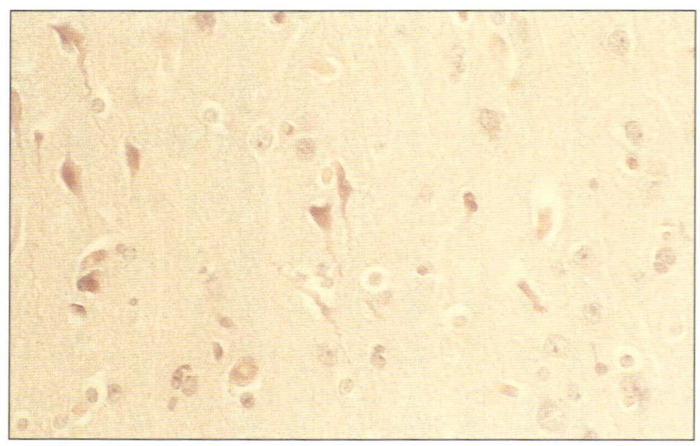

2.47 Dark cell change – artefact. Neurons near the surface of a surgical biopsy may appear shrunken, with darkly staining nuclei and twisted corkscrew axons and dendrites. (H & E)

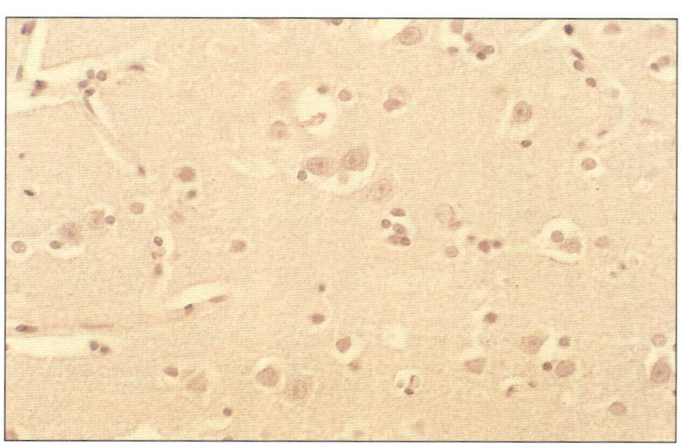

2.48 Perineuronal and perivascular spaces – artefact. This is commonly seen in paediatric material embedded in paraffin wax, and can be reduced or abolished by prolonging the duration of each stage of dehydration, clearing and embedding. (H & E)

bodies, cytoplasmic inclusions in Pick's disease, and Lewy bodies (*see Chapter 7*).

Abnormalities are also seen in various metabolic disorders (*see Chapter 8*). Using light microscopy, it is sometimes possible to identify various intracytoplasmic or nuclear inclusion bodies. Ferrugination is another feature in which neurons become encrusted with iron and calcium, particularly in the vicinity of old vascular lesions (**2.49**). Pigment deposits are characteristically found in the Hallervorden–Spatz syndrome (*see Chapter 7*), in the basal ganglia in cases of striatonigral degeneration (*see Chapter 7*), and after severe birth hypoxia (*see Chapter 9*). Neuronophagia is the term used to describe the process by which microglial cells surround dead or dying nerve cells, which may still be recognisable by their outlines. Apoptosis or programmed cell death is quite different from neuronophagia and is particularly evident during development of the CNS and in tumours.

Reactions to axonal transection

These include both the response in the nerve cell body termed central chromatolysis and the response in the distal myelinated axon referred to as Wallerian degeneration.

Central chromatolysis

Central chromatolysis occurs in both central and peripheral neurons. It may be followed either by regeneration or may proceed to degeneration and ultimate death of the nerve cell. The changes occur more rapidly and to a greater degree if the axonal damage is close to the cell body, and are particularly well seen in the cell bodies of neurons whose axons project out of the nervous system into cranial or peripheral nerves. Histologically, central chromatolysis is characterised by swelling of the cell body, with displacement of the nucleus to the periphery of the cell and enlargement of the nucleus. The centre of the cell body becomes cleared as a result of dispersion of the Nissl substance – chromatolysis (**2.50**). This change is particularly well seen in preparations stained by cresyl violet, while electron microscopy shows that it is due to fragmentation and dispersion of the granular endoplasmic reticulum and ribosomal rosettes.

Wallerian degeneration

Wallerian degeneration, also known as anterograde axonal degeneration, results from disruption of an axon. The severed ends of both the proximal and distal stumps swell to form axonal bulbs. These bulbs are attributed to anterograde and retrograde axoplasmic flow, and can be identified by light microscopy in routine human material about 15–18 hours after injury. They are not infrequently seen adjacent to infarcts or haematomas as well as in certain types of head injury, where they may form part of the complex of diffuse axonal injury. The bulbs may swell to 50μm diameter, and it is from these bulbs that fibre regeneration may occur. If regeneration does not occur, then the distal portion of the transected axon will undergo progressive degeneration. Within 3–4 days, the whole of the axon distal to the site of transection will become irregular in outline and then fragmented. These features can be identified in H & E-stained preparations, but are particularly well seen after silver impregnation preparations. In certain diseases, there is a slowly progressive degeneration of axons from their distal ends back to the cell bodies. Bulbous swellings develop on the degenerating axon, the cell body of which does not show chromatolysis. This is thought to represent a 'dying-back' process which

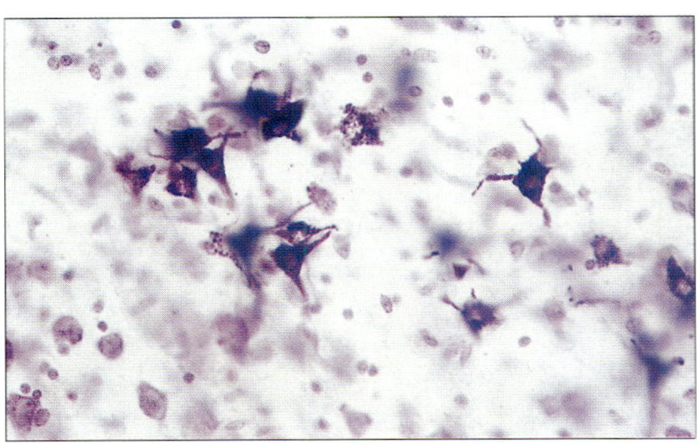

2.49 Ferruginated neurons. The cell bodies and processes of dead neurons are encrusted by granules of iron and calcium salts. (Celloidin: cresyl violet)

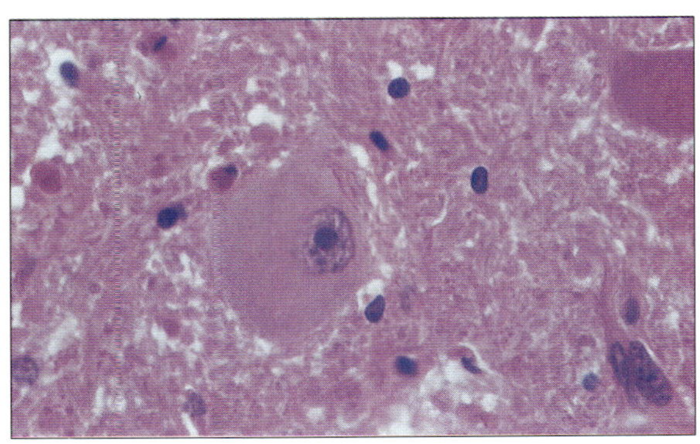

2.50 Central chromatolysis of the ventral horn cell of the spinal cord. The cell body is rounded, with clearing of Nissl substance from the central part of the perikaryon and an eccentrically placed nucleus. (H & E)

may occur in systemic disorders *(see Chapter 7)* and in toxic axonopathies of both the CNS (**2.51**) and peripheral nervous system.

Following axotomy, changes take place within the terminal innervation fields of the affected axons – a characteristic feature of which is the formation of degenerating boutons terminaux. These are also well-demonstrated in silver impregnation preparations. Both the axonal debris and the degenerating terminals are removed rapidly by phagocytosis. If the process has occurred in a motor nerve, then the changes of neurogenic atrophy in muscle will consequently develop *(see Chapter 7)*. Commensurate with the changes in axons, myelin breaks down into ovoid bodies. This process occurs more quickly in the peripheral nervous system than in the CNS and can be recognised by a variety of staining procedures. During the process of myelin degradation, cholesterol esters are produced which stain red with Sudan dyes and black with osmium as in the Marchi technique. The loss of myelin can also be demonstrated by so-called negative stains in which normal myelin is black – loss of myelin can therefore be identified by lack of staining.

ASTROCYTES

Damage to the CNS is usually accompanied by hypertrophy and hyperplasia of astrocytes. The process of astrocytosis is usually associated with the production of large numbers of glial fibres stainable by PTAH (**2.52**) or for GFAP (**2.53**). At this point, it is worth noting that GFAP is intracellular, whereas collagen, which is the equivalent product from fibroblasts, is extracellular. The process occurs rapidly within about 48 hours of tissue damage. As the process develops, the tissue becomes firmer than normal and acquires a translucent appearance, which is seen characteristically in plaques of multiple sclerosis and in the walls of syringomyelia cavities. The glial fibres are usually laid down in an irregular manner, but occasionally, particularly in the molecular layer of the cerebellum, they assume a regular and

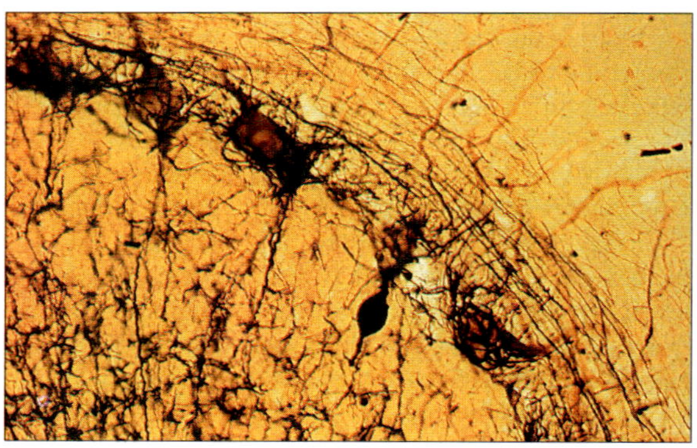

2.51 Axonal balloons. There is a terminal swelling (balloon or torpedo) on the axon of a Purkinje cell from a patient with alcoholic encephalopathy. (Palmgren silver)

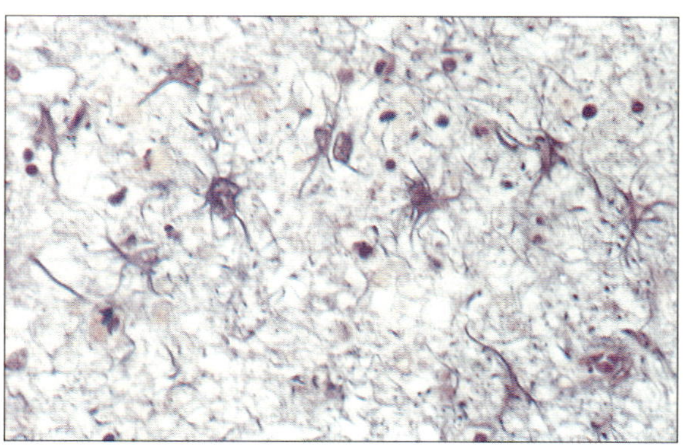

2.52 Astrocytosis. There is hypertrophy and hyperplasia of fibre-forming astrocytes. (PTAH)

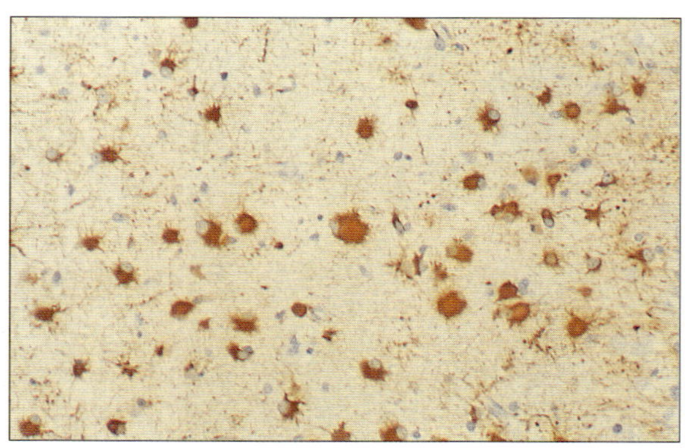

2.53 Astrocytosis. (ICC for GFAP)

parallel arrangement known as isomorphic gliosis (**2.54**).

In longstanding astrocytosis, in some gliomas (*see Chapter 10*) and in certain types of leucodystrophy (*see Chapter 8*), Rosenthal fibres may be found (**2.55**). These are irregular, darkly eosinophilic structures, which have no other particular staining affinities. Often, a mixed glial and fibroblastic response, referred to as the gliomesodermal reaction, is seen in the capsule around intracerebral abscesses. Astrocytes in oedematous white matter become enlarged and acquire eosinophilic homogeneous cytoplasm and an eccentric nucleus (**2.56**). Such cells are known as gemistocytic astrocytes, and with resolution of the lesion they become fibre-forming astrocytes. In various metabolic disorders, but principally in hepatic encephalopathy and associated with portocaval shunts, the nuclei of protoplasmic astrocytes become enlarged, reniform in shape, and acquire one or more prominent nucleoli. They are then known as Alzheimer type 2 astrocytes.

OLIGODENDROCYTES

Damage to oligodendrocytes may be a consequence of viral infection, radiotherapy, chemotherapy, or various immunological mechanisms. It results in demyelination, the features of which are described above as part of Wallerian degeneration.

MICROGLIA

As already noted, there is a microglial reaction in encephalomyelitis, and microglia also take part in neuronophagia. When reactive, as in syphilis, they become elongated and assume the features of rod

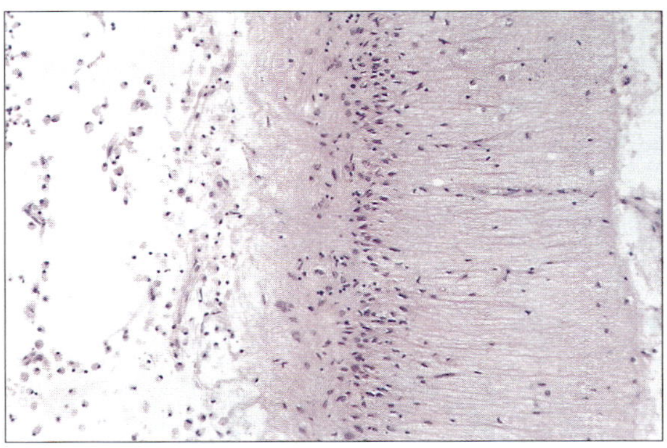

2.54 Isomorphic gliosis, showing an old infarct in the cortex of cerebellum. Note the regular and parallel arrangement of the fibre-forming astrocytes in the molecular layer. (H & E)

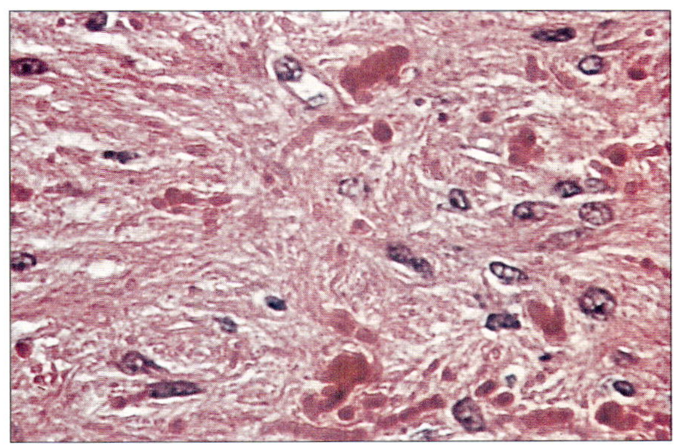

2.55 Rosenthal fibres. These are eosinophilic structures which may be round, oval, or enlongated. The nature of the centre of these structures is uncertain but their periphery consists of glial fibres which are GFAP positive. (H & E)

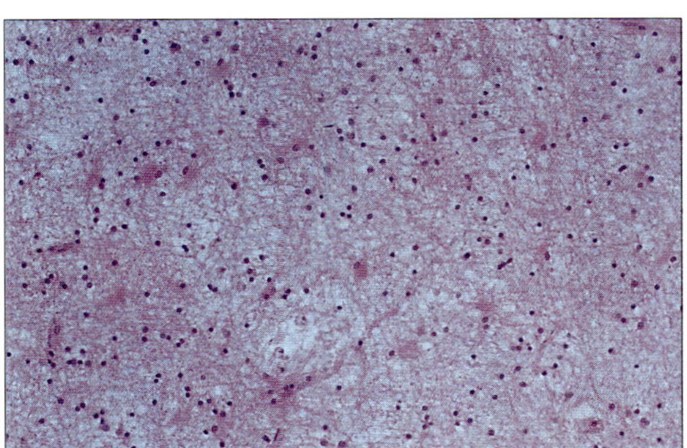

2.56 Oedematous white matter. In contrast with normal myelin (*see* **2.26**), there is loosening of the white matter with paler staining due to separation of myelinated fibres and an astrocytosis. (H & E)

cells (**2.57**). When brain tissue has been destroyed, the rod cells become enlarged and rounded with eccentric nuclei and vacuolated cytoplasm as a result of the phagocytosis of the breakdown products of myelin. These lipid phagocytes are commonly seen in plaques of demyelination *(see Chapter 6)* and at the edge of cerebral infarcts. Such phagocytes may be pigmented and are referred to as siderophages when they stain positively with Perl's prussian-blue reaction. In several disease processes, particularly after trauma, clusters of microglia may be seen in white matter. These are thought to represent reactions to foci of axonal damage. Similar changes are also seen in cases of bacteraemia.

EPENDYMAL CELLS

The most common change is that of granular ependymitis as a consequence of either hydrocephalus or chronic inflammation. It consists of small nodules on the surface of the ventricles (**2.58**). Histologically, the nodules are collections of proliferating subependymal astrocytes and are often not covered by ependyma.

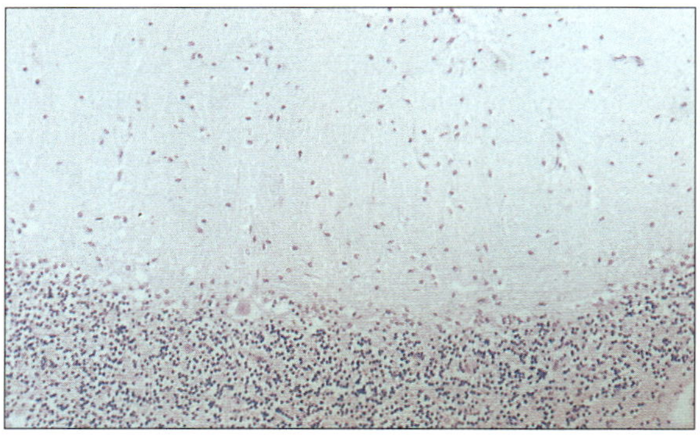

2.57 Reactive microglia. These appear as rod-shaped nuclei in areas of recently damaged brain, e.g. ischaemic damage in cerebellum. (H & E)

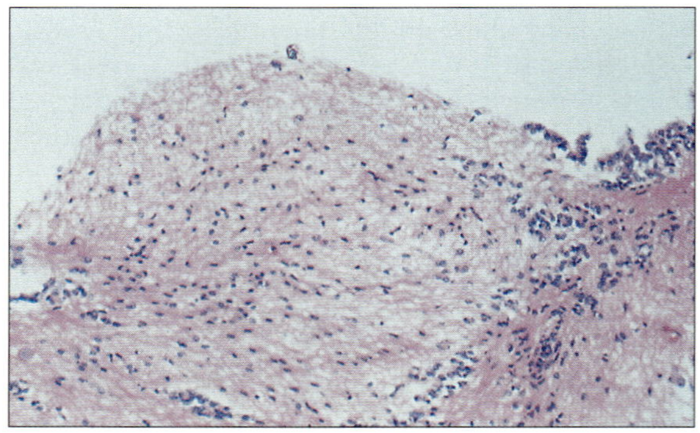

2.58 Granular ependymitis. This consists of small collections of reactive subependymal astrocytes, often devoid of a covering of ependymal cells. (H & E)

Neuropathological features of raised intracranial pressure due to unilateral mass lesion
Narrowing of sulci and flattening of gyri
Reduction in size of ipsilateral ventricle
Midline shift
Supracallosal hernia
Tentorial hernia
Compression of ipsilateral oculomotor nerve
Tonsillar hernia
Brainstem haemorrhage/infarction, including Kernohan notch
Medial occipital lobe infarction

2.59 Neuropathological features of raised intracranial pressure due to unilateral mass lesion.

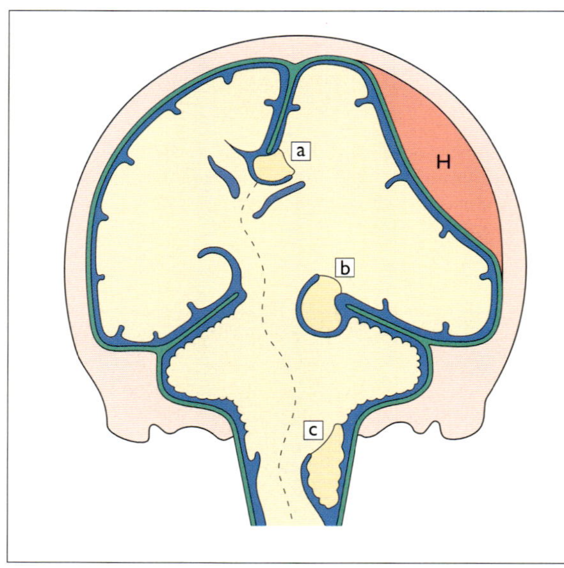

2.60 Raised intracranial pressure, showing the intracranial compartments and the result of a mass lesion on the right hand side. In addition to a shift of the midline structures and distortion of the ventricular system, there is: (a) a supracallosal hernia; (b) a tentorial hernia; (c) a tonsillar hernia.

RAISED INTRACRANIAL PRESSURE

SUPRATENTORIAL MASS LESION

Unilateral supratentorial mass lesions of whatever nature results in the development of several characteristic features (**2.59, 2.60**). As a supracallosal (subfalcine or cingulate) hernia develops, the ipsilateral cingulate gyrus becomes displaced beneath the falx.

A tentorial hernia develops as the medial part of the ipsilateral temporal lobe becomes displaced through the tentorial incisura (**2.61**). This results in stretching and distortion of the ipsilateral IIIrd nerve, producing characteristic dilation of the pupil on the side of the expanding lesion.

As these conditions advance, the hypothalamic structures become displaced backwards and downwards, and come to lie below the level of the tentorial opening. This is accompanied by certain clinical signs and symptoms (**2.62**). Also, the midbrain is narrowed in its transverse axis, the aqueduct is compressed, and the contralateral cerebral peduncle is pushed against the opposite free edge of the tentorium – the Kernohan notch (**2.63**). This brain distortion and

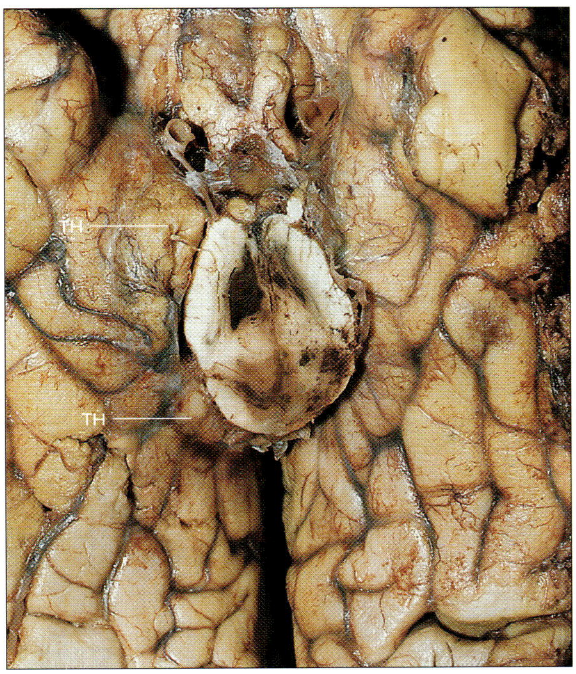

2.61 Tentorial hernia. There was an expanding lesion in the right cerebral hemisphere. Note the conspicuous tentorial hernia (TH), haemorrhagic compression of the ipsilateral oculomotor nerve, and extensive secondary haemorrhage into the upper brainstem.

Neurological features associated with progressive elevation of intracranial pressure

Reduction in level of consciousness

Dilation of pupil ipsilateral to mass lesion

Bradycardia, increase in pulse pressure and increased mean arterial pressure

Cheyne–Stokes respiration

2.62 Clinical features associated with progressive elevation of intracranial pressure.

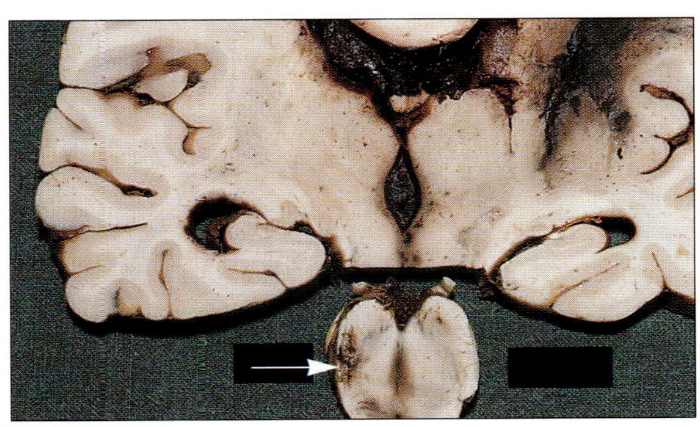

2.63 Kernohan notch. A mass lesion in the right cerebral hemisphere has induced an ipsilateral tentorial hernia and a contralateral peduncular lesion (arrow head).

internal herniation may cause severe impairment of blood circulation through the pericallosal, anterior choroidal and posterior cerebral arteries (**2.64**). As a result, widespread infarction may occur in the structures they supply.

A tonsillar hernia may also occur in association with a supratentorial mass lesion. It is the downward displacement of the cerebellar tonsils through the foramen magnum. If herniation is due to a supratentorial lesion, there is often a combination of tentorial and tonsillar herniation.

Occasionally, the posterior inferior cerebellar arteries may be compressed to such an extent that infarction occurs in the cerebellar hemispheres. The cerebellum may also be displaced upwards through the tentorial opening to produce the so-called reversed tentorial hernia.

The main feature indicating that intracranial pressure has been high during life is a wedge of pressure necrosis in the parahippocampal gyrus (**2.65**).

SWELLING AND OEDEMA

BRAIN SWELLING

The term brain swelling describes a localised or generalised enlargement of the brain, while congestive brain swelling tends to be diffuse, affecting one or both hemispheres. The arteriolar network is dilated and the capillary bed is flooded with stagnant blood.

The precise pathogenesis is unknown, but it can develop very quickly, particularly in children following a head injury and in patients after evacuation of an acute subdural haematoma (*see Chapter 5*).

CEREBRAL OEDEMA

This term is used to describe an increase in the water content of brain tissue, which in turn leads to an increase in the volume of all or part of the brain. The normal water content of grey matter is 80% of the wet weight, and of white matter 68% of wet weight: the content in cerebral oedema would be about 81–82% and 77–79%, respectively. There are several types of cerebral oedema and the increased water content may be either extracellular or intracellular. In vasogenic oedema, the blood–brain barrier is defective, and water, sodium and protein are extravasated into the extracellular space. This occurs particularly in white matter. On histological examination, there is pallor of myelin staining, with the myelin sheaths being rather vacuolated and beaded (**2.56**). Gemistocytic astrocytes are conspicuous. If the oedema persists for several weeks or months, there is a loss of myelin, particularly in periventricular white matter.

In cytotoxic oedema, the commonest type of which is due to ischaemia, the changes are essentially intracellular and are a result of energy failure within neurons. A similar type of oedema may result from the actions of such toxins as triethyltin and hexachlorophane. In hydrostatic oedema, the passage of

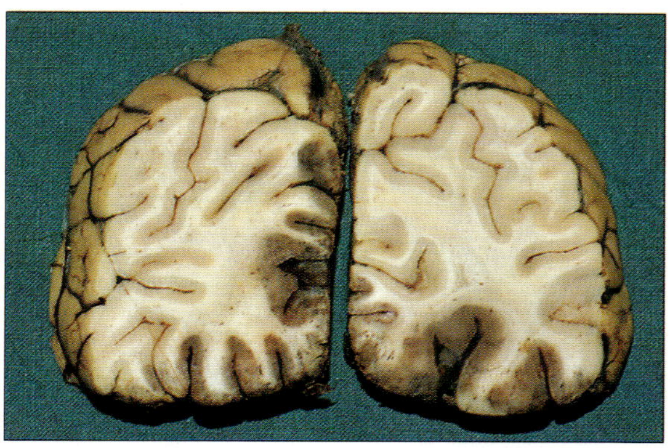

2.64 Medial occipital lobe infarction. There is haemorrhagic infarction in the cortex of the medial and inferior surfaces of each occipital lobe within the distribution of the posterior cerebral arteries.

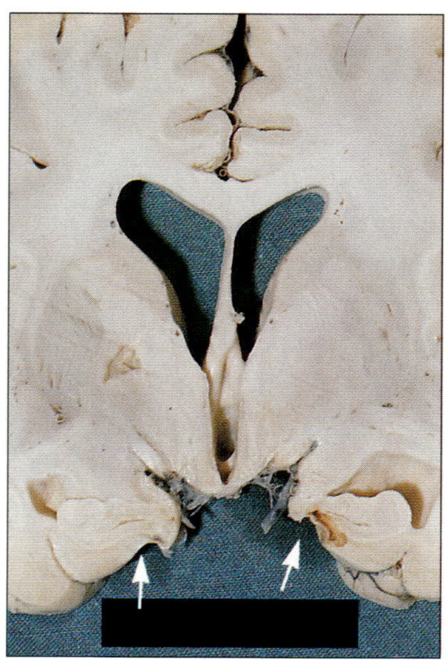

2.65 Pressure necrosis. A previous episode of raised intracranial pressure is characterised by a wedge in the medial part of the parahippocampal gyrus (arrows).

protein-poor fluid into the extracellular space is followed by a sudden increase in the intravascular pressure, which forcibly dilates the capillary bed. This type of oedema is seen in hypertensive encephalopathy. In interstitial oedema, the water content of the periventricular tissue increases in acute obstructive hydrocephalus, as fluid is forced into the periventricular white matter through damaged ependyma. Finally, in hypo-osmotic oedema, swelling occurs as a result of a large reduction in serum osmolality.

HYDROCEPHALUS

FORMATION AND CIRCULATION OF CSF

This process is depicted in **2.66**. The majority of CSF is produced in the choroid plexuses of the lateral, third and fourth ventricles. CSF leaves the lateral ventricles, via the interventricular foramina of Monro, and passes through the aqueduct of Sylvius to enter the fourth ventricle. It then exits via the foramina of Luschka (lateral) and Magendie (midline) to enter the subarachnoid space of the posterior fossa. Some CSF passes through the foramen magnum into the spinal subarachnoid space where it is absorbed in the prolongations of the subarachnoid space along the spinal nerve roots. However, most CSF circulates through the posterior fossa, from where it reaches the supratentorial space through the tentorial incisura. It then flows over the cerebral hemispheres to be absorbed via arachnoidal granulations in the superior sagittal sinus (**2.1**). The volume of CSF is about 120ml and has a turnover of some 3–5 times per day. Samples of CSF are usually obtained by lumbar puncture, but in neurosurgical units, specimens may be taken via catheters placed within the lateral ventricles.

DESCRIPTION OF HYDROCEPHALUS

The term hydrocephalus means an increased volume of CSF within the cranial cavity. In internal hydrocephalus, the increased volume of CSF is within the ventricular system, whereas in external hydrocephalus the excess CSF is in the subarachnoid space. The hydrocephalus is said to be communicating if CSF can flow freely from the ventricular system to the subarachnoid space; if it cannot it is non-communicating. Compensatory (*ex-vacuo*) hydrocephalus occurs when the increased volume of CSF is due to loss of brain tissue (*see Chapter 7*). The most common causes of ventricular enlargement are secondary to cerebral atrophy, itself due to ageing or to neurodegenerative disease. In these circumstances, the intracranial pressure is not elevated.

Obstructive hydrocephalus

Acutely developing hydrocephalus with an increased intracranial pressure is usually caused by obstruction to the free flow of CSF. The ventricles enlarge and

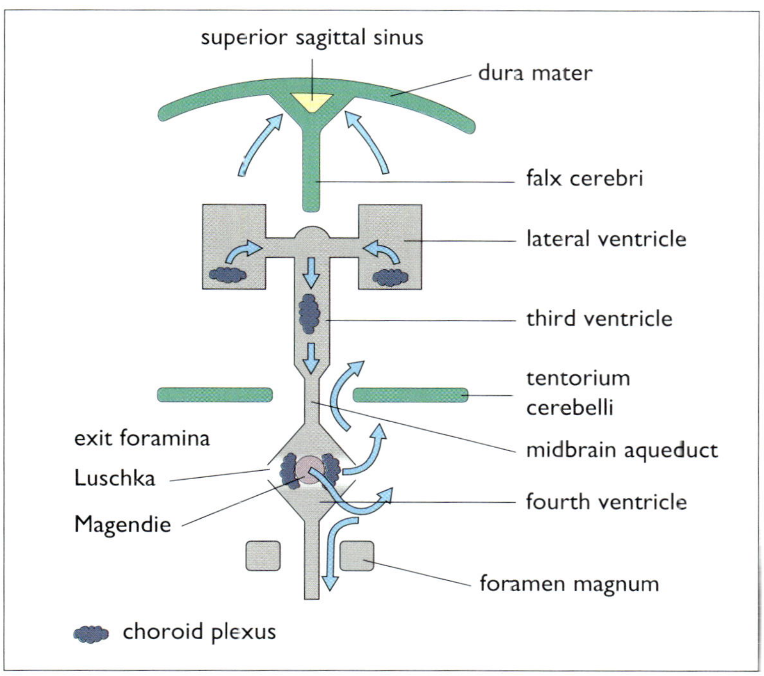

2.66 The formation and circulation of CSF. The bulk of CSF is produced in the choroid plexuses of the lateral, third and fourth ventricles. The direction of flow is indicated by the arrows.

interstitial oedema develops in periventricular white matter. Death can occur rapidly unless effective treatment is instituted promptly. There is usually time, however, to establish ventricular drainage to remove CSF; this results in rapid reduction in size of the ventricles. In obstructive hydrocephalus, it is the site of the lesion rather than its nature which is of importance. Thus, a small lesion adjacent to an interventricular foramen or the aqueduct in the midbrain is of much greater significance than a large expanding lesion in a frontal or occipital lobe.

Congenital or acquired lesions of the posterior fossa are particularly prone to the development of obstructive hydrocephalus. The free flow of CSF may also be impeded by obliteration of the subarachnoid space following meningitis or subarachnoid haemorrhage. The site of the obstruction can usually be identified fairly readily by the enlargement of the ventricular system proximal to the obstruction:

- if the obstruction is at an interventricular foramen, one lateral ventricle enlarges;
- if it is in the third ventricle or the aqueduct both lateral ventricles enlarge;
- if it is at the exit foramina of the fourth ventricle, the entire ventricular system enlarges.

Normal pressure hydrocephalus

This condition is characterised by ventricular enlargement and a clinical syndrome consisting of progressive dementia, disturbance of gait, and urinary incontinence or urgency. It is possible to demonstrate episodes of moderate intracranial hypertension, particularly during sleep, which may be improved by a ventriculoperitoneal shunt.

Benign intracranial hypertension

It is not clear if this represents a single entity or is merely one of several different disease processes which cause raised intracranial pressure. It occurs more frequently in women than in men. Patients present with high intracranial pressure, and radiologically the ventricular system is not enlarged. Steroid treatment is often helpful in relieving symptoms.

TRAUMA BY NON-MECHANICAL FORCES

The most important of these are the effects of irradiation and of chemotherapy.

IRRADIATION

The type, frequency and extent of post-radiotherapy complications depend on many factors. These include the total dose of irradiation, the number of fractions, the dose per fraction, total treatment time, the volume irradiated, the elimination of 'hot spots' by the use of multiple fields, and the use of other treatments, such as steroids, radiosensitisers or antineoplastic chemotherapy.

The most serious effects are those of the late-delayed reactions caused either by diffuse damage to white matter (leucoencephalopathy) or a space-occupying glial vascular reaction (delayed radionecrosis). These features tend to occur from about one year to many years after treatment, and have been described following irradiation of intracranial or intraspinal tumours.

Delayed radionecrosis

The macroscopic appearances of radionecrosis are similar to those of a malignant glioma. The white matter becomes expanded and replaced by focally cystic waxy pale-yellow tissue (**2.67**) in which there

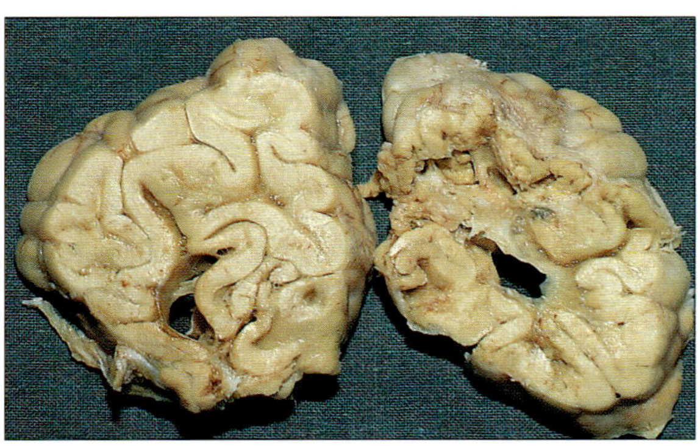

2.67 Delayed radiation necrosis. There is yellow-brown discoloration and marked loss of the white matter in the occipital lobes.

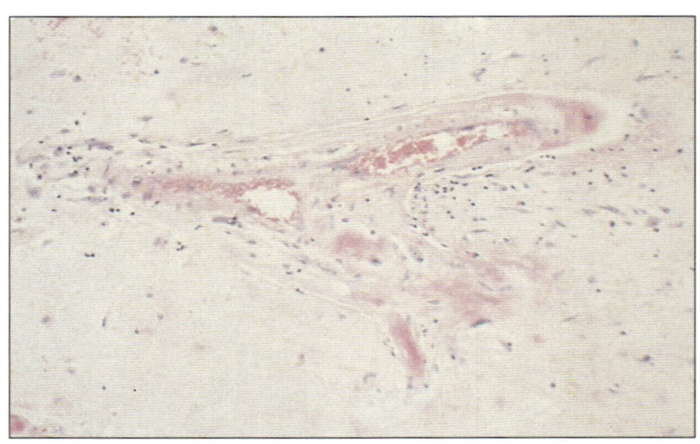

2.68 Delayed radiation necrosis. There is disintegration of tissue with fibrinoid necrosis of small blood vessels (H & E).

may be petechial haemorrhages. Histologically, the process is characterised by appearances that range from coagulative necrosis, around which there is no, or minimal reactive changes, to foci of demyelination, loss of axons and infiltration by macrophages, lymphocytes and plasma cells. The most important change is fibrinoid necrosis and hyalinisation of blood vessel walls (**2.68**), which may be sufficient to cause obliterative endarteritis and thrombotic occlusion of small vessels.

Additional features include the formation of telangiectatic vessels, proliferation of perivascular fibroblasts, and an associated astrocytosis, often with bizarre multinucleated cells resembling those seen in progressive multifocal leucoencephalopathy, which does not however show abnormal blood vessels (*see Chapter 6*).

The pathogenesis of radionecrosis remains uncertain, but in general the incidence of necrosis is progressively greater with higher irradiation doses. Below 57Gy, this complication is rarely seen; between 57Gy and 65Gy, it may develop in up to 3% of patients; above 65Gy, the incidence may be as high as 18–20%.

Leucoencephalopathy

A diffuse leucoencephalopathy, which may be necrotizing, is also associated with radiotherapy. However, it is most likely to be a complication of drug treatments. Additional complications include impairment of cognitive function, hypothalamo-pituitary dysfunction, and occasionally irradiation-induced damage to both large extracranial and intracranial arteries.

Brain tumours

An uncommon complication of cranial irradiation may be the induction of brain tumours, the commonest examples being meningeal fibrosarcomas and meningiomas. There have also been an increasing number of reports of a second neuroectodermal tumour developing in children with intracranial tumours, particularly cerebral deposits of leukaemia treated by radiotherapy. Most of these second tumours are glioblastoma and have appeared within the first three decades of life.

CHEMOTHERAPY

Complications in the CNS are usually due to a direct effect of the drug being used, but infection may occur secondary to the leucopenic effect of treatment. Complications include an acute or chronic encephalopathy or myelopathy and an acute cerebellar syndrome. A chronic encephalopathy has been described following methotrexate administration and has since been recognised as a disseminated necrotising leucoencephalopathy. Abnormalities tend to be limited to white matter and the histological features are distinctive, comprising foci of disseminated coagulative necrosis that appear to be unrelated to blood vessels. There is loss of myelin and extensive damage to axons with bulb formation and astrocytosis, but all in the apparent absence of either an inflammatory cell or macrophage response. These changes sometimes occur in the absence of any vascular damage.

FURTHER READING

Adams JH, Graham DI. *An Introduction to Neuropathology*. 2nd edn. Edinburgh, Churchill–Livingstone, 1994.

Adams JH, Murray MF. *Atlas of Post-Mortem Techniques in Neuropathology*. Cambridge, Cambridge University Press, 1982.

Advisory Committee on Dangerous Pathogens. HIV: *The Causative Agent of AIDS and Related Conditions. 2nd Revision of Guidelines.* London, HMSO, 1990.

Advisory Committee on Dangerous Pathogens. *Precautions for Work with Human and Animal Transmissible Spongiform Encephalopathies.* London, HMSO, 1994.

Esiri MM, Oppenheimer DR. *Diagnostic Neuropathology.* Oxford, Blackwell Scientific, 1989.

Health and Safety Commission's Health Services Advisory Committee. *Safe Working and the Prevention of Infection in Clinical Laboratories.* London, HMSO, 1991.

Health and Safety Commission's Health Services Advisory Committee. *Safe Working and the Prevention of Infection in the Mortuary and Post-Mortem Room.* London, HMSO, 1991.

Polak JM, Van Noorden S (eds). *Immunocytochemistry: Modern Methods and Applications.* 2nd edn. Bristol, John Wright, 1986.

Weller RO. *Colour Atlas of Neuropathology.* London, Harvey Miller, 1984.

3. Infections

Several factors combine to reduce the risk of CNS infection, including the:

- dura mater;
- blood–brain barrier;
- microglia;
- pericytes;
- blood cells;
- lymphatic drainage of the CNS.

The tough dura mater lines the skull and spinal canal, and completely encloses the CNS. It provides an effective physical barrier, preventing invasion by microorganisms from local foci of infection. The unique properties of the blood–brain barrier (*see Chapter 1*) also reduce the ingress of particles, proteins and fluid to a considerable extent compared with other tissues.

Within the parenchyma of the nervous system, the resident population of microglial cells has macrophage functions and a possible role in immunosurveillance, though the full range of activities of these cells is poorly understood. Pericytes are a specialised collection of cells which are part of the outer vascular walls. They express some lymphoid and macrophage cell markers and may play a role in normal protective mechanisms. Under normal circumstances, there is a traffic of blood monocytes (and possibly lymphocytes) through the cerebral endothelium. However, the part played by these cells in either combating infection or allowing the entry of microorganisms, such as human immunodeficiency virus (HIV), is not clear.

Traditionally, the CNS has been regarded as an immunologically privileged site, and the parenchyma as having no lymphatic channels. It has been shown recently, however, that some parts of the CNS have lymphatic clearance, with drainage to cervical nodes in particular. Thus, the special immunological status of the CNS may be more apparent than real and may be restricted to a limited tolerance of grafts. Circulating CSF may actually serve as a dispersal mechanism for microorganisms once they have entered the nervous system, and they may spread rapidly by this mechanism.

Selective involvement of CNS

The CNS often shows patterns of selective involvement, particularly with viruses such as poliovirus and herpes simplex virus. This suggests that neurotropic mechanisms may operate in some cases; it is possible these are receptor mediated.

Pathogenetic mechanisms

Bacteria may produce powerful exotoxins which damage or kill cells directly. Viral infections may also lyse cells. In some infections, however, the pathogenesis of damage is far from clear. For example, HIV infects microglia and it is thought that neurons may be damaged secondarily by cytotoxic molecules released by activated macrophages.

CNS reactions to infection

The CNS is capable of a brisk appropriate response to penetration by microorganisms. Bacterial infections evoke a polymorphonuclear leucocyte reaction, and viruses evoke a lymphocytic response. These reactions are characteristically seen in the subarachnoid space (**3.1**) and the Virchow–Robin perivascular spaces (**3.2**) in the parenchyma, particularly in the early stages of infection. Other special forms of inflammation seen in the CNS suggest a particular diagnosis, as follows:

- A granulomatous reaction is found in tuberculosis, fungal infections, syphilis and sarcoidosis.
- Cerebral malaria is characterised by small areas of demyelination centred on a vessel distended with parasitised erythrocytes.

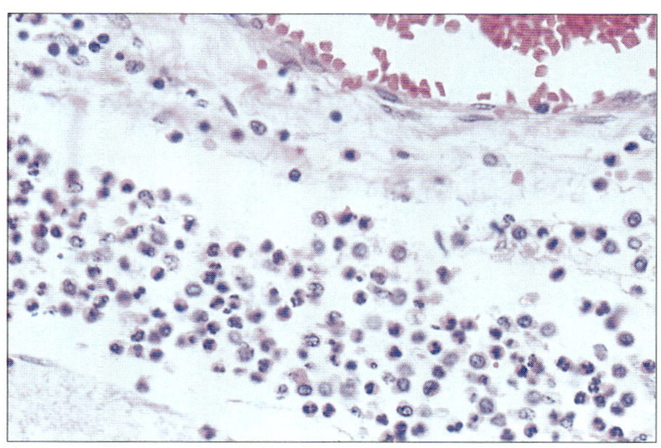

3.1 Acute inflammatory infiltrate in the subarachnoid space from a 29-year-old man with bacterial meningitis.

- Microglial cells may show a diffuse response, becoming visible as rod cells as in syphilis, or may be focally aggregated as in viral encephalitis. Since microglial responses occur in many disease processes, however, these may be nonspecific phenomena.

It should be remembered that the patterns and distribution of CNS responses may be considerably modified by treatment.

RISK FACTORS FOR CNS INFECTION

Although the intact nervous system may fall victim to virulent organisms that overcome its normal defence mechanisms, certain circumstances increase its vulnerability to all types of infection.

Disruption of normal coverings

This usually occurs as a result of accidental and non-accidental trauma. The risk of infection varies according to the degree of exposure of CNS tissues, and the circumstances in which this occurs. For example, while it is expected in compound fractures, it is a rare complication of neurosurgical procedures or of lumbar puncture. Congenital malformations such as encephaloceles and spina bifida, are very prone to postnatal infection.

Local sources of infection

Any source of infection in the tissues adjacent to the CNS may serve as an entry point for microorganisms. Particular hazards include localised foci in the skull, such as sinusitis and otitis media. Until fairly recently, mastoiditis was a frequent forerunner of CNS infections in the developed world, and is still common in some parts of the world.

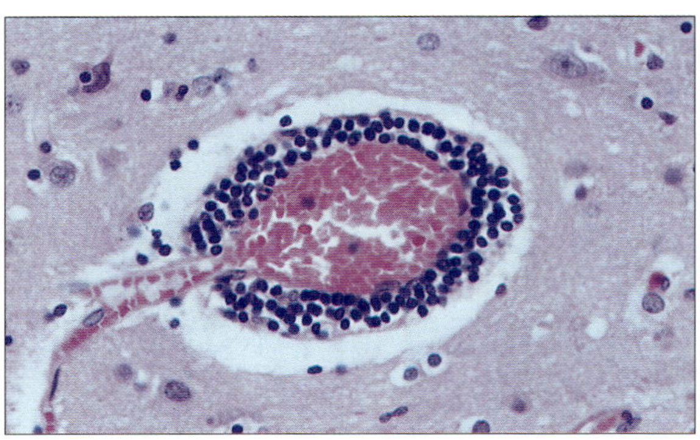

3.2 Perivascular cuff of lymphocytes in the Virchow–Robin space in a 39-year-old woman with viral encephalitis.

Bloodborne infections

If the blood carries a significant number of organisms, as in septicaemia, or in infected thrombotic emboli originating from a source such as endocarditis, there is a considerable risk of microorganisms entering the brain. Mycotic aneurysms may result from thrombotic emboli, with the attendant risk of infection and haemorrhage. However, breakdown of the blood–brain barrier in the vicinity of infarcts or tumours does not usually lead to infection of brain tissue unless there is accompanying septicaemia.

General immunodeficiency status

If the immune competence of the individual as a whole is reduced for whatever reason, the CNS is more vulnerable than usual to infection, particularly with opportunistic agents. Examples of impaired immunological status are discussed below.

CLINICAL SIGNS AND SYMPTOMS OF INFECTION

The microorganisms that attack the CNS are usually bacteria or viruses, while fungi, protozoa and metazoa are also important but less common. The diagnosis of CNS infections may be clinically straightforward or extremely challenging. The clinical presentation depends not only on the type of organism, but also on the age of the patient and the tissue compartment predominantly infected. Infections occurring in infants or in the elderly may be difficult to diagnose, and CNS infections occurring during fetal life may not show their effects until weeks or months after birth. The signs and symptoms of meningitis are rather different from those of encephalomyelitis. Infections may be classified according to their site:

- osteomyelitis of skull or vertebral column;
- extradural infection;
- subdural infection;
- subarachnoid infection;
- parenchymal infection;
- ventriculitis and choroid plexitis.

Infective processes may involve the bone or meninges at the vault of the skull, at the base, or in the vertebral column. Epidural (**3.3**) and subdural (**3.4**) abscesses can arise from local spread to these compartments. Some viral infections show considerable variation in the interval between infection and the onset of clinical illness, and also in the duration of illness. A few viruses have the ability to lie dormant for years in the nervous system without causing ill-health. Clinical signs and symptoms of acute infection of the nervous system include:

- headache;
- neck stiffness;

- photophobia;
- raised temperature;
- general malaise.

If untreated, CNS infections may lead to a disturbance of consciousness and a fatal outcome.

Investigations

Investigation of possible cases of CNS infection includes examination of the CSF, though lumbar puncture is a potentially hazardous investigation in the presence of raised intracranial pressure. This may accompany CNS infections if these are in the form of mass lesions or of obstructive hydrocephalus. The characteristic CSF findings in different forms of infection are shown in **3.5**. Early confirmation of suspected diagnosis and identification of the infecting organism are necessary for effective treatment in bacterial infections, and in those non-bacterial infections which are potentially responsive. Examination of the patient should include details of occupation and recent travel, and the possibility of tropical or unusual infections of the nervous system should be considered in patients with a relevant history. HIV infection may be suspected in any unusual neurological illness, particularly in patients in the recognised risk groups.

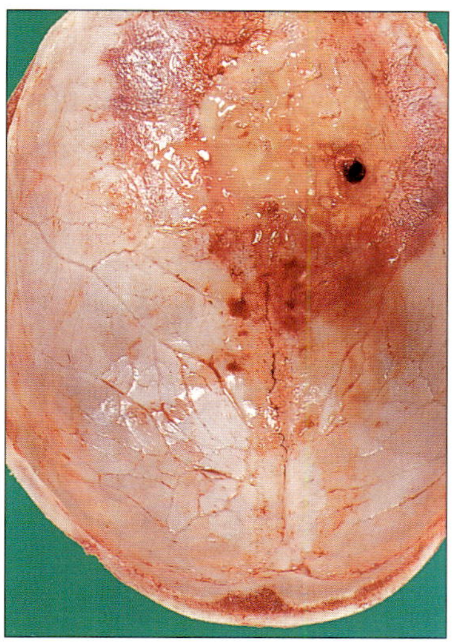

3.3 Epidural abscess originating from the vault of the skull.

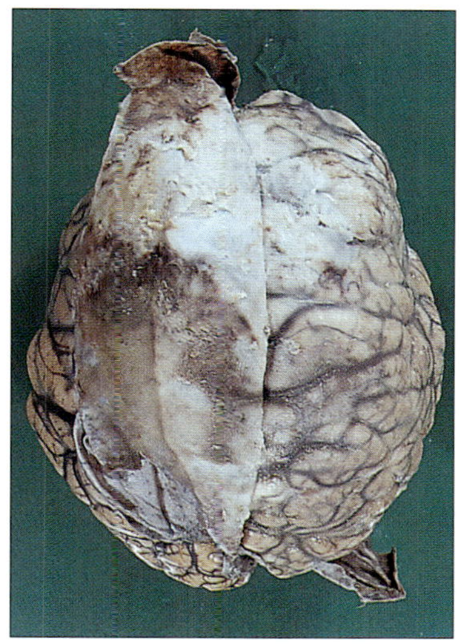

3.4 Subdural empyema (abscess) shown by reflection of the dura mater.

Comparison of CSF findings in CNS infections and multiple sclerosis

Condition	Glucose (mmol/l)	Protein (g/l)	Cytology
Normal	2.5–4.0	0.1–0.45	Up to 5x10⁶/l lymphocytes
Bacterial meningitis	0–2.0	0.5–5.0	Polymorphs++
Abscess	Normal	0.5–1.0	Polymorphs and lymphocytes
Viral meningitis	Normal	0.5–1.5	Polymorphs early, lymphocytes later
Tuberculosis	1.2–2.0	0.5–3.0	Polymorphs early, lymphocytes later
Multiple sclerosis	Normal	0.5–1.0 (Oligoclonal IgG on electrophoresis)	Lymphocytes (plus plasma cells in active phases)

3.5 Comparison of CSF findings in CNS infections and multiple sclerosis.

BACTERIAL INFECTIONS

Bacterial infections of the nervous system may arise *de novo* when a virulent organism attacks the nervous system in an otherwise healthy individual, or as a complication of a spreading local or bloodborne infection. Severe bacterial infections may occur in relation to the dura mater, but the leptomeninges (bacterial meningitis) and brain (abscess) are the most important sites of infection.

BACTERIAL MENINGITIS

Acute inflammation of the leptomeninges is a serious and potentially life-threatening form of infection (**3.6**). It affects all people of all ages, with individual bacterial species showing a predilection for certain age groups (**3.7**).

Bacteria may be isolated from the CSF (**3.8**), which contains large numbers of polymorphonuclear leucocytes (**3.9**) in the early and acute stages. These are later accompanied by macrophages, plasma cells and lymphocytes as the inflammatory reaction evolves. The presence of acute inflammation in the subarachnoid compartment may result in rapid brain swelling leading to sudden death by herniation (**3.10**). This may occur before the accumulation of visible exudate, and so the meninges may appear merely congested on gross examination. Bacterial meningitis may involve the blood vessels in the subarachnoid space, leading to inflammation and thrombosis, and may involve both the cranial and spinal nerve roots causing a radiculitis (**3.11**).

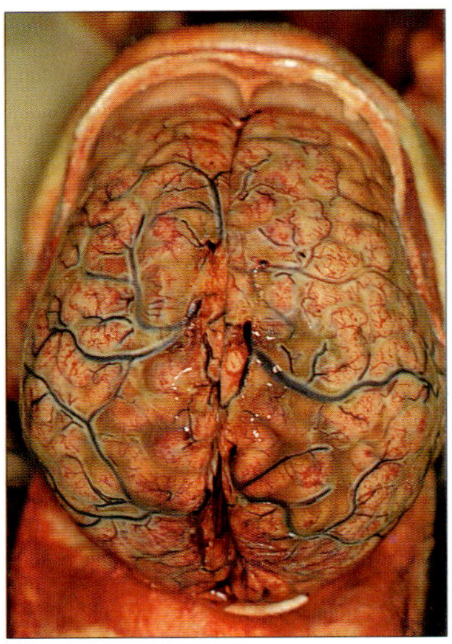

3.6 Acute bacterial meningitis with pus tracking along vessels in the subarachnoid space. Case viewed in the autopsy room after removal of the dura mater.

Bacterial meningitis in different age groups	
Neonatal	*Escherichia coli* *Listeria monocytogenes*
Infant	*Haemophilus influenzae*
Adolescent	Meningococcus (*Neisseria meningitidis*)
Adult	Meningococcus (*N. meningitidis*) Pneumococcus (*Streptococcus pneumoniae*)

3.7 Bacterial meningitis in different age groups.

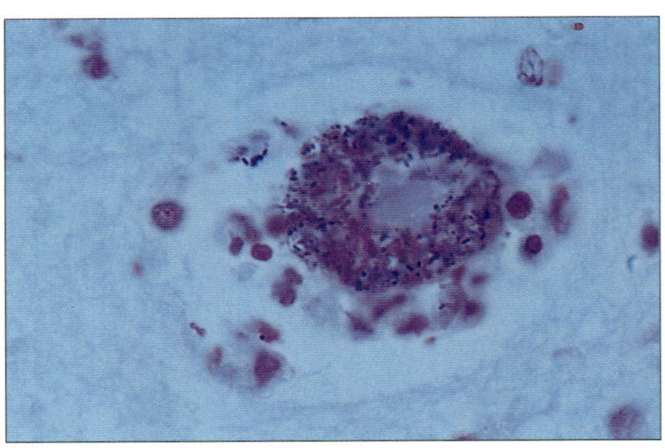

3.8 Gram-positive cocci in the inflammatory infiltrate in a case of bacterial meningitis. (Gram stain)

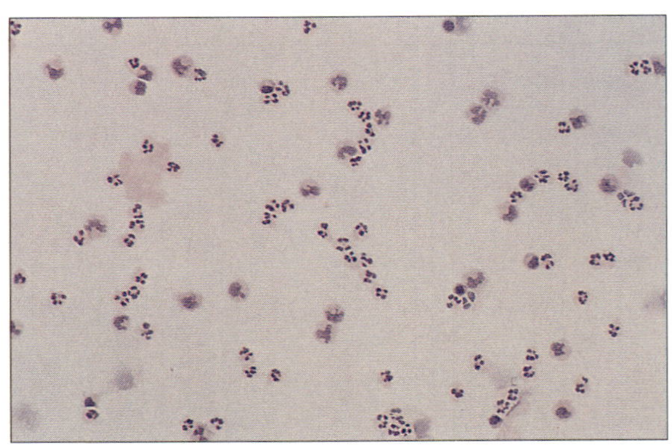

3.9 Cerebrospinal fluid cytospin preparation showing numerous polymorphonuclear leucocytes together with macrophages, monocytes and occasional lymphocytes. Case of acute bacterial meningitis.

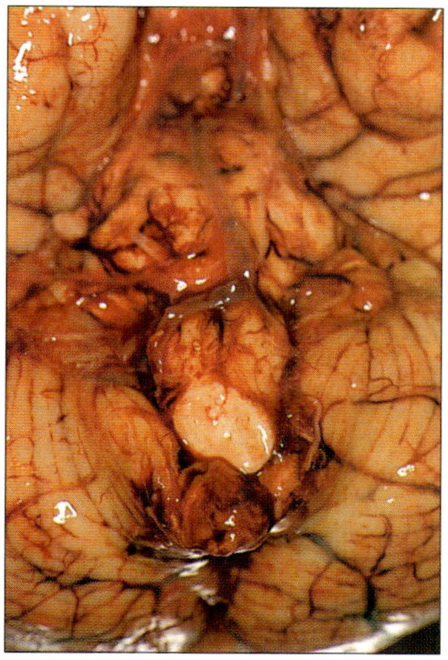

3.10 Ventral view of the brain shown in **3.6**. The medulla oblongata is compressed and distorted by herniated and partially necrotic cerebellar tonsils.

Spread of infection to involve the CNS parenchyma occurs either directly in subpial tissue or along the Virchow–Robin spaces. Choroid plexuses and ventricular lining cells may become infected, leading to an acute plexitis and ventriculitis (**3.12**). The combination of brain swelling and inflammatory thrombosis of vessels particularly veins, in the subarachnoid space may lead to the further serious complication of infarction (**3.13**). If fibrosis occurs during resolution of bacterial meningitis, the resulting impairment of CSF circulation may lead to hydrocephalus (**3.14**).

CEREBRAL ABSCESS

A cerebral abscess may arise in the absence of a significant bacterial meningitis and may be single or multiple. Single abscesses usually have a local cause, while multiple abscesses result from septicaemia

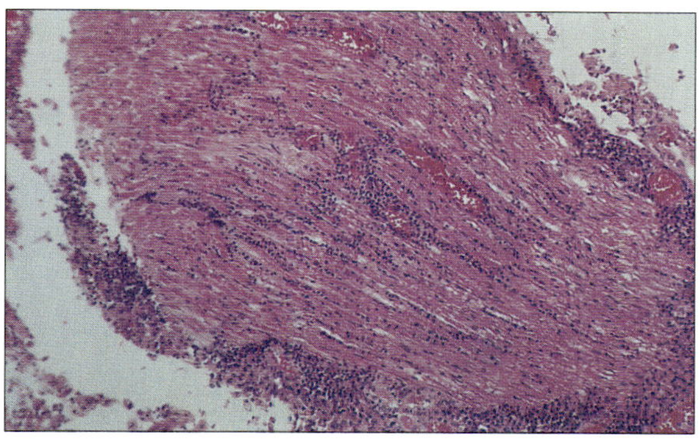

3.11 Cranial nerve root infiltrated with polymorphs and lymphocytes within the subarachnoid space, confirming radiculitis in a case of bacterial meningitis of five days' duration.

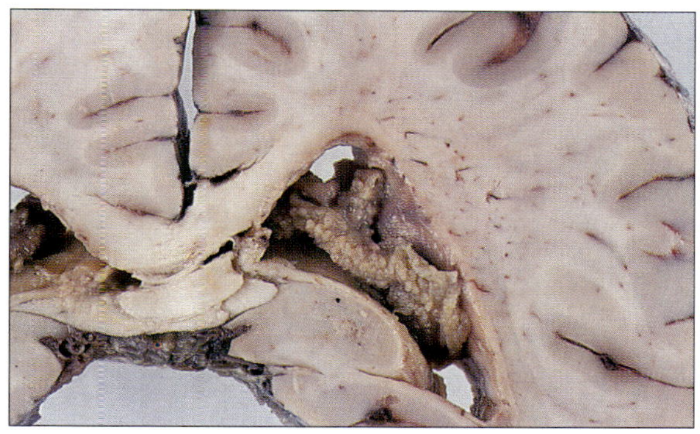

3.12 A slice of brain from a case of established meningitis showing the presence of ventriculitis and choroid plexitis.

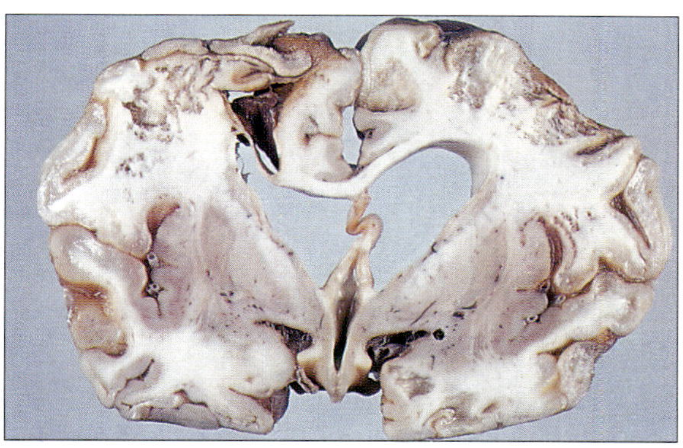

3.13 A slice of brain showing extensive cortical and white matter infarction which has occurred in the presence of bacterial meningitis. The patient had survived for some weeks after the primary infection.

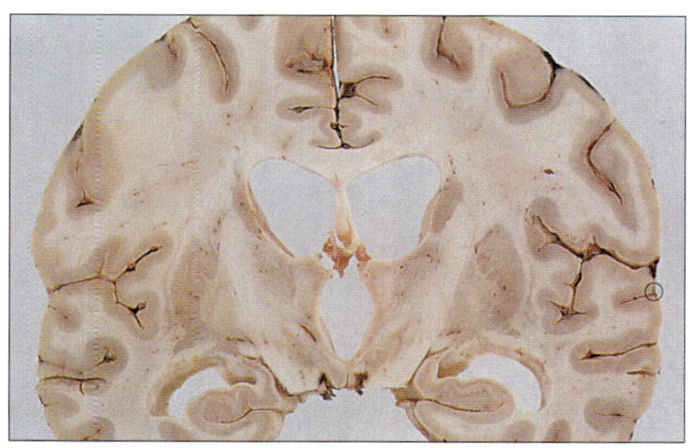

3.14 A slice of brain showing hydrocephalus which has resulted from recent bacterial meningitis. Symmetrical dilatation of the lateral ventricles (including the temporal horns) and the third ventricle is present. The meninges, particularly in the right Sylvian fissure, appear thickened and the ventricular lining is also irregular in the temporal horns.

(**3.15**). The various causes of cerebral abscess are given in **3.16**. Cerebral abscesses are a more common form of intracranial mass lesion than neoplasms in less affluent countries. The formation of a cerebral abscess causes swelling (**3.17**), at least in the early stages, and because it is a space-occupying lesion, it carries the risk of brain shifts and herniation (*see Chapter 2*). In the longer term, a chronic abscess may cause epilepsy. Significant bacterial causes of CNS abscesses include streptococcal species, *Staphylococcus aureus*, *Bacteroides* spp. and *Escherichia coli*.

CNS TUBERCULOSIS

Tuberculosis is a major problem worldwide and its incidence is increasing, even in non-immunocompromised populations of industrialised countries. It is endemic in poorer countries and is a common complication in some cohorts of acquired immunodeficiency syndrome (AIDS), particularly in Africa.

Tuberculosis of the nervous system is secondary to a primary infection elsewhere in the body and reaches the CNS by means of the bloodstream. Tuberculous meningitis (**3.18**) is characterised by an initially polymorphonuclear leucocyte inflammatory response, which is soon replaced by a lymphocytic and macrophage infiltrate. Untreated cases develop a classic granulomatous reaction with giant cells (**3.19**). The potential for fibrosis in the leptomeninges is particularly high with this form of inflammation.

The differential diagnosis includes all other granulomatous reactions, particularly sarcoidosis, and diagnosis depends on identification or isolation of

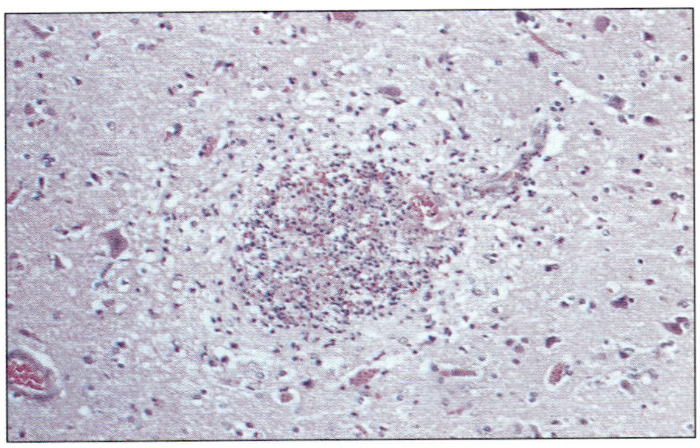

3.15 Early acute cerebritis in a section of cerebral cortex. Inflammatory infiltrate is spreading out from a pyaemic focus related to a small blood vessel.

Causes of cerebral abscess	
Local causes of cerebral abscess	otitis media sinusitis nasal, facial and dental infections skull fracture penetrating injury neurosurgical procedures
Haematogenous causes of cerebral abscess	acute bacterial endocarditis bronchiectasis and lung abscess cyanotic heart disease intravenous drug abuse

3.16 Causes of cerebral abscess.

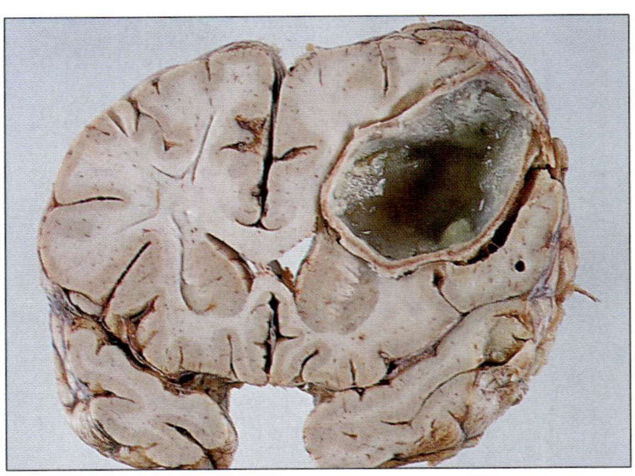

3.17 Chronic cerebral abscess in the right parietal lobe showing a thick fibrotic wall and greenish contents. This patient had suppurative lung disease.

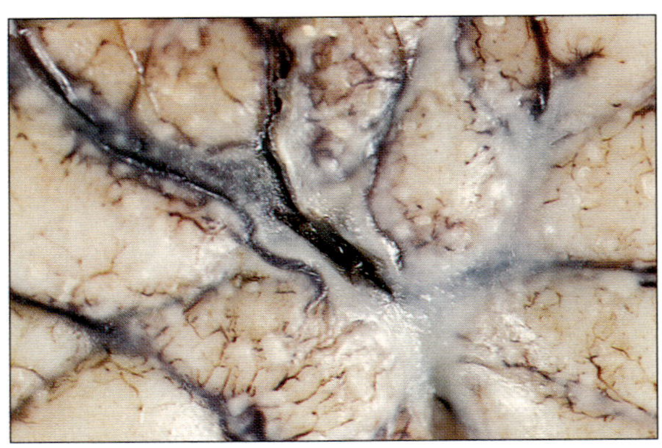

3.18 Case of tuberculous meningitis showing opacity of the leptomeninges, together with numerous pale nodules indicating the presence of subarachnoid granulomata.

tubercle bacilli (**3.20**). These may be exceedingly sparse and difficult to find, but CSF culture should be undertaken in all suspected cases.

CNS tuberculoma

Focal tuberculous infections are known as tuberculomas. These lesions may occur within the CNS, either with or without accompanying tuberculous meningitis. They vary from small chronic inflammatory foci consisting of small granulomas to large caseating abscesses, which cause mass effects (**3.21**). Lesions may be single or multiple (**3.21**).

In countries where tuberculosis is common, tuberculomas are often the commonest form of intracranial mass. In the presence of tuberculosis of the vertebral column, compression of the spinal cord or nerve roots may occur either as a result of vertebral collapse (classically seen in Pott's disease, as in **3.22**), or more insidiously from infection and caseation spreading in the epidural space.

Other granulomatous conditions of the nervous system

Other granulomatous conditions of the nervous system include sarcoidosis and leprosy, the first being a multisystem disorder of unknown cause. When present in the nervous system, sarcoidosis is found predominantly in the meninges and hypophyseal

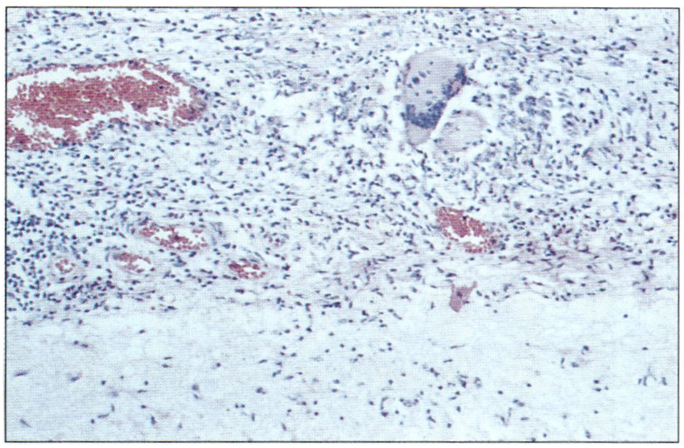

3.19 Section of the cerebral cortex and leptomeninges from a case of tuberculous meningitis showing chronic inflammatory infiltrate with a central giant cell.

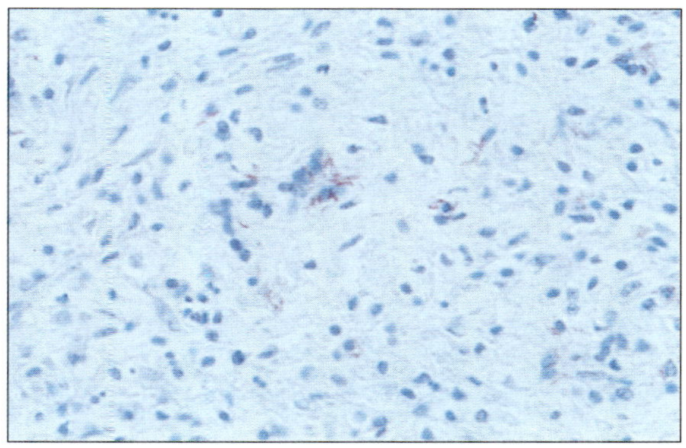

3.20 Section of tuberculous meningitis showing the presence of acid-fast and alcohol-fast bacilli in the meningeal infiltrate (Ziehl–Neelson stain).

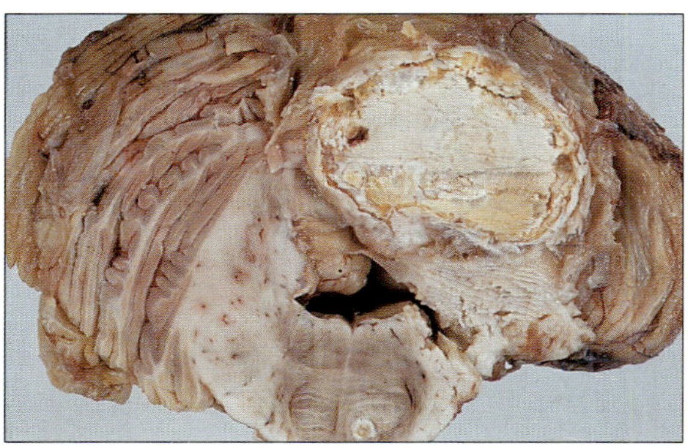

3.21 Two tuberculomas are present, a large one in a cerebellar hemisphere and a very small one in the pons. Typical caseous material fills the cavity of the larger lesion.

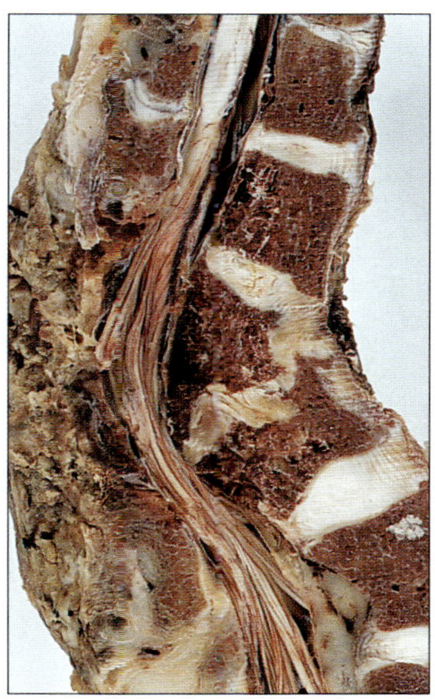

3.22 Section through a vertebral column in which some of the vertebral bodies and spines are distorted by tuberculous infection. Angulation of the spinal canal is shown with pressure on the nerve roots. Spinal epidural caseous material is also present surrounding the lower roots.

region of the brain (**3.23**), typically as non-caseating granulomas (**3.24**). Leprosy is largely confined to the skin and peripheral nerves.

SYPHILIS

Involvement of the nervous system by *Treponema pallidum* is a late complication of the systemic disease. It is rarely seen in affluent countries because effective antibiotic treatment of primary and secondary stages of syphilis prevents progression to neurosyphilis and other tertiary manifestations. It is possible that syphilis may again become common in the context of AIDS. The diagnosis of neurosyphilis may be suspected in patients with positive serology and a clinically relevant history. Three forms of neurosyphilis are found:

- Meningovascular syphilis – this granulomatous inflammation of the meninges is accompanied by characteristic intimal thickening of blood vessels within the subarachnoid compartment (**3.25**).
- General paralysis of the insane (GPI) – widespread parenchymal infection causes dementia and histological examination shows a widespread and diffuse rod cell infiltrate (**3.26**) in response to the presence of *T. pallidum*. Vasculitis may also be present. Spirochaetes may be demonstrated using silver stains (**3.27**) or antibody techniques.
- Tabes dorsalis – in this form of neurosyphilis, the posterior columns and dorsal root entry zone of the spinal cord are the main target of disease

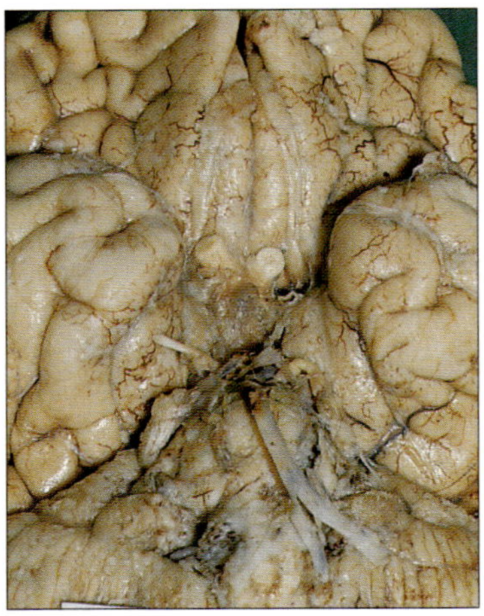

3.23 The base of the brain from a case of CNS sarcoidosis. The leptomeninges are more opaque than normal and display a rather granular appearance, particularly on the inferior surface of both frontal lobes, adjacent to the optic chiasm.

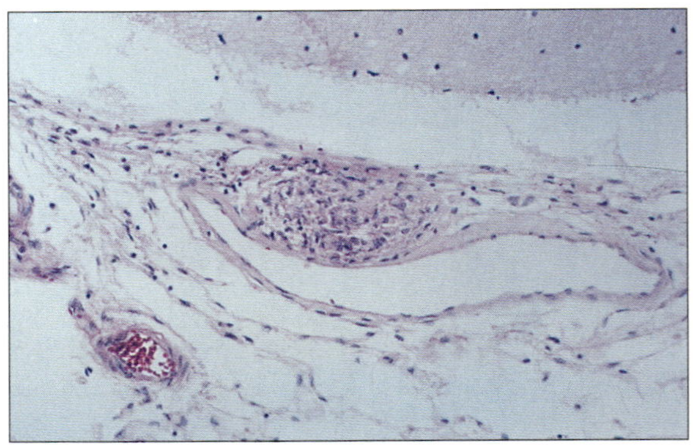

3.24 A section of the leptomeninges showing a small granuloma in the wall of a subarachnoid vein in CNS sarcoidosis.

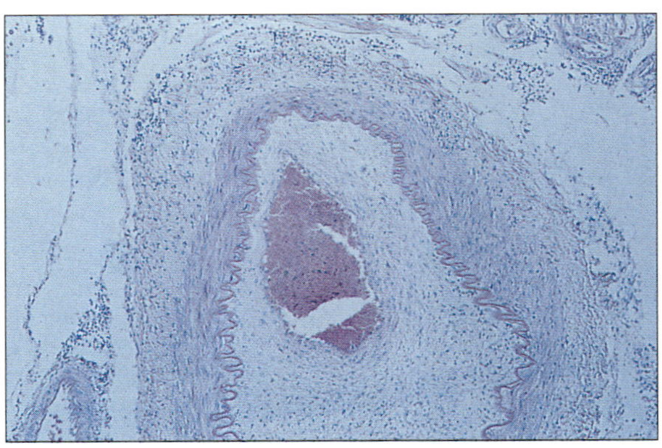

3.25 Leptomeningeal artery from a case of meningovascular syphilis. Chronic inflammatory infiltrate is present in the outer wall of the vessel and gross intimal thickening is seen, which narrows the lumen of the vessel.

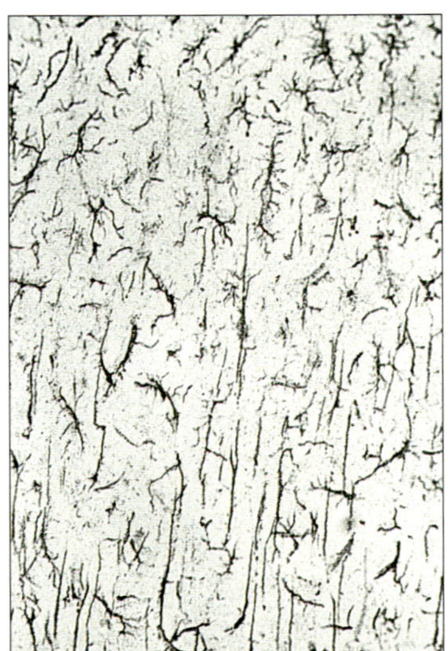

3.26 Rod cell infiltrate (activated microglial cells) in the cortex of a case of general paralysis of the insane. (Hortega silver carbonate stain)

(**3.28**). Severe axonal loss and secondary demyelination occur. These correspond to the clinical presentation of profound loss of joint position and vibration sense, with the consequent risk of peripheral tissue damage.

WHIPPLE'S DISEASE

In this condition, infection of the brain may be isolated or part of a systemic disease. Characteristic collections of periodic-acid Schiff (PAS)-positive macrophages, containing gram-positive bacilli, are found particularly in the basal regions of the brain (**3.29, 3.30**), including the mamillary bodies and the region of the hypothalamus.

LYME DISEASE

This spirochaetal infection is transmitted by tick bites and may involve the nervous system, as well as non-CNS organs, causing a lymphocytic meningitis and intimal proliferation in blood vessels.

VIRAL INFECTIONS

Risk factors for viral infections of the nervous system include systemic and respiratory viral illnesses. The mode of entry is likely to be haematogenous, though some viruses, such as rabies virus, enter the nervous system by retrograde axonal transport from the point of entry at an infected bite. Viruses vary in their

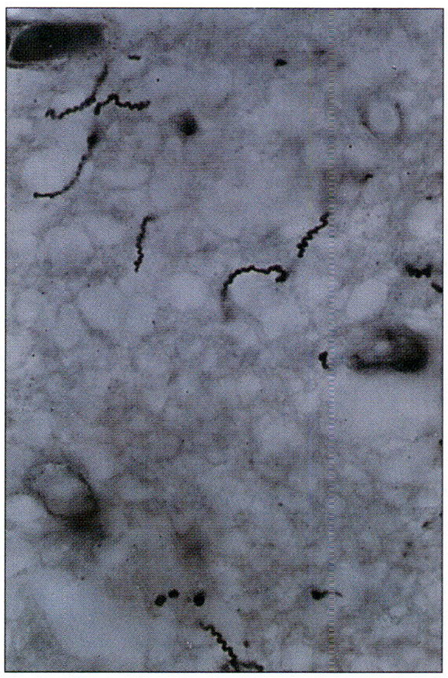

3.27 Section of cerebral cortex from a case of general paralysis of the insane showing the presence of spirochaetes. (Levaditi's stain)

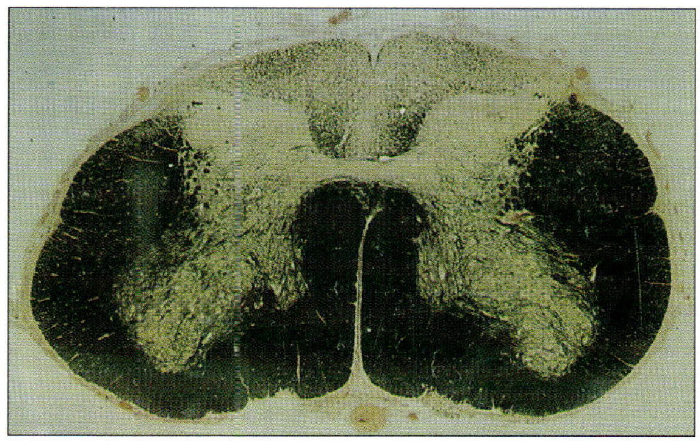

3.28 Spinal cord from a case of tabes dorsalis, stained for myelin, and showing damage in the posterior columns and dorsal nerve root entry zones. (Loyez stain)

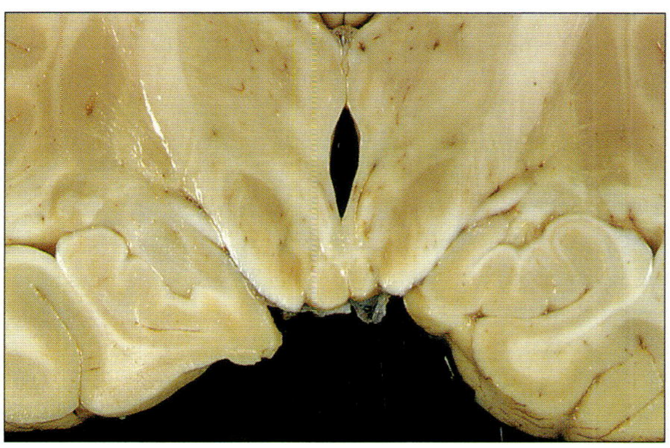

3.29 Discoloration of the mamillary bodies and adjacent structures at the base of the brain from a case of cerebral Whipple's disease.

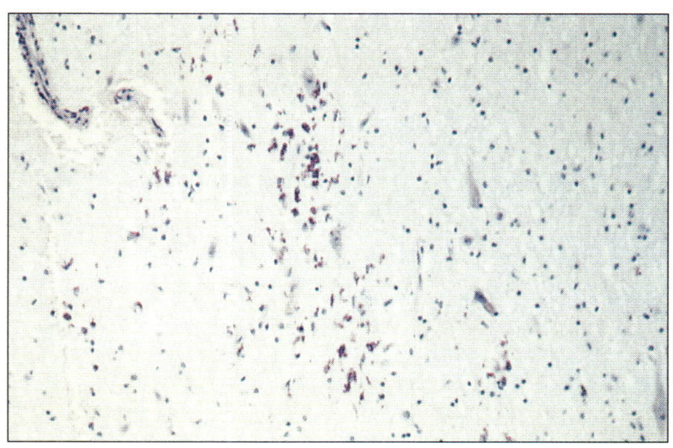

3.30 Section of brain tissue in a case of Whipple's disease showing infiltration of grey matter by PAS-positive macrophages. (Periodic acid–Schiff stain)

selected targets, presumably as a result of particular interactions between virus and individual cell surfaces. Some viruses, such as cytomegalovirus (CMV), can proliferate in many CNS cell types including endothelium, while others, such as polioviruses, have a predilection for particular cell types and target motor neurons (**3.31**). Few viral infections are amenable to therapy, though prevention by immunisation is a useful strategy in protecting the CNS.

The major viral causes of infection are listed in **3.31**, which also shows the principal targets of each virus. The marked differences between viruses in this respect suggest that selective neurotropism is important. The effects of CNS viral infections are wide-ranging and more complex than those of CNS bacterial infections.

Mild or severe infections

Some forms of viral infection, particularly viral meningitis, may cause only a shortlived and rapidly resolving illness. Others are life-threatening or almost invariably fatal, e.g. rabies encephalitis.

Immediate (acute) or delayed (subacute, reactivated) infections

Viral entry to the CNS may cause immediate (acute) illness with an early inflammatory response and variable degrees of tissue damage. Alternatively, there may be a latent period of months or years between the time of initial infection and the manifestation of CNS disease. For example, the measles virus may give rise to an acute encephalitis during the primary illness, while a much more insidious measles-related illness, subacute sclerosing panencephalitis, may occur years after the primary infection. Another example of reactivated viral infection is varicella–zoster.

Infections mediated directly or indirectly

Neural tissue may be damaged directly by viruses or only secondarily involved during an immune process, which is itself a response to viral infection. Examples of immunologically mediated (but virally induced) diseases are postinfectious encephalitis and Guillain–Barré syndrome. In postinfectious encephalitis, small perivenous patches of demyelination occur in the central white matter during the convalescent period after a general viral illness (*see Chapter 6*). In contrast, in Guillain–Barré syndrome, Schwann cell myelin is destroyed after a systemic viral illness causing peripheral nerve demyelination. In both cases, the inflammation in neural tissue is sterile, does not contain virus, and is immunologically mediated by antibodies reacting against myelin basic protein and other sheath components.

CNS target of particular viruses	
Meninges	Mumps virus Enteroviruses Coxsackieviruses Human immunodeficiency virus
Motor neurons	Polioviruses Enteroviruses
Neurons and glia	Herpes simplex virus (primarily temporal lobe) Rabies virus Measles virus
Neurons, glia and endothelium	Cytomegalovirus (in immunocompromised subjects)
Oligodendroglia	Papovavirus (usually in immunocompromised subjects)
Microglia	Human immunodeficiency virus
Dorsal root ganglia	Herpes zoster–varicella
Fetal nervous system	Rubella Cytomegalovirus

3.31 The CNS targets of particular viruses.

PATHOLOGY OF CNS VIRAL INFECTIONS

CNS viral infections, as with bacterial infections, may be somewhat compartmentalised as viral meningitis and viral encephalomyelitis. In practice, the meninges are often involved in the process of viral encephalitis, leading to meningoencephalitis.

Viral meningitis

In viral meningitis (**3.32**), the presence of the virus provokes a lymphocytic response. This includes the production of specific antibodies, such as immunoglobulins IgM and IgG, which may help to identify the infection. Viral causes of meningitis include mumps virus, coxsackieviruses and enteroviruses. CSF analysis and culture are helpful diagnostic procedures (**3.5**).

Viral infections of the brain and spinal cord

Viral infections of the brain and spinal cord often cause very severe tissue damage which may be fatal (**3.33**). They are generally associated with more virulent viruses (**3.31**). Histological examination of biopsy or autopsy tissues usually discloses the presence of viral inclusions in infected cells. Inclusions may be identified by specific immunocytochemical staining. They may be:

- sparse or numerous;
- intranuclear, as in measles (**3.34**);

- intracytoplasmic, such as the Negri body of rabies (**3.35**);
- both intranuclear and intracytoplasmic, as in CMV infection (**3.36**).

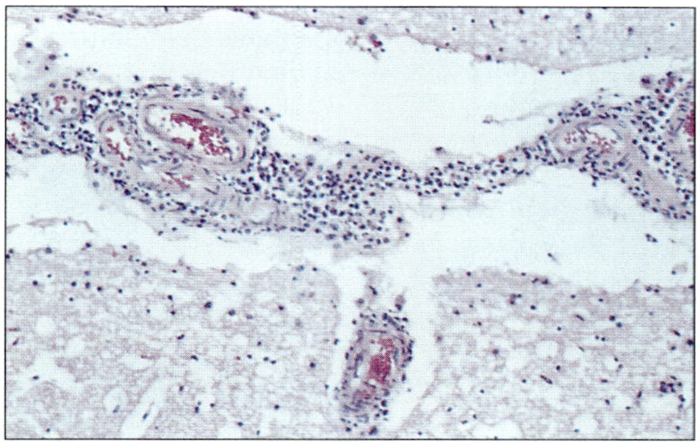

3.32 Lymphocytic infiltrate of the subarachnoid space in a case of viral meningitis.

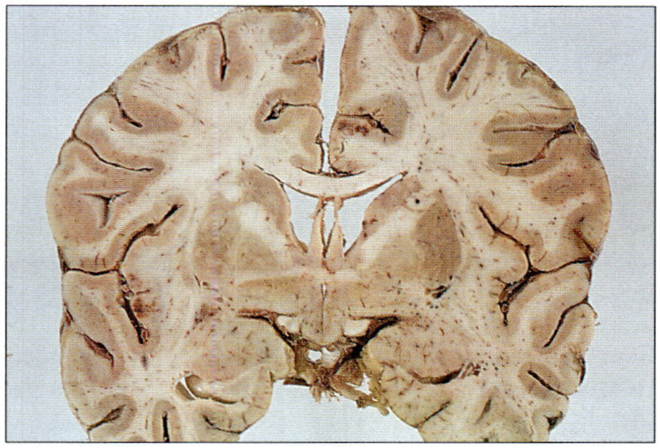

3.33 Brain slice showing the changes of acute viral encephalitis (virus not identified). The brain is slightly swollen and congested, and shows haemorrhagic lesions in the right cingulate gyrus and the left insular cortex.

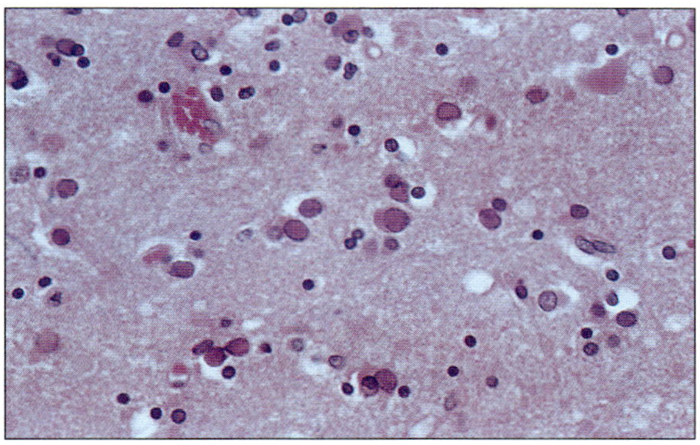

3.34 Section of cerebrum from a case of acute measles encephalitis. Many of the cells show distended nuclei-containing inclusions.

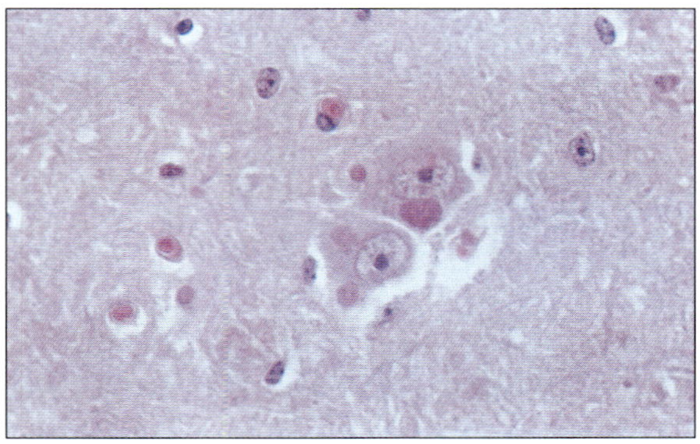

3.35 Spinal cord from a case of rabies with cytoplasmic inclusions both in neurons and in glial cells.

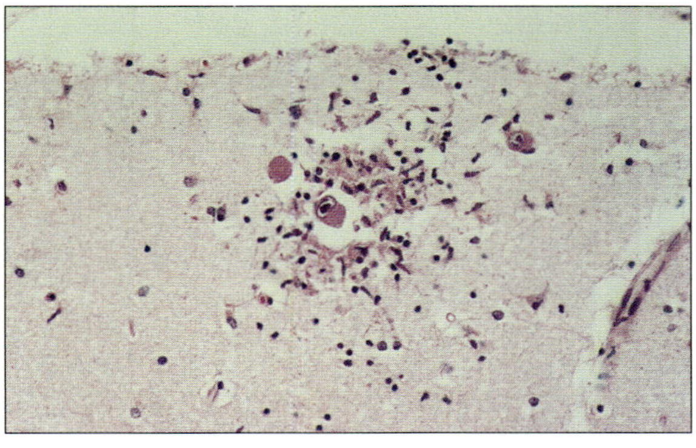

3.36 Typical owl-eye intranuclear inclusions are seen in cytomegalovirus encephalitis, together with distention of the cytoplasm by viral particles.

Viral infections are associated with a characteristic lymphocytic infiltrate, which is predominantly perivascular and made up of mixed T cells and B cells (**3.37**). Plasma cells and macrophages occur in varying numbers and glial and microglial responses are usually present. Focal demyelination is a feature of infections which target oligodendrocytes, the classic example being progressive multifocal leucoencephalopathy (*see Chapter 6*). Frank necrosis may occur and may be curiously focal, as in the temporal lobe damage of herpes simplex encephalitis (**3.38**). In some cases of presumed viral encephalitis, inclusions are extremely hard to identify despite the inflammatory reaction. Occasionally, this reaction is characterised by microglial nodules rather than by lymphocytic infiltrates and this is particularly true in the brainstem.

Other conditions which should be considered in the differential diagnosis of florid inflammatory reactions are listed in **3.39**. They include the rare paraneoplastic phenomenon of limbic encephalitis (**3.40**) and certain conditions that mimic Leigh's syndrome (*see Chapter 8*), which occur sometimes in immunosuppressed patients. These can be differentiated from infective conditions by a peculiar and characteristic endothelial proliferation.

Pathological patterns

Particular viruses cause characteristic patterns of pathology within the nervous system (**3.31**). They include:

- polioviruses;
- herpes simplex virus;
- rabies virus;

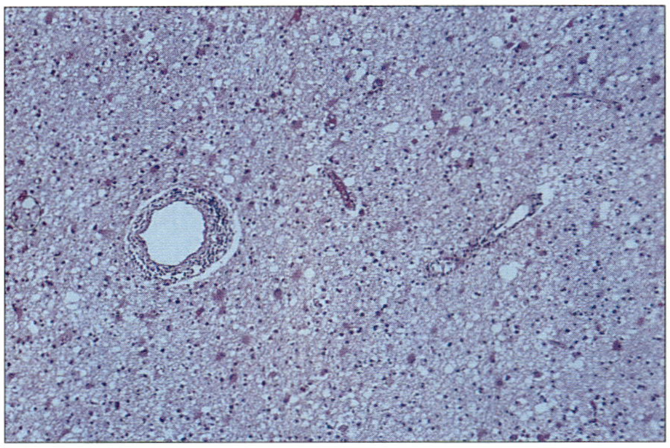

3.37 Section of cerebral tissue in a case of viral encephalitis showing oedema, reactive gliosis and perivascular lymphocytic cuffing.

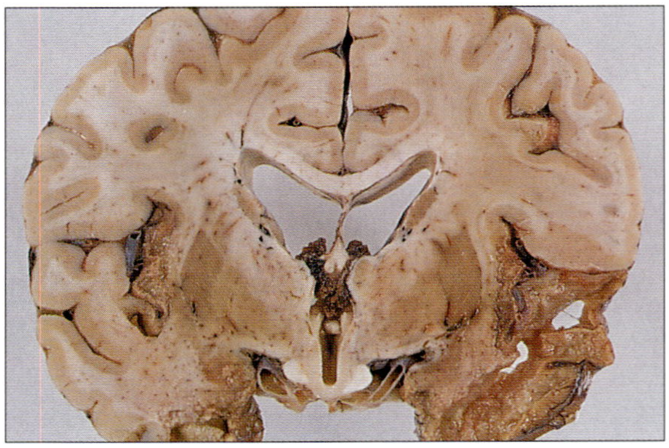

3.38 Appearances of the brain in chronic herpes simplex encephalitis. Both temporal lobes are profoundly damaged and show cystic degeneration.

Conditions displaying perivascular lymphocytic cuffing
acute viral encephalitis
early HIV infection (but not full-blown AIDS)
postinfectious encephalitis
acute multiple sclerosis
limbic encephalitis

3.39 Conditions that show perivascular lymphocytic cuffing.

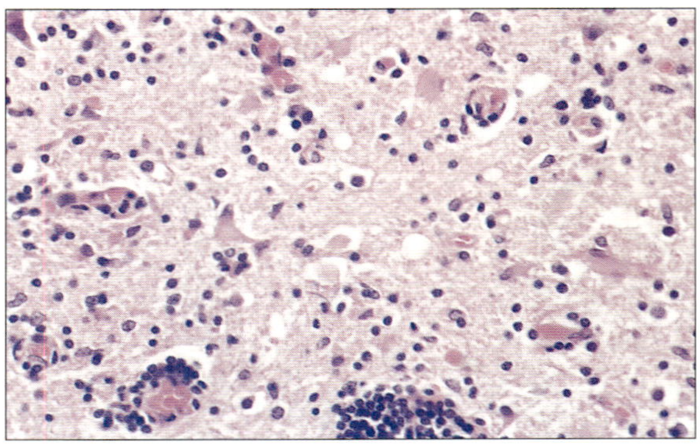

3.40 Section of grey matter from a case of limbic encephalitis. Degenerative changes are seen in relation to an inflammatory infiltrate which is predominantly perivascular. This condition usually occurs in the presence of a distant malignant process.

- measles virus;
- herpes varicella–zoster virus;
- Epstein–Barr virus.

The polioviruses attack motor nerve cells, particularly in the spinal cord (**3.41**) and the brainstem. In acute poliomyelitis, infected nerve cells undergo neuronophagia (dissolution with microglial assistance) and are associated with microglial clusters. These disappear with the subsidence of the acute phase of illness, and in the longer term, neuronal loss may be the only hallmark of the infection.

The endstage of old poliomyelitis has a superficial similarity to motor neuron disease, prompting search for a viral aetiology for this neurodegenerative condition. Herpes simplex virus causes an encephalitis which predominantly affects the limbic system, including the temporal lobes, and sometimes the frontal lobes (**3.38**). Acute infection is associated with extensive tissue destruction and necrosis, and if the patient survives, temporal lobe function is usually impaired. Acyclovir is an effective antiviral therapy in the early stages of herpes encephalitis. Rabies infection causes widespread encephalitis with characteristic cytoplasmic inclusions in different cell types (**3.35**).

The measles virus may damage the CNS in one of two forms – in the acute phase as measles encephalitis, or in the more protracted but devastating form of subacute sclerosing panencephalitis. In both cases, intranuclear inclusions (**3.34**) may be detected, though they are far commoner in the former condition.

The inflammatory reaction may be surprisingly slight. A link between measles virus and multiple sclerosis has been sought following detection of measles antibody in CSF samples from patients with multiple sclerosis, but this association remains tenuous. In herpes varicella–zoster, the virus remains latent in the dorsal root and trigeminal ganglia after an initial chickenpox infection, with the virus having travelled apparently along sensory nerves from the skin lesions.

After a latent period lasting possibly for decades, viral reactivation occurs and skin lesions develop in the dermatome supplied from the infected sensory ganglion. An inflammatory infiltrate is present within the affected dorsal root ganglia and reactivation may occur more readily with immunosuppression and in old age.

Finally, the Epstein–Barr virus does not primarily affect the nervous system, but is sometimes detected because of its association with lymphomas, including CNS lymphomas. The incidence of such tumours is rising in the context of AIDS.

HUMAN IMMUNODEFICIENCY VIRUS INFECTION OF THE NERVOUS SYSTEM

Although AIDS is a comparatively new disease, the CNS has been a focus of considerable study following the recognition that the nervous system is abnormal in up to 90% of cases of full-blown AIDS. Clinically, patients may present with dementia, motor impairment, hallucinations, paraparesis, peripheral neuropathy or myopathy. The virus is able to infect microglial cells of the nervous system by means of the CD4-receptor expressed at low level on their surface. The characteristic histological hallmark of HIV encephalitis is the presence of multinucleated giant cells (**3.42**), particularly in the central white matter of the brain. This may be accompanied by

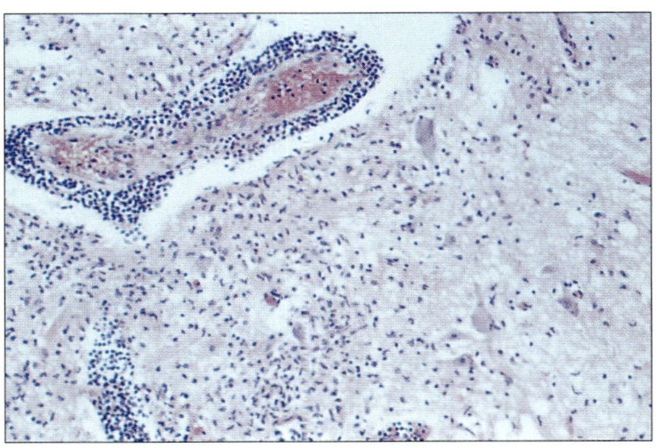

3.41 Section from the spinal cord of a case of acute poliomyelitis. Perivascular lymphocytic cuffing is present. Microglial cells are prominent in the parenchyma and surround one of the large neurons present in this section.

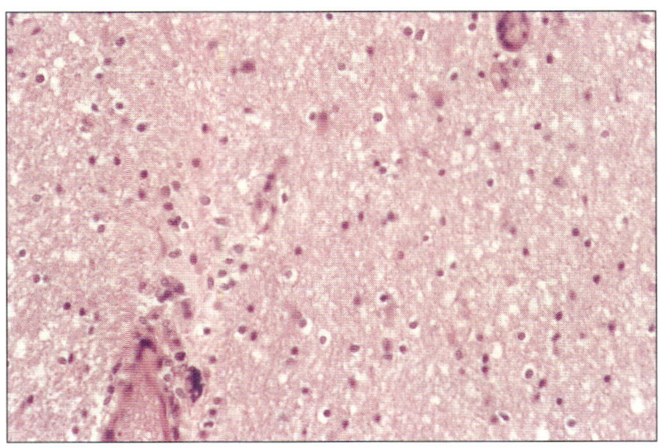

3.42 Section of white matter from a case of AIDS, showing multinucleated giant cells, which are the histological hallmark of HIV encephalitis. The giant cells are frequently perivascular in location.

widespread white matter damage, including gliosis, macrophage accumulation and myelin pallor (**3.42**). HIV encephalitis is significantly associated with high viral load and is more common in drug abusers than in homosexuals. Virus may be detected immunocytochemically both within giant cells (**3.43**) and in morphologically normal microglial cells (**3.44**).

As a result of profound immune suppression, the CNS is vulnerable in AIDS to a variety of opportunistic infections and to CNS lymphoma. The most common opportunistic infections include *Toxoplasma* (**3.45**, **3.46**), cytomegalovirus (**3.47**), *Cryptococcus* (**3.48**), and papovavirus. Herpes simplex, atypical mycobacteria, and fungi, other than *Cryptococcus*, are less

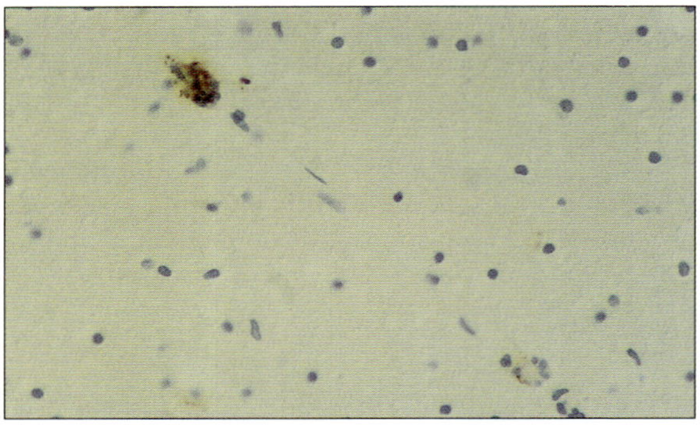

3.43 The presence of HIV within giant cells from a case of AIDS is confirmed by immunocytochemical positivity for viral protein (p24 antigen).

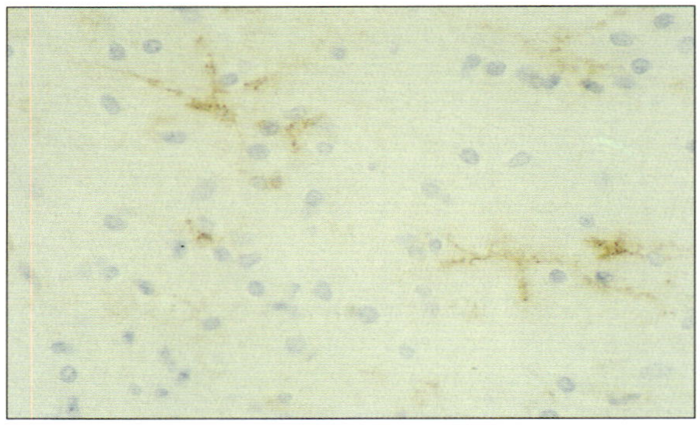

3.44 HIV infection of apparently normal microglial cells is confirmed in this case of AIDS by the presence of HIV p24 immunopositivity.

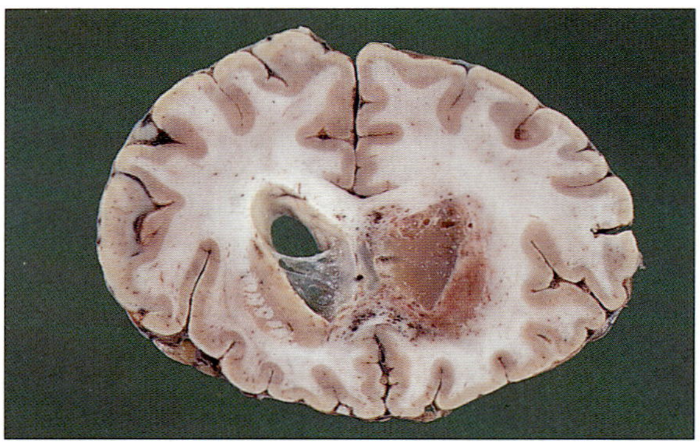

3.45 Toxoplasma ventriculitis causing an intraventricular coagulum and periventricular necrosis in a case of AIDS.

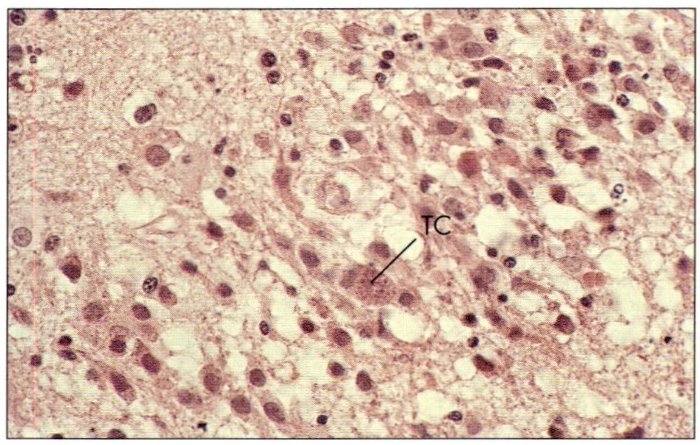

3.46 Toxoplasma cyst (TC) with sparse inflammatory infiltrate present in the dentate gyrus of a case of AIDS.

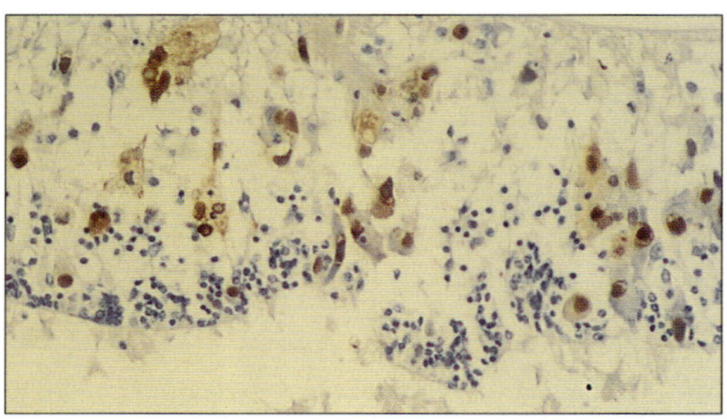

3.47 Cytomegalovirus frequently infects the retina as well as the brain in AIDS. (CMV antibody)

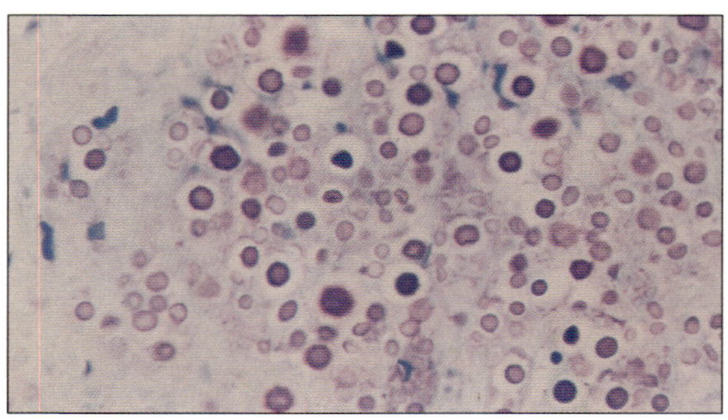

3.48 *Cryptococcal* meningitis in a patient with AIDS. (PAS)

common. None of these are dependent on the co-presence of HIV encephalitis. In some AIDS patients, vacuolar myelopathy is present within the corticospinal tracts (**3.49**), and often in the posterior columns, of the spinal cord. This vacuolar change is present within myelin sheaths and is associated with macrophage infiltration. Whether HIV is the cause of these lesions, which mimic subacute combined degeneration of the cord, remains unresolved.

Before the onset of AIDS, HIV-positive patients who come to autopsy for other reasons often display a low-grade lymphocytic meningitis. The lymphocytic infiltrate is largely made up of T cells and may represent a response to low-level early infection of the nervous system. It is generally considered that HIV enters brain tissue early in the course of infection and remains latent until the onset of AIDS. However, polymerase chain reaction (PCR) studies of brain tissue in the pre-AIDS stage are often negative, suggesting that HIV is not present or is effectively suppressed before the onset of AIDS.

Since some opportunistic infections, such as toxoplasmosis, may be amenable to treatment, their early diagnosis is a matter of importance. Differentiation between lymphoma and *Toxoplasma* can be difficult even with neuroimaging, and therapeutic trials of antitoxoplasma therapy may be necessary. Biopsy may be considered in patients who present diagnostic problems.

Proper histological assessment of small fragments of cerebral biopsy tissue in AIDS cases presents a considerable challenge given that more than one pathology may be present. It should be remembered that unfixed or frozen biopsy or autopsy tissues from HIV-positive patients are still infective and should be handled accordingly as category 3 risk tissues.

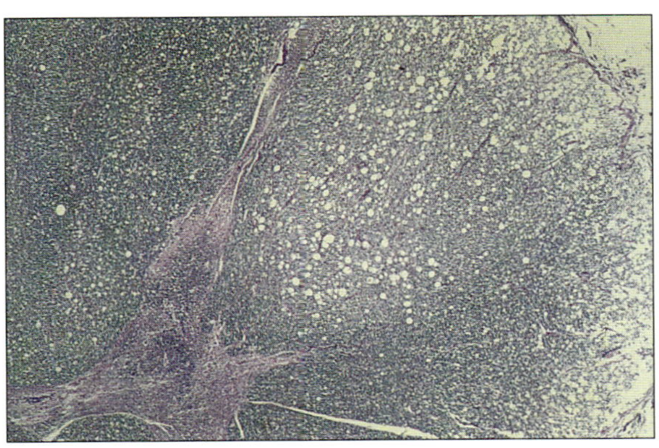

3.49 A section of the spinal cord stained for myelin. It shows vacuolation of the corticospinal tract in a case of vacuolar myelopathy of AIDS. (Luxol fast blue)

CNS INFECTIONS IN OTHER IMMUNOCOMPROMISED PATIENTS

Although AIDS patients comprise the largest group of immunocompromised patients worldwide, there are other groups at risk because of spontaneous or iatrogenic immunosuppression. Transplant recipients sometimes succumb to CNS infections, particularly fungal infections (*see below*). Viral infections such as CMV and papovavirus seem to be less common in these other groups of immunocompromised adult patients and this may reflect subtle differences in the pattern of immunosuppression or may merely reflect different environmental exposure. Splenectomised patients are vulnerable to pneumococcal infection.

Other categories of immunocompromised patients include those with haematological and lymphoid disorders, diabetes and autoimmune diseases, and those undergoing treatment with radiotherapy or chemotherapy. Old age also suppresses natural immunity, while immune function is immature in the fetus leading to a risk of CNS damage following infection with toxoplasma, cytomegalovirus or rubella, acquired transplacentally from the mother (*see Chapter 9*). Patients with diabetes mellitus are susceptible to infections, including an unusual but characteristic transnasal infection with mucormycosis.

PRION DISEASES

This group of rare transmissible dementias includes Creutzfeldt–Jakob disease, kuru and Gerstmann–Straussler–Scheinker syndrome. They are characterised by spongiform change in the grey matter with neuronal loss and astrocytosis. Although a marked microglial response is present, which has been overlooked previously, there is no other manifestation of inflammatory reaction, despite the presence of a transmissible agent.

The natural history of the disease and evidence from experimental and iatrogenic transmission suggest that there is a long latent period between acquisition of the infective agent and development of symptomatic disease. However, exhaustive study has failed to reveal any viral nucleic acid in infective extracts and the agent is now thought to be a perverted form of a normal cellular protein called prion protein. The pathology of prion diseases is considered in more detail in *Chapter 7*.

FUNGAL INFECTIONS

Fungal infections usually occur only in immunocompromised individuals. Fungi which may colonise the

CNS include *Candida* (**3.50**), *Cryptococcus*, *Aspergillus* (**3.51**), *Mucor* and *Histoplasma*. The fungi are bloodborne from some non-CNS source of infection, generally in the respiratory tract. Fungi colonise the walls of blood vessels (**3.52**) and cause thrombosis before spreading into parenchymal tissues. They are readily demonstrated in tissue section by PAS-positivity and by their affinity for silver stains (**3.52**). Their presence provokes an active chronic inflammatory reaction (**3.53**), which includes some polymorphs and which may be granulomatous in the later stages of infection. Giant cells may be prominent in some fungal meningitides. Staining reactions demonstrate the morphology of the fungi. *Aspergillus* is made up of septate hyphae which tend to branch in an acutely angular fashion (**3.52**). *Candida* has similar appearances but branching is close to the perpendicular.

PROTOZOAL CNS INFECTION

TOXOPLASMOSIS

An established toxoplasma infection of the CNS (**3.45**) causes inflammation and necrosis, in which free trophozoites and encysted forms (**3.46**) of the protozoan may be detected at the viable tissue margins either by routine staining or by immunocytochemical techniques. Treated toxoplasma infections may show only scarring and mineralisation.

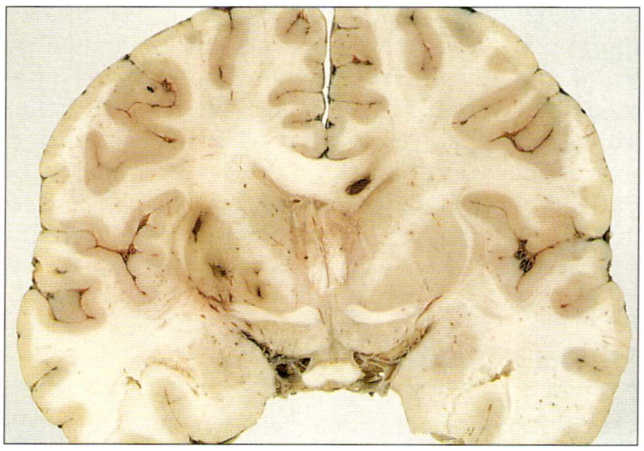

3.50 Fungal (candida) encephalitis in a transplant patient. The brain is swollen and ventriculitis obliterates the ventricular cavities. Haemorrhagic lesions are present in the corpus callosum and left lentiform nucleus.

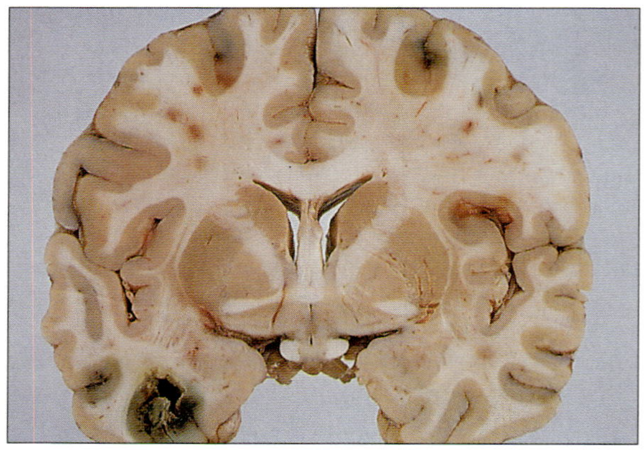

3.51 Aspergillosis of the CNS. A fungal abscess is present in the left temporal lobe.

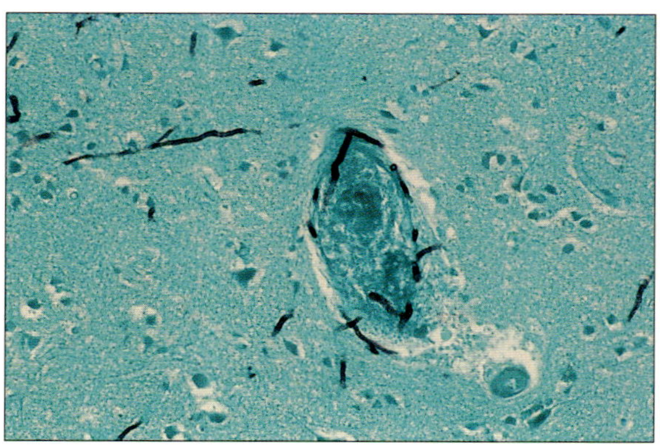

3.52 Fungal hyphae, demonstrated by a silver stain, in the wall of a parenchymal vessel and spreading into the neuropil. Angular branching suggests that this fungus is *Aspergillus*. (Grocott methenamine silver stain)

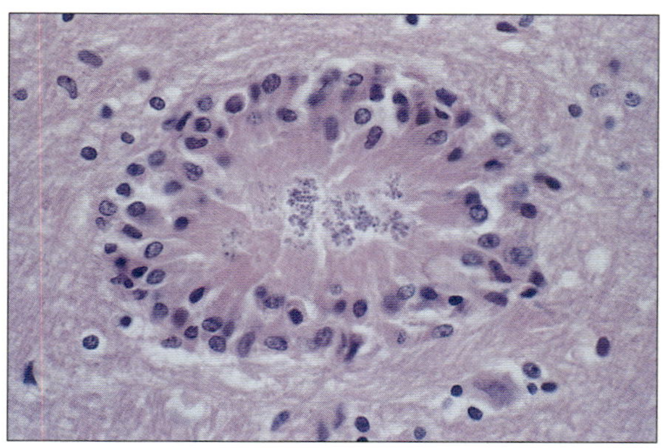

3.53 Inflammatory focus in a case of fungal cerebritis shows the presence of *Histoplasma* in the centre of a collection of macrophages and microglial cells. The patient was being treated for leukaemia.

Toxoplasma CNS infection may be congenital or acquired/reactivated in later life in immunocompromised individuals.

TRYPANOSOMIASIS

Invasion of the nervous system by this protozoan causes active chronic inflammatory foci which are often perivascular (**3.54**) and associated with a florid plasma cell reaction. Some plasma cells may be distended by immunoglobulin deposits and the presence of these bosselated eosinophilic cells called morula (**3.54**) provides a rather distinctive feature.

AMOEBIASIS

Amoebic CNS infection may take the form of an acute meningitis or encephalitis characterised by polymorphs and haemorrhage. The organisms have an appearance simulating macrophages. Amoebic abscesses may also occur. Different forms of amoeba, including *Entamoeba histolytica* and *Naegleria* spp., may all give rise to amoebiasis of the CNS.

MALARIA

Cerebral malaria is a complication of the systemic form of the disease, in which small cerebral blood vessels are distended with parasite-infected red blood cells. Circulation through such distended blood vessels becomes impaired, with resulting small infarcts, predominantly in white matter. Haemorrhage may also occur (**3.55**). Small foci of demyelination are found around infested blood vessels.

The presence of small areas of infarction with a central occluded blood vessel provokes both a microglial and glial reaction, and these small lesions are called Durck granulomas. Patients dying of acute cerebral malaria do not necessarily show the presence of these lesions and the diagnosis depends on identification of parasites within red blood cells (**3.56**). Malaria pigment within blood vessels mimics formalin pigment

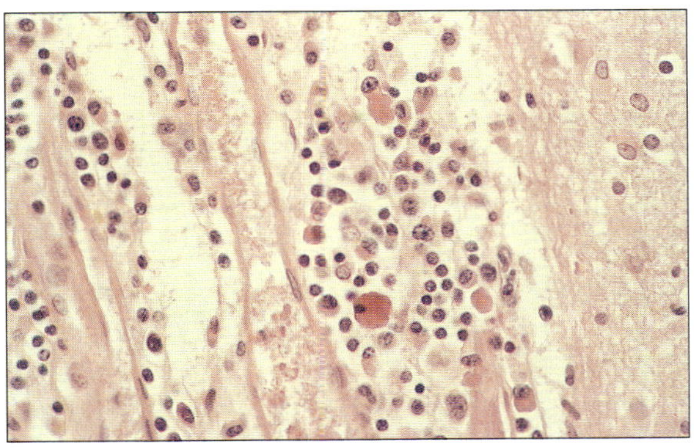

3.54 In trypanosomiasis, morular cells, distended with immunoglobulin, are present within the perivascular chronic inflammatory infiltrate.

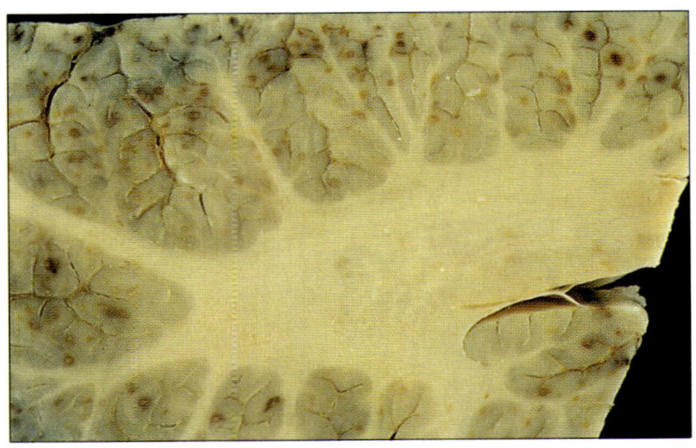

3.55 Petechial haemorrhages in the cerebellum from a case of cerebral malaria.

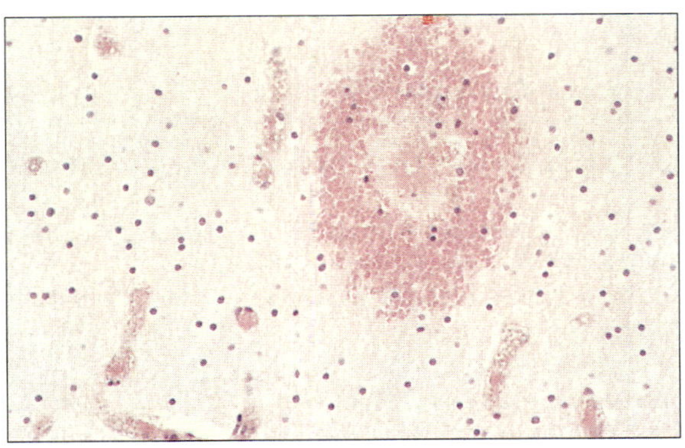

3.56 Section from a case of malaria showing a small cerebral haemorrhage, centred on an occluded blood vessel. Parasitised red cells can be seen in all of the small blood vessels of this section.

METAZOAL CNS INFECTION

The larval forms of some parasites may gain entry to the CNS where they become encysted. Inflammatory reactions may contain many eosinophils. The diseases are usually acquired by eating partially cooked infected meat or foodstuffs contaminated by animal faeces. The most significant forms are hydatid disease (*Taenia echinococcus*) (**3.57**) and cysticercosis (*Taenia solium*) (**3.58**). Cysts may be multiple and occur in any area of the brain (**3.58**). The wall of the cyst is made up of secreted larval products, which form a hyaline chitinous coat (**3.57**) surrounded by glial reactions. Larval remnants may be found within the cyst cavity. Nematodes (*Strongyloides*) may form similar focal lesions (**3.59**) within the CNS. These parasitic cysts may remain dormant (**3.60**) or may increase in size with swelling and mass effects.

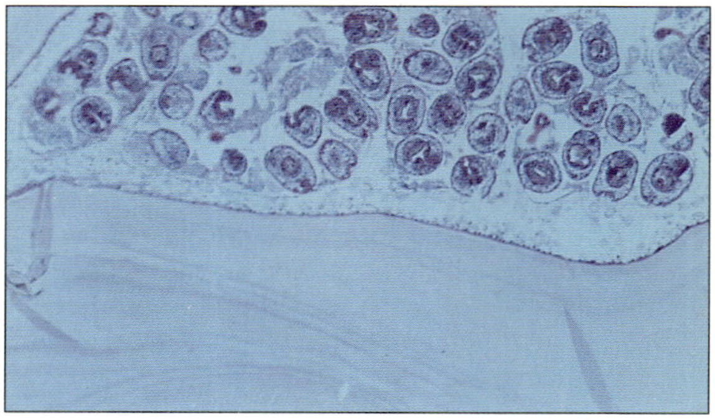

3.57 Echinococcal cyst showing larvae (above) contained within a chitinous wall (below).

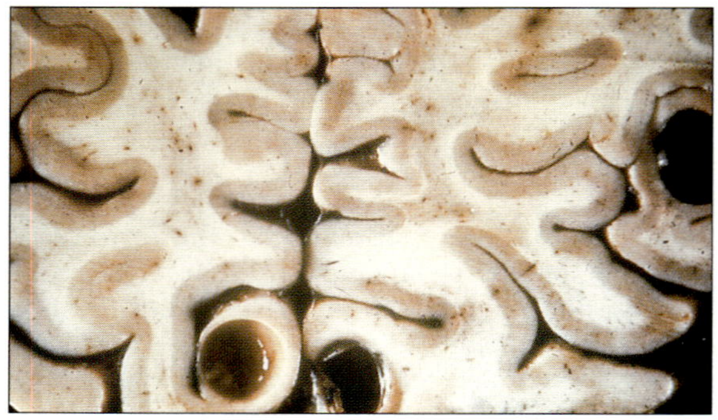

3.58 Cysts of cysticercosis in the brain.

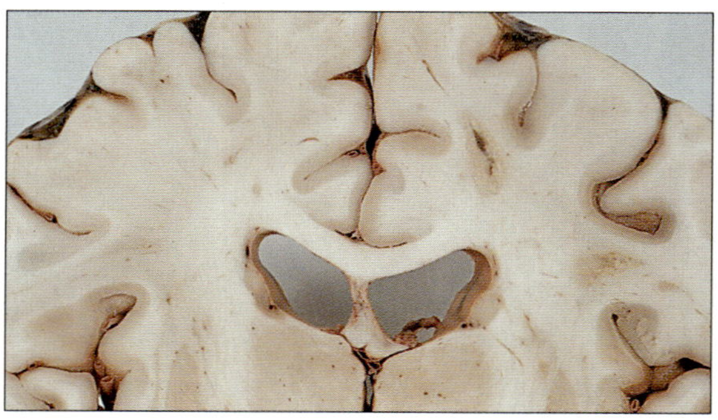

3.59 Partially cystic central white matter lesions in a case of cerebral strongyloidosis.

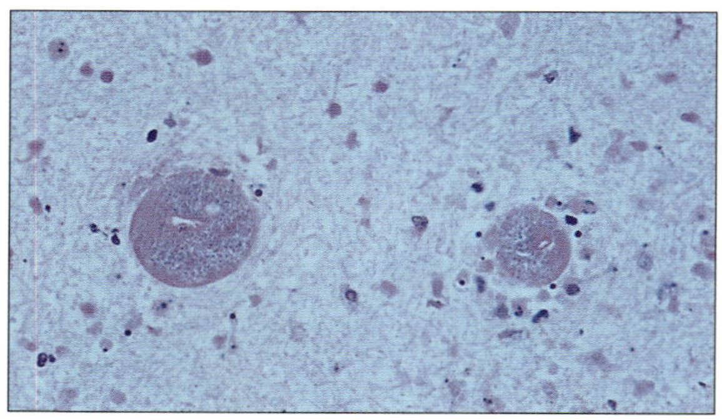

3.60 Degenerate *Strongyloides* larvae in brain tissue. Little reaction is noted in the surrounding neuropil.

FURTHER READING (see also Further Reading for Chapter 2)

Esiri MM, Kennedy PGE. Virus Diseases. In: Adams JH , Duchen LW (eds). Greenfield's *Neuropathology.* 5th edn. London, Edward Arnold, 1992, pp 335–399.

Kirkpatrick JB. Neurologic Infections due to Bacteria, Fungi and Parasites. In: Davis RL, Robertson DM (eds). *Text Book of Neuropathology.* 2nd edn. Baltimore, Williams and Wilkins, 1991, pp 719–803.

Leestma JE. Viral Infections of the Nervous System. 2nd edition. In: Davis RL, Robertson DM (eds). *Text Book of Neuropathology.* Baltimore, Williams and Wilkins, 1991, pp 804–903.

Scaravilli F. *The Neuropathology of HIV Infection*. London, Springer-Verlag, 1993.

Weller RO. Bacterial and Fungal Infections and Granulomatous Diseases. In: Symmers W St C (ed). *Nervous System, Muscle and Eyes: Systemic Pathology*. 3rd edn. Vol. 4. London, Churchill–Livingstone, 1990, pp 151–179.

4. Vascular Disease and Hypoxic Brain Damage

In the UK, as in other developed countries, cerebrovascular disease ('stroke') accounts for some 10% of all deaths, being surpassed only by heart disease and cancer. It has been estimated that about 500,000 new 'strokes' occur annually in the USA, about half of which result in death. In those patients who survive, about 50% are permanently disabled, and only 10% return to normal activity.

'Strokes' are most common in the elderly, but also occur in patients of other ages, including neonates, infants, children and young adults. Prospective epidemiological studies suggest that about 84% of 'strokes' are due to infarction and about 16% are due to haemorrhage (**4.1**). A number of factors that increase the risk of both cerebral infarction (**4.2**) and spontaneous (non-traumatic) haemorrhage (**4.3**) have been identified.

BLOOD SUPPLY OF THE BRAIN AND SPINAL CORD

The distribution of the arterial supply and the venous drainage are very important in determining the position of vascular lesions and their neurological sequelae (*see Chapter 2*).

Type	Frequency (%)
Infarction (non-haemorrhagic)	
Thrombotic	53
Embolic	31
Haemorrhagic	
Intracerebral	10
Subarachnoid from saccular aneurysm	6
Bleeding into infarct	1

4.1 Types and frequency of cerebrovascular disease.

Risk factors for cerebral infarction
Atheroma
Hypertension
Serum lipids Obesity Diet
Diabetes mellitus
Heart disease
Disease of neck artery
Medication
Cigarette smoking
Hypothyroidism
Metabolic disorders (MELAS)

4.2 Risk factors for cerebral infarction.

Risk factors of intracranial haemorrhage	Frequency (%)
Hypertension	50
Rupture of saccular aneurysm	20
Thrombocytopenia	8
Mycotic aneurysm	6
Vascular malformation	5
Tumour	2
Reperfusion of area of infarction	–
Amyloid (congophilic) angiopathy	–

4.3 Risk factors and frequency of intracranial haemorrhage.

STRUCTURAL CHANGES RESULTING FROM VASCULAR DISEASE AND HYPOXIA

These may be limited to neurons (selective neuronal necrosis) or may also involve glia and blood vessels (infarction).

SELECTIVE NEURONAL NECROSIS

In selective neuronal necrosis, structural damage is limited to neurons. Neurons are particularly susceptible to hypoxia because of their obligative aerobic glycolytic metabolism. However, the occurrence of histological artefacts often makes it difficult to identify changes in neurons attributable to ischaemia (*see Chapter 2*). Nevertheless, selected material has shown that there is an identifiable sequence of events, namely the ischaemic cell process, which is the neuropathological common denominator in all types of hypoxia.

When a neuron is irreversibly damaged, the first changes to occur are those of ischaemic cell change, in which the cell body and nucleus become simultaneously shrunken and triangular in shape. The cytoplasm stains intensely with eosin, and from bright blue to dark mauve with Luxol fast blue, while the nuclei stain intensely with cresyl violet. The next change to occur is the development of incrustations. These are dense profiles of neuronal cytoplasm formed from the cell surface, which is dented and distorted by swollen astrocytic processes. The small dense granules of incrustations lie on, or close to, the surface of the neuron. Finally, the neuron undergoes homogenising cell change in which the cytoplasm becomes progressively paler and the nucleus smaller. The time course of ischaemic cell change is relatively constant for neurons, depending on their size and shape. This means the interval between an hypoxic episode and death can be assessed with reasonable accuracy, provided the time lapsed since hypoxia is no less than two hours and no more than 24 hours (**4.4–4.6**).

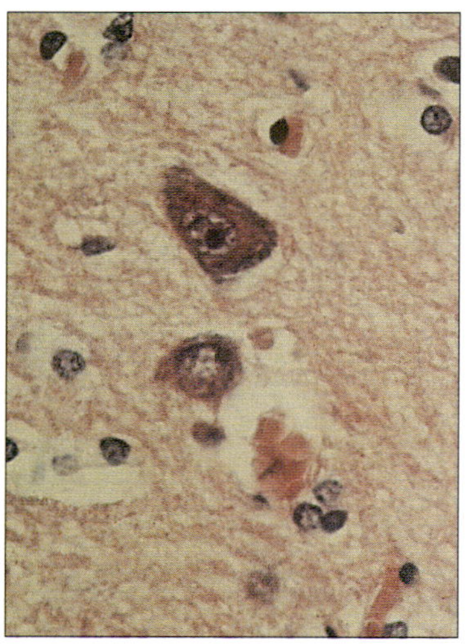

4.4 Normal pyramidal neurons in the neocortex. (H & E)

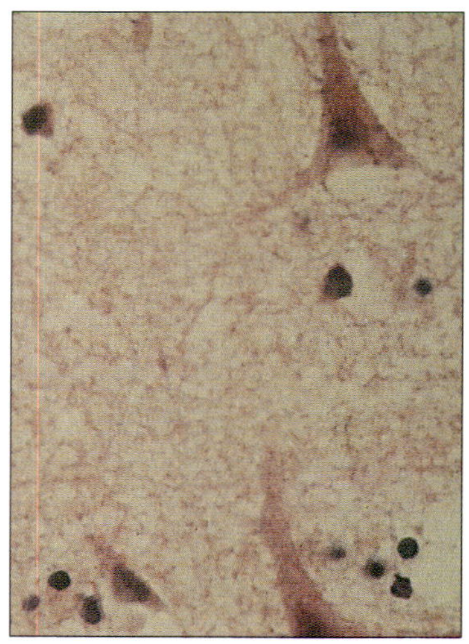

4.5 Ischaemic cell process in the neocortex, showing neurons that are triangular in shape with condensed darkly staining nuclei and eosinophilic cytoplasm. (H & E)

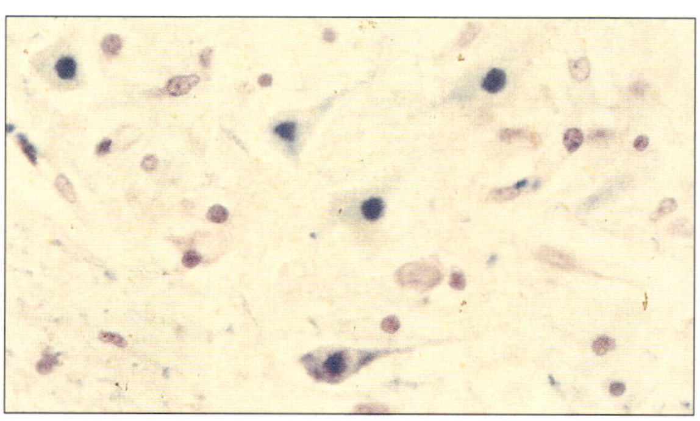

4.6 Ischaemic cell process in the neocortex, showing ischaemic neurons with condensed triangular nuclei and blue/mauve cytoplasm. (Combined Luxol fast blue and cresyl violet)

INFARCTION

In infarction, as well as neuronal necrosis, there is also involvement of the glia and blood vessels. Infarction is due to a local arrest or severe reduction in cerebral blood flow. It can affect an entire arterial territory, or if there is some collateral circulation in the adjacent arterial territories, it may be restricted to the central portion of the arterial territory (**4.7–4.10**). Infarcts may be 'anaemic' or 'haemorrhagic'. The affected tissue is often soft to touch, and if the infarct is haemorrhagic the cortex or the basal ganglia will

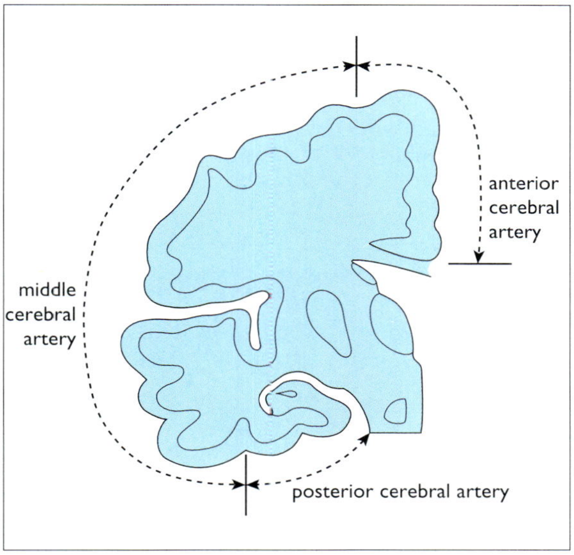

4.7 Line diagram showing the distribution of arterial blood supply to one cerebral hemisphere.

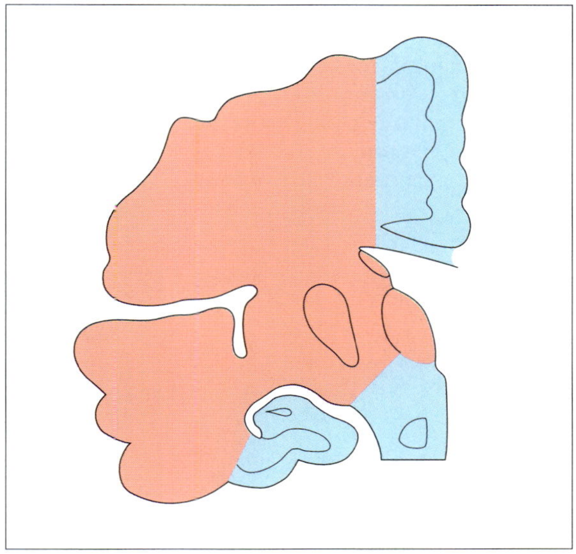

4.8 Line diagram showing a large infarct (red area) in the whole distribution of the middle cerebral artery.

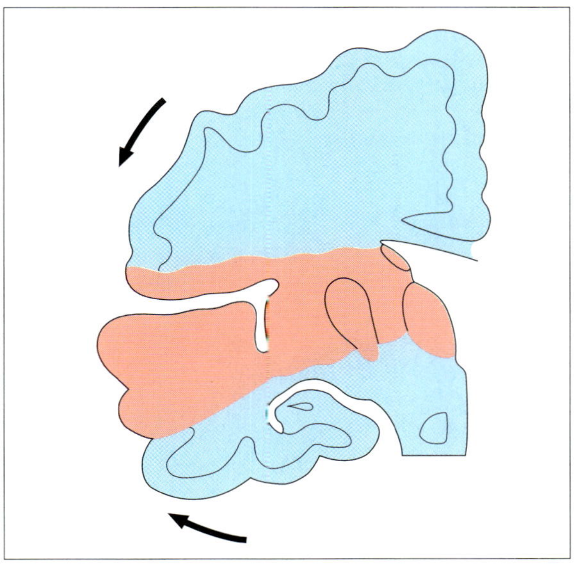

4.9 Line diagram showing an infarct limited to the central distribution of the middle cerebral artery because of increased symmetrical collateral circulation from the anterior and posterior cerebral arteries. (Red = Distribution of infarct.)

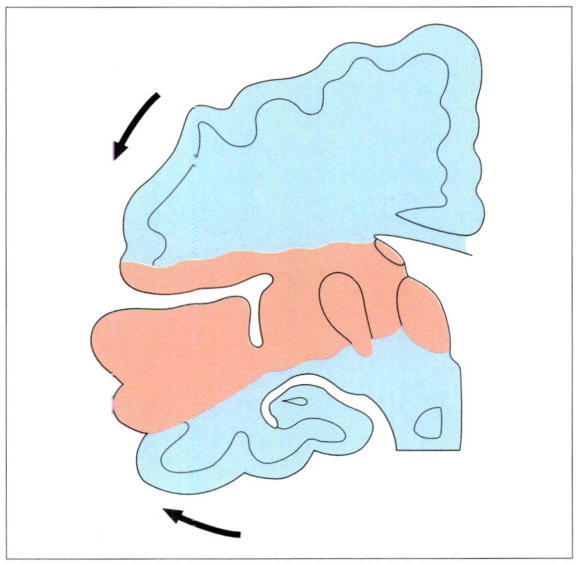

4.10 Line diagram showing an infarct, the pattern of which has been determined by asymmetrical collateral supply from the anterior and posterior cerebral arteries.

show dusky discolouration (**4.11**). Particularly in young patients, an infarct may become so swollen that death from raised intracranial pressure may occur within 24–30 hours of onset (**4.12**). Occasionally, a haematoma may develop in what was initially an 'anaemic' infarct. Such transformation is more likely after embolic infarction and after thrombolytic therapy. If the infarct is in a cerebral hemisphere, the subsequent changes usually include shrinkage of tissue and enlargement of the adjacent lateral ventricle (**4.13, 4.14**). Longstanding infarction, as within the distribution of one posterior cerebral artery, is easy to see from external examination of the brain (**4.15**). Wallerian degeneration will occur in any nerve fibres that have been destroyed. Thus, if the infarct involves the internal capsule, there will be progressive degeneration and shrinkage of the corresponding pyramidal tract in the brainstem and in the spinal cord (**4.16**). In the cerebellum, old infarcts retain a thin strip of molecular layer and central white matter with loss of Purkinje and granular cells.

Histologically, brain tissue that has undergone recent infarction has the appearance of coagulative necrosis, and within the cortex the outlines of dead neurons are recognisable (**4.4, 4.5**). This picture is followed by patchy, decreasing stainability in both grey and white matter (**4.17, 4.18**), and with time an infarct undergoes a series of changes, the time course

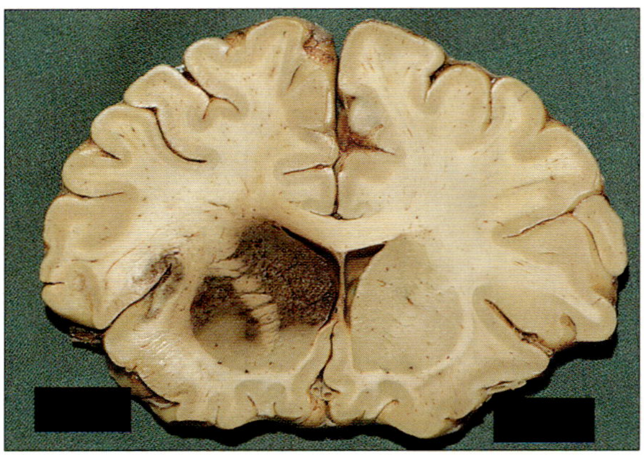

4.11 Cerebral infarction: seven day survival. There is infarction of the striatum, most likely due to embolism. Whereas the cortical lesion is largely 'anaemic', the lesion in the basal ganglia is 'haemorrhagic'. The patient died from myocardial infarction.

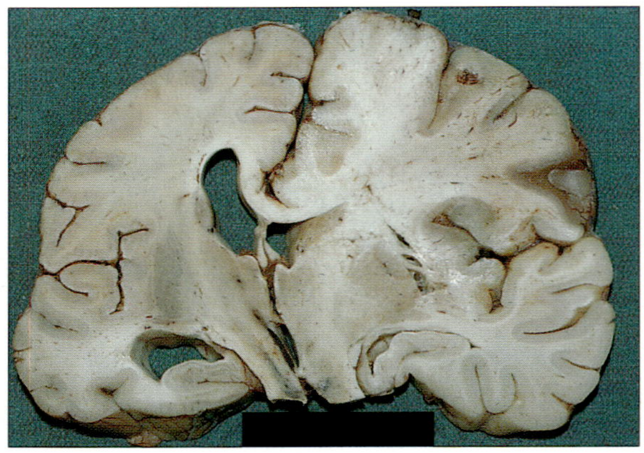

4.12 Cerebral infarction: 30-hour survival. There is a large infarct in one cerebral hemisphere due to occlusion of the internal carotid artery. There are internal herniae and asymmetry of ventricles due to midline shift and the effects of raised intracranial pressure.

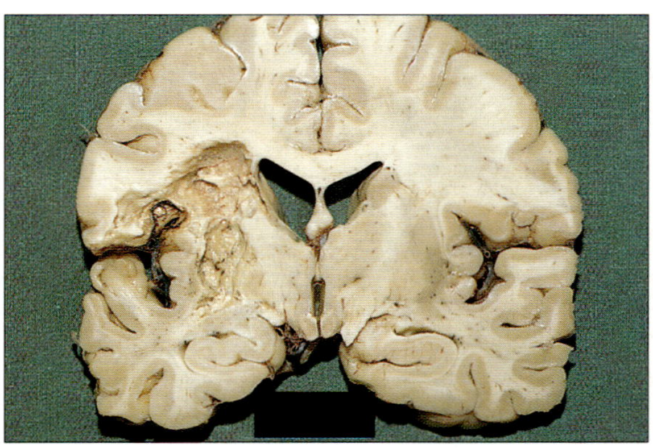

4.13 Cerebral infarction: three months' survival. There is an infarct in the central distribution of one of the middle cerebral arteries. The lesion affects superficial and deep grey matter, and white matter.

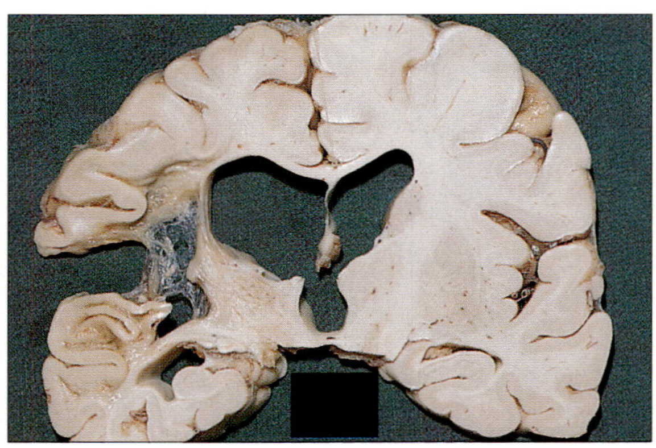

4.14 Cerebral infarction: four years' survival. There is a longstanding infarct in the central distribution of one of the middle cerebral arteries: both grey and white matter have been affected. Note the asymmetrical hydrocephalus (*ex-vacuo*).

of which can be assessed with some accuracy (**4.19**). In so-called 'evolving' or 'progressive' infarction, structural changes of different ages may be seen at the edge of the lesion. The margin of tissue between infarcted tissue and normal brain is an area of haemodynamic instability, known as the penumbra.

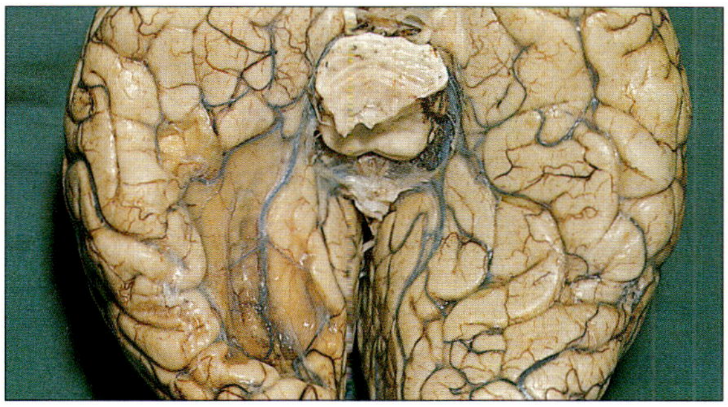

4.15 Cerebral infarction: three years' survival. There is a longstanding infarct on the under aspect of one temporal and occipital lobe in the distribution of the posterior cerebral artery.

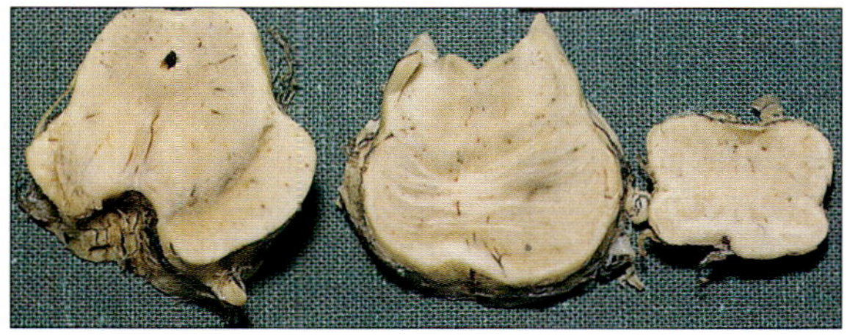

4.16 Hemiatrophy of brainstem: long survival. There is hemiatrophy at all levels of the brainstem due to longstanding Wallerian degeneration in one corticospinal tract below the level of an old infarct.

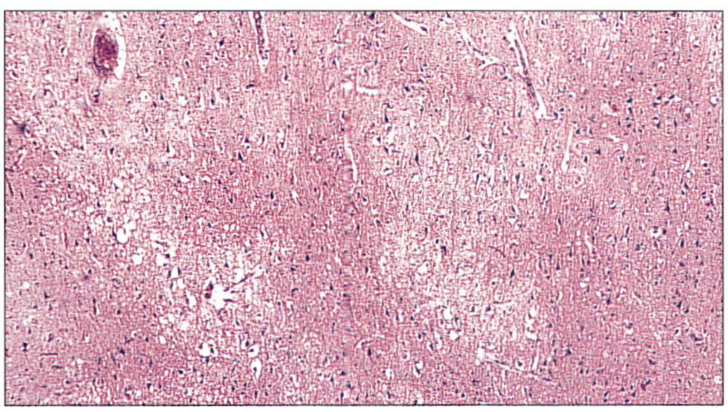

4.17 Cerebral infarction: 18 hours' survival. There is irregular pallor of staining of the neocortex in which necrotic neurons can be seen. (H & E)

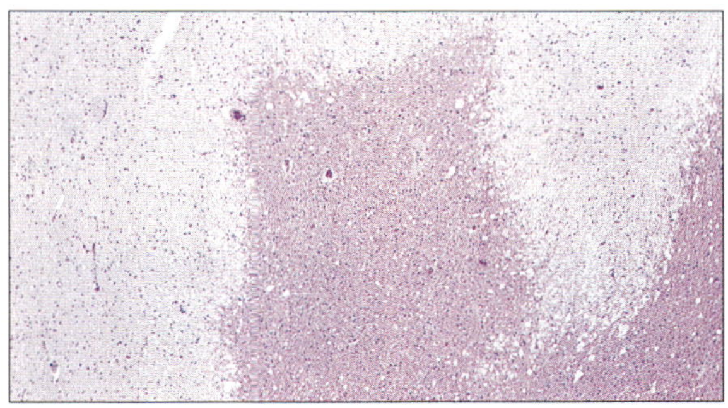

4.18 Cerebral infarction: 18 hours' survival. There is a definite boundary between normal white matter and the infarct. (H & E)

Time after infarction	Histological changes
15–20 hours	Defined margin between ischaemic and normal brain Spongy neuropil due to swelling of astrocytes and neuronal necrosis Pallor of myelin staining
24–30 hours	Early appearance of polymorphs in meninges and in small blood vessels at margin of lesion; endothelial enlargement; extravasation of RBCs
24–36 hours	Activation of microglia and astrocytes
36–48 hours	Appearance of macrophages and early separation of infarct from normal brain
1–2 weeks	Liquefaction of tissue; gliosis
Months	Cavitation and completion of glial scar; decrease in size and number of astrocytes; atrophy of damaged tissue

4.19 Histological changes and time course of cerebral infarction.

ARTERIAL INFARCTION

The most common causes of cerebral arterial infarction are atheroma, embolism, hypertension and cerebral arteritis.

ATHEROMA

In developed countries, this is the most common and important arterial disease in adults. As the plaques enlarge, they may be complicated by calcification and ulceration. Stenosis may progress to complete occlusion of the vessel, either due to bleeding in the base of the plaque or atheroma, or more often due to the formation of thrombus.

Usually, atheroma of the cerebral arteries is associated with atheroma in other parts of the body. However, a patient with marked atheroma in the aorta and coronary arteries may have little or no disease in the cerebral arteries; the reverse may also occur. At normal blood pressure, the internal cross-sectional area of an artery must be reduced by up to 90% before blood flow is impaired. Therefore, extensive atheroma of the neck or intracranial arteries does not necessarily lead to cerebral infarction, unless there is an episode of cardiac arrest or hypotension occurring in surgical or medical shock.

Stenosis and occlusion of the extracranial neck arteries

Atheroma is particularly common at the lower end of the internal carotid artery, but there are many subjects with severe stenosis or thrombosis of one (**4.20**), or even both, internal carotid arteries, who do not necessarily develop a cerebral infarct. Other causes of carotid artery stenosis and occlusion are listed in **4.21**.

Occlusion of an internal carotid artery may occur without any symptoms or signs. If infarction does occur, it may take several forms:

- massive infarction within the entire territory supplied by the middle cerebral artery, which sometimes involves anterior cerebral arterial territory as well (**4.12**);
- infarction of the cortex around the Sylvian fissure, with or without involvement of the basal ganglia and the internal capsule;
- infarction restricted to the internal capsule (so-called 'capsular' infarct, **4.22**);

Causes of stenosis and occlusion of the extracranial neck arteries
Atheroma
Thrombosis
Embolism
Dissecting aneurysm
Trauma
Fibromuscular dysplasia
Infection at base of skull
Aortic arch syndrome
Moya Moya disease

4.21 Causes of stenosis and occlusion of the extracranial neck arteries.

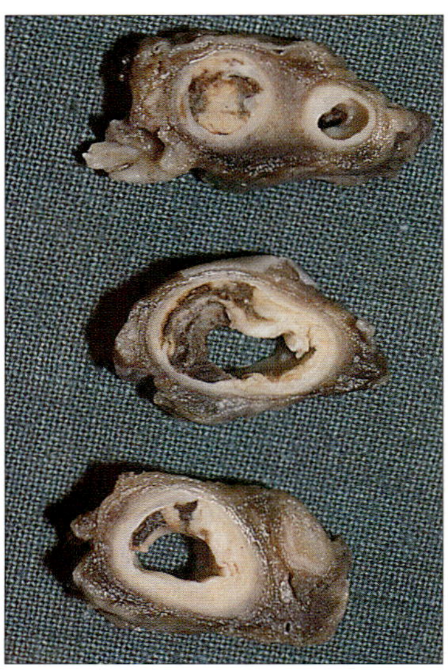

4.20 Occlusion of common carotid artery: seven days' survival. There is thrombotic occlusion superimposed upon 'complicated' atheroma which has propagated into the internal carotid artery. This has caused a large infarct in the territory of the middle cerebral artery.

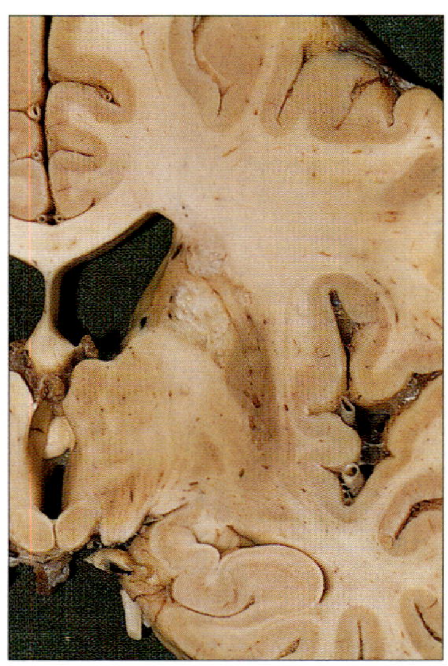

4.22 'Capsular' infarct: nine days' survival. There is a band of infarction (capsular infarct) that straddles the internal capsule and affects the caudate nucleus and the putamen. The internal carotid artery was occluded.

- small infarcts throughout the white matter;
- infarction within the boundaries between the territories supplied by the anterior and middle cerebral arteries (*see below*).

Stenosis, ectasia or occlusion of the vertebral and basilar arteries (**4.23**) may result in infarction in the brainstem, in the cerebellum (**4.24**), or in the territories of the posterior cerebral arteries (**4.25**).

Occlusion of intracranial arteries

Embolism and thrombosis are the most common causes of occlusion of these vessels, and the middle cerebral artery is occluded most often (**4.26**). Infarction within the distribution of the posterior cerebral artery is a common incidental post-mortem finding in the elderly (**4.15**). The most common causes of occlusion of the vertebral artery are listed in **4.27**.

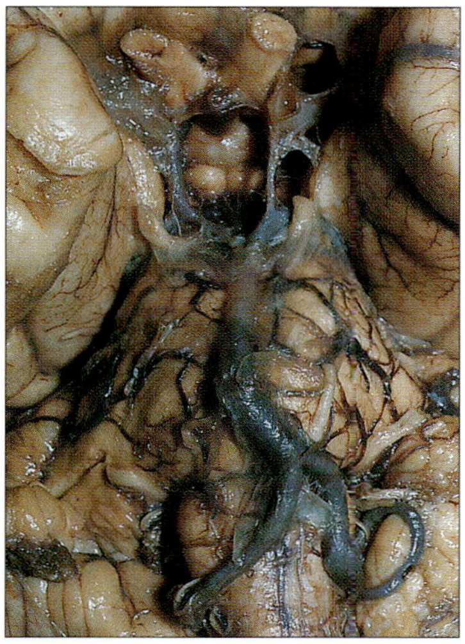

4.23 Thrombotic occlusion of basilar artery: nine days' survival. The basilar artery is prominent and was firm to touch. There is minimal atheroma, though the patient was hypertensive.

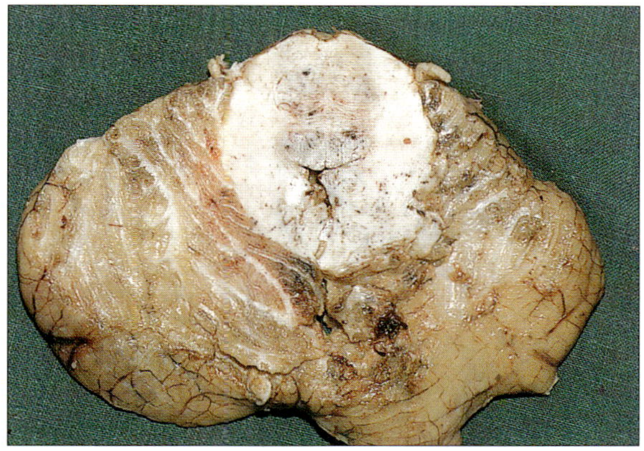

4.24 Infarction of hindbrain: 11 days' survival. Extensive infarction of the brainstem and cerebellar hemispheres due to occlusion of the vertebrobasilar arterial tree.

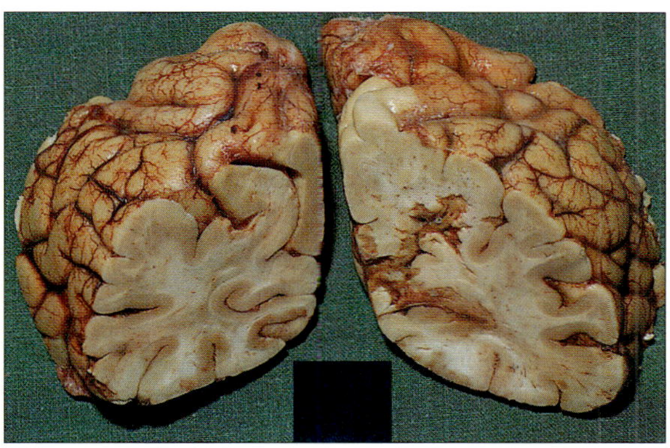

4.25 Infarction of each calcarine cortex: six days' survival. In addition to recent infarction of each medial occipital cortex, there is more longstanding infarction in the same distribution on the right. At post mortem, there was thrombotic occlusion of an extensively atheromatous basilar artery.

Causes of occlusion of a middle cerebral artery
Embolism (from heart, aorta, or neck arteries)
Thrombosis (formed on atheroma)
Vasospasm (saccular aneurysm)
Arteritis
Blood dyscrasia

4.26 Causes of occlusion of a middle cerebral artery.

Causes of occlusion of a vertebral artery
Thrombosis (formed on atheroma)
Deformation by osteophytes
Certain neck movements, viz. hyperextension, manipulation, intubation for anaesthesia
Rheumatoid arthritis with subluxation of atlanto-occipital joint
Birth injury following assisted or breech presentation

4.27 Causes of occlusion of a vertebral artery.

Occlusion of the spinal arteries

Occlusion of the anterior spinal artery is usually secondary to trauma, subluxation of the spine, cervical spondylosis, syphilis or embolism. It is also a common complication of an aortic aneurysm (**4.28, 4.29**). The pattern of infarction varies depending on the location of vascular disease. Damage may be limited to the ventral horns, more often to the ventral two-thirds of the cord; rarely the entire cord is involved.

EMBOLISM

There is a two- to fivefold increase in the incidence of 'stroke' in patients with ischaemic heart disease. The embolus may arise from thrombus formed on endocardium overlying an infarct (**4.30**). In two-thirds of cases, this complication develops within the first three weeks after acute myocardial infarction. Other causes of embolism include endocarditis (**4.31**).

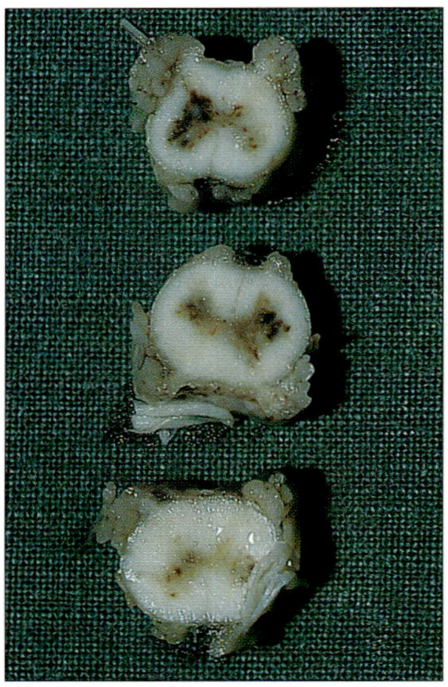

4.28 Infarction of spinal cord: two days' survival. There is haemorrhagic necrosis of the grey matter of the thoracic segments due to atheromatous dissection of the abdominal aorta.

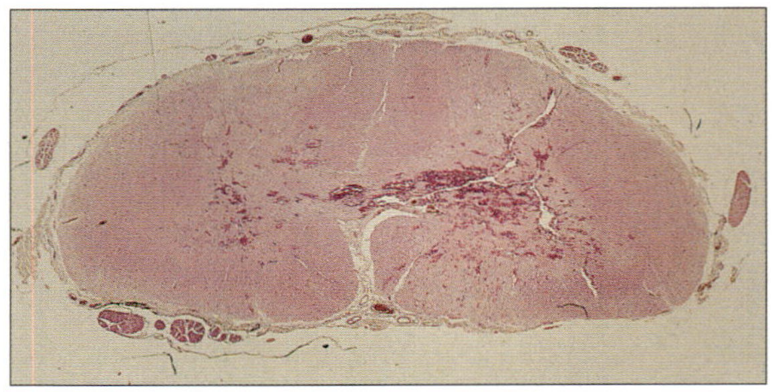

4.29 The same case as in **4.28**, confirming that necrosis is largely confined to grey matter of the dorsal and ventral horns. The anterior spinal artery was patent. (H & E)

Cerebral embolism	
Features	Between 30 and 60% of 'strokes' are embolic in nature For anatomical and haemodynamic reasons most emboli pass into the middle cerebral artery Most produce transient occlusion only
Sources	Heart disease (infarction, endocarditis, calcific aortic stenosis, rheumatic heart disease, prolapsed mitral valve, cardiomyopathy, arrhythmias) Disease of extracranial neck arteries and arch of aorta Cardiac surgery Paradoxical Systemic embolism of fat or various gases

4.30 Cerebral embolism.

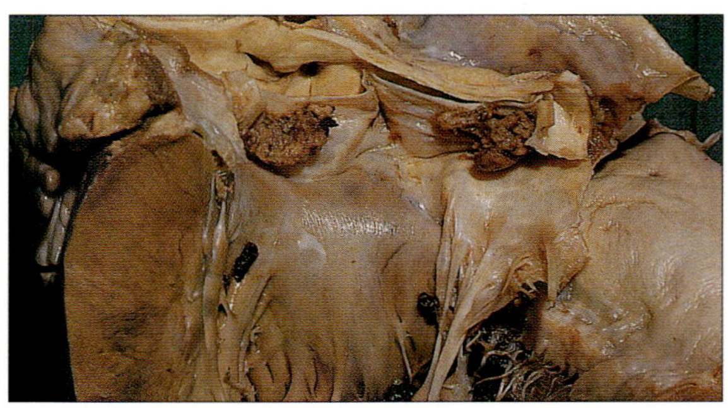

4.31 Bacterial endocarditis: eight days' survival. This patient presented with a sudden onset hemiparesis having been 'unwell' for three weeks with fever and weight loss. At post mortem there was a bacterial endocarditis. This had given origin to a number of emboli, one of which had occluded a middle cerebral artery.

Fat embolism

Fat embolism may develop as a complication of fracture of the long bones. Most of the fat will be trapped in the lungs, but very rarely, emboli will enter the systemic circulation. If, as a result, death occurs within 3–4 days, the white matter of the brain will be diffusely studded with petechial haemorrhages (**4.32**). Many globules of fat are seen in the small arterioles, and the walls of the small blood vessels are often necrotic.

Air embolism

Air embolism may develop during abortion, neurosurgical procedures in a sitting position, catheterisation procedures and subatmospheric decompression. Under these circumstances, infarction is commonly found within the arterial boundary zones.

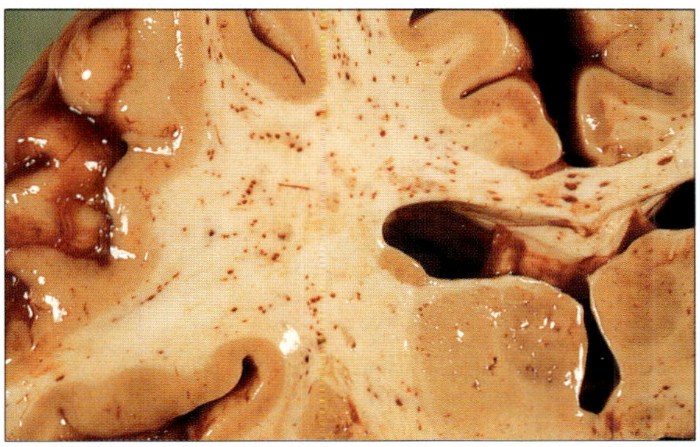

4.32 Fat embolism: five days' survival. There are multiple petechial haemorrhages in the white matter of the cerebral hemisphere.

Nitrogen embolism

This may occur if there is a sudden reduction of atmospheric pressure from an elevated level to normal, as encountered by underwater divers and workers in caissons. In these circumstances, dissolved gases in the blood come out of solution, and nitrogen forms small bubbles that cause the 'bends' and 'chokes'. The principal neuropathological findings are multiple foci of ischaemic damage, particularly in the grey matter of the cerebral hemispheres or in the spinal cord. The lesions have been attributed to a mixture of gases and fat embolism combined with hypotension. With survival, both ascending and descending Wallerian degeneration may be seen.

HYPERTENSION

Hypertension is a major risk factor for 'stroke' (**4.33**). Not only is atheroma of the larger cerebral arteries more severe in hypertensive than in normotensive subjects, but atheroma can also be found in the penetrating arteries of the internal capsule, basal ganglia and pons. Hypertension also causes hyaline arteriosclerosis, a change similar to that seen in the elderly and in patients with diabetes mellitus.

Hypertension is also associated with lacunes, which are small cavities measuring up to about 10mm diameter found in the basal ganglia, thalami and pons in the brains of elderly subjects or hypertensives (**4.34**). About 90% of lacunes are associated with hypertension. Some appear as expanded perivascular spaces, while others are small infarcts or resolving haemorrhages. The terms état lacunaire and état crible are used to describe the presence of numerous lacunes in grey and white matter, respectively.

Hypertension and the brain	
Features	Altered response of cerebral blood vessels to chronic hypertension with a shift of autoregulatory curve to the right Increased amount of atheroma Hyaline arteriosclerosis
Pathology	Lacunes: infarction Intracerebral haematoma formation, viz. basal ganglia, cerebellum, pons Multi-infarct dementia Leucoariosis (Binswanger's disease) Hypertensive encephalopathy

4.33 Hypertension and the brain.

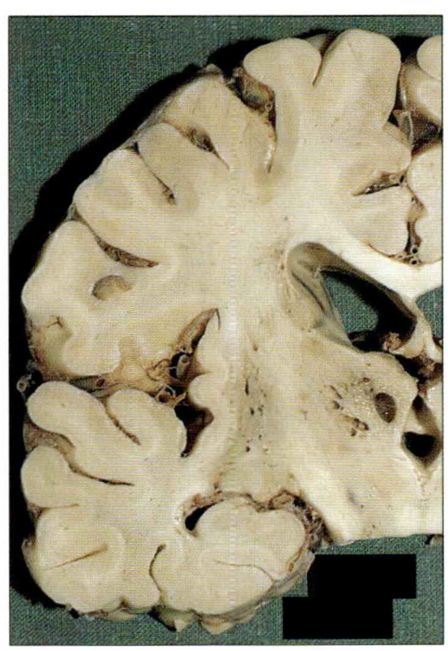

4.34 Lacunes. There are several smooth-walled cysts in the thalamus occurring as incidental findings in a known hypertensive patient.

There is also an association between hypertension (**4.35, 4.36**) and a slowly developing dementia (e.g. subcortical arteriosclerotic encephalopathy, Binswanger's disease, leucoariosis, or multi-infarct dementia). In leucoariosis, CT imaging shows a periventricular lucency, which is pathologically due to the loss of myelin and the thinning of axons in the deep white matter of the cerebral hemispheres. Severe hypertension may also be complicated by hypertensive encephalopathy. This is a disorder in which the upper limit of autoregulation is exceeded by forced cerebral hyperperfusion, induced by eclampsia or malignant-phase hypertension.

CEREBRAL ARTERITIS

There are many types of vasculitis which result in cerebral infarction. These include:

- bacterial, fungal and viral diseases;
- systemic vasculitides such as polyarteritis nodosa, Wegener's granulomatosis, and giant cell or temporal arteritis (**4.37, 4.38**);
- collagen vascular disease such as systemic lupus erythematosus;
- a miscellaneous group of disorders that includes Takayasu's disease, granulomatous angiitis (**4.39**), and radiation arteritis.

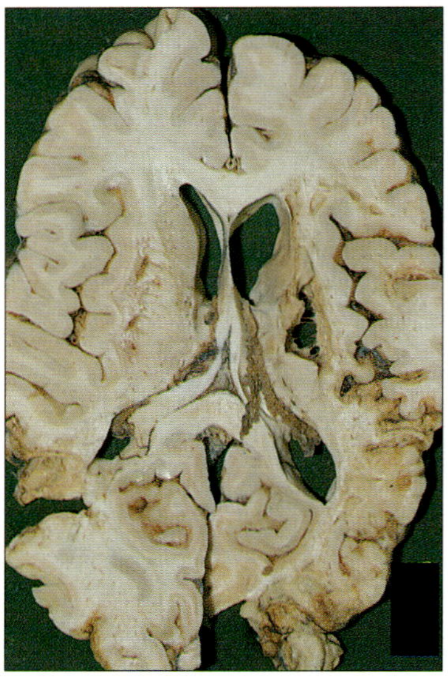

4.35 Multiple cerebral infarcts: two years' survival. This hypertensive patient experienced a number of 'cerebrovascular accidents'. The specimen was cut in the horizontal plane to match neuroimaging. Note the several bilateral infarcts.

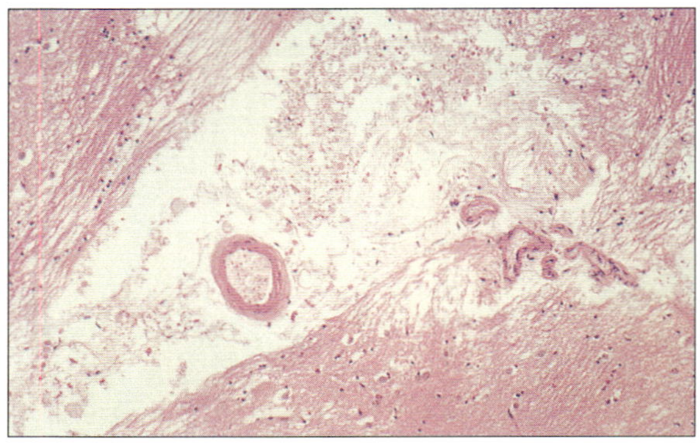

4.36 In the same case as **4.35**, an old infarction can be seen due to hyaline thickening of blood vessels. (H & E)

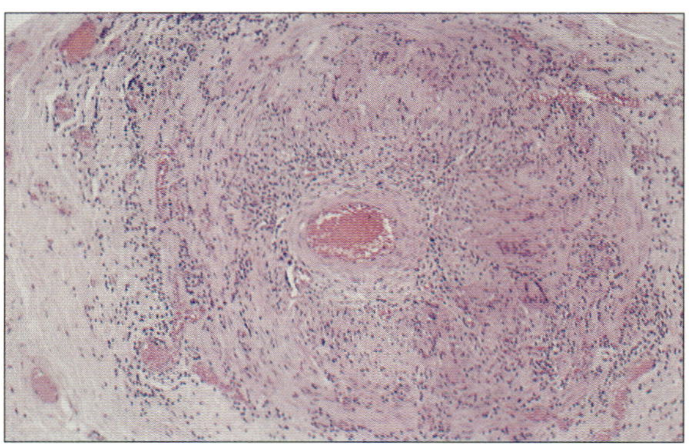

4.37 Giant cell arteritis of a meningeal artery, showing endothelial proliferation and a cellular infiltrate including multinucleated giant cells. (H & E)

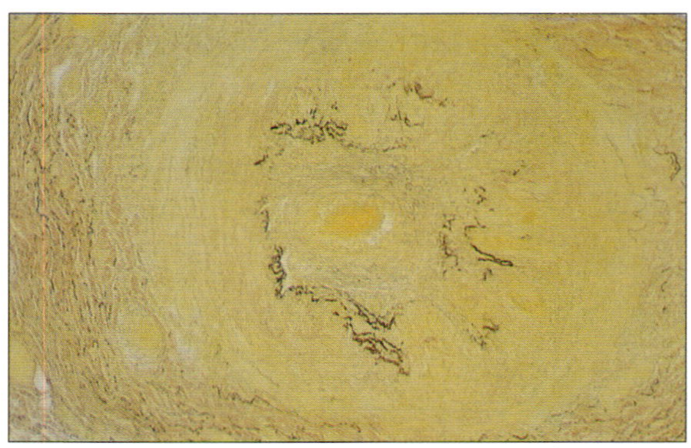

4.38 In the same case as **4.37**, fragmentation of internal elastic lamina can be seen. (Miller's elastica.)

MISCELLANEOUS CAUSES OF CEREBRAL INFARCTION

Dissection

Dissection of the carotid artery in the neck is the most frequently reported site of dissection, occurring most commonly in middle-aged adults. It is either spontaneous or associated with trauma. Spontaneous cervical carotid dissection usually occurs in otherwise healthy subjects, but is associated with fibromuscular dysplasia or Marfan's syndrome in 20% of cases. Traumatic dissection may follow direct puncture of the carotid artery for arteriography, or may develop following a neck injury caused by an over-the-shoulder restraining harness in a road traffic accident (**4.40**). Sometimes, the trauma is trivial. Traumatic dissection has been associated with most sporting activities, coughing, chiropractic manipulation and vigorous neck turning.

Dissection of the intracranial carotid system is rarely due to trauma, and more commonly occurs in association with cystic medial necrosis, fibromuscular dysplasia, atheroma or homocystinuria.

Other causes

Other causes of cerebral infarction include the aortic arch syndrome (pulseless disease or Takayasu's arteritis), which follows a progressive reduction of blood flow in the territories of the innominate, left common carotid and left subclavian arteries. There are many causes of this condition, some of which have features of a collagenosis.

In Moya Moya disease, cerebral angiography shows an unusual network of small blood vessels – likened to a 'puff of smoke' at the base of the brain. This condition predominates in the Japanese. Pathologically, there is a stenosis or occlusion of the terminal portions of the internal carotid arteries and proximal portions of the anterior and middle cerebral arteries. The aetiology is unclear.

In recent decades, associations have been established between cerebral infarction and various drugs, including, in the 1960s, an association between 'stroke' and oral contraceptives. More recently, there has been increasing awareness of the role of drugs of abuse in younger patients, including opiates, amphetamine, cocaine and LSD. There is also an association between 'stroke' and alcohol abuse.

There is also a group of young patients with mitochondrial cytopathies with combined involvement of skeletal muscle and the CNS. These include **M**itochondrial (myopathy), **E**ncephalopathy, **L**actic **A**cidosis and **S**troke-like episodes (MELAS). In most patients, the disorder is attributed to a single-point mutation in mitochondrial DNA. The pathogenesis of the cerebral infarction is not clear, but suggestions include the endothelial accumulation of abnormal mitochondria and the effects of the mitochondrial defect on secondary mediators of cerebral ischaemia.

Cerebral infarction is also associated with pregnancy and the puerperium. Other causes include raised intracranial pressure (*see Chapter 2*), and infarction due to vasospasm secondary to rupture of a saccular aneurysm.

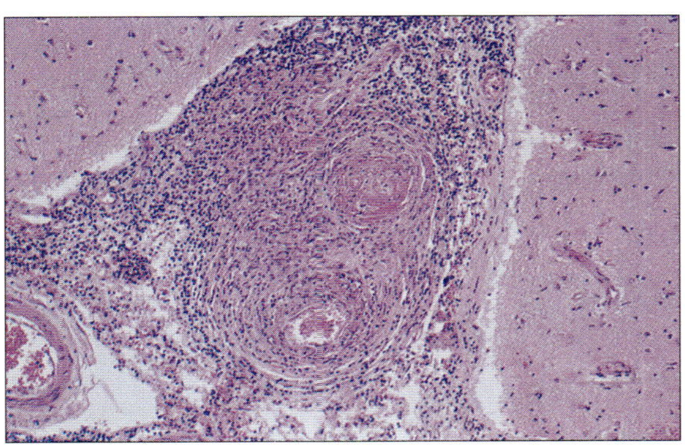

4.39 Granulomatous angiitis. Note the marked mononuclear cell infiltrate of the meningeal blood vessels, in one of which there is necrosis. A giant cell is also seen. (H & E)

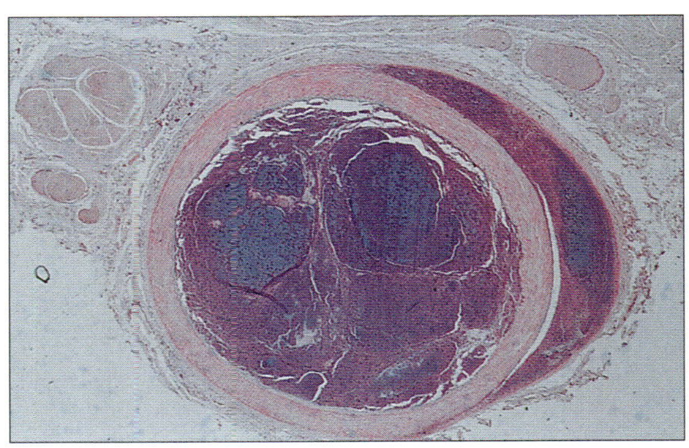

4.40 Dissection: three days' survival. There is thrombotic occlusion of an internal carotid artery following traumatic dissection in the wall of the artery. (H & E)

VENOUS INFARCTION

There are two principal types of thrombotic occlusion, namely primary (non-infectious) and secondary (due to pyogenic infection). Primary thrombosis may complicate pregnancy or the puerperium, various haematological disorders, the use of oral contraceptives and extreme dehydration in children (marasmus).

Secondary thrombosis is most often found as a complication of pyogenic infection, e.g. the superior sagittal sinus may become thrombosed if infection spreads from the frontal sinuses or from a compound fracture of the skull. Similarly, the lateral and cavernous sinuses may become occluded if infection spreads from either the middle ear or the central part of the face, respectively.

In both primary and secondary thrombosis, the brain has distended thrombosed cortical veins adjacent to the thrombosed sinus. On section, there is haemorrhagic infarction of the cortex (**4.41**), with petechial haemorrhages in the subcortical white matter. When the central or great vein of Galen is thrombosed, there is infarction of the basal ganglia and cingulate gyri.

MICROINFARCTION

There is also an association between multiple microinfarcts and haematological disorders such as sickle-cell disease, polycythaemia rubra vera, leukaemia and thrombotic thrombocytopenic purpura.

SPONTANEOUS (NON-TRAUMATIC) INTRACRANIAL HAEMORRHAGE

Bleeding occurs either into brain substance, or into the subarachnoid space. Traumatic haemorrhage is considered in *Chapter 5*.

INTRACEREBRAL HAEMORRHAGE

This is particularly common in Afro–Caribbeans, the Japanese and in the UK, especially in late middle-aged males with hypertension. In four-fifths of cases, the haematoma is in the region of the basal ganglia – the so-called 'capsular' or thalamic haematoma (**4.42**), with about 14% of cases occurring in the pons (**4.43**),

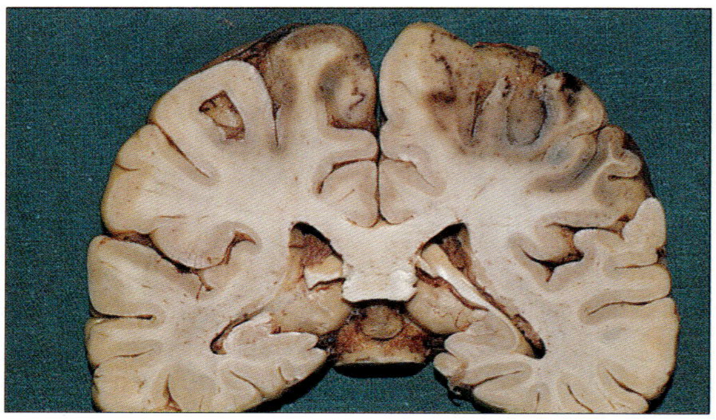

4.41 Venous infarction: three days' survival. There was idiopathic occlusion of the superior sagittal sinus at post mortem in an elderly patient. Note asymmetrical duskily haemorrhagic infarction of the supramedial cortex of each cerebral hemisphere.

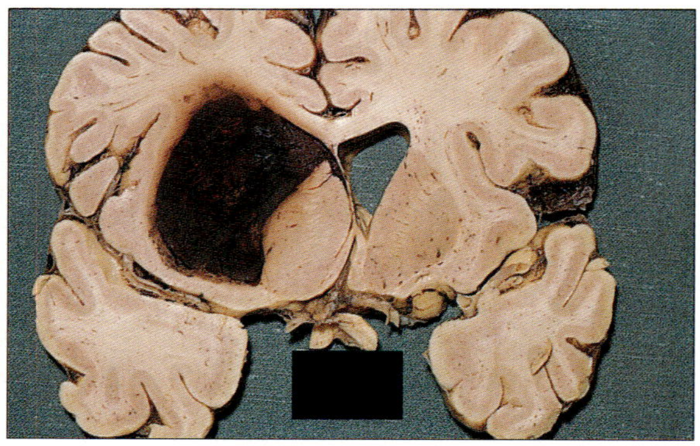

4.42 Spontaneous intracerebral haematoma: six days' survival. There is a large recently formed haematoma centred on the basal ganglia. Note that the overlying cortex is intact and the blood has tracked medially to present within the ventricular system.

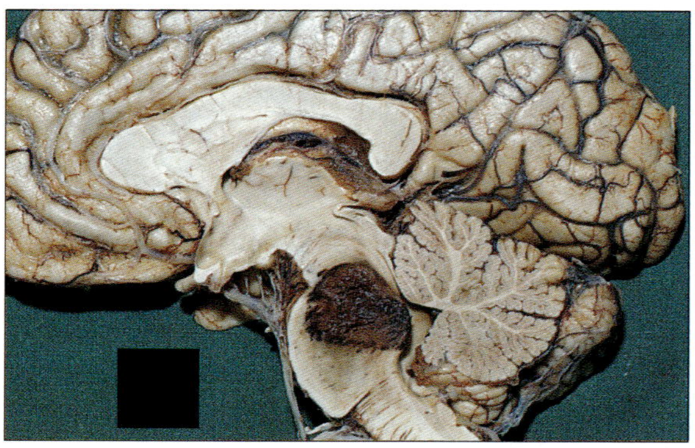

4.43 Spontaneous pontine haematoma: three weeks' survival. Mid-sagittal slice to show haematoma in the upper part of the brainstem.

and about 6% in the cerebellum (**4.44**). The haematoma usually enlarges rapidly and causes considerable damage. Due to the rapidity of the expanding lesion and the resultant distortion and herniation of the brain, death often occurs within 24–36 hours, as a result of raised intracranial pressure. The use of antihypertensive drugs has led to a considerable reduction in deaths from cerebral haemorrhage.

The haematoma often ruptures into the ventricles or through the surface of the brain into the subarachnoid space. Sometimes the haematoma is relatively small: the lesion becomes brown in colour and the clot is ultimately absorbed and replaced by xanthochromic fluid – the so-called apoplectic cyst (**4.45**).

The principal risk factor is hypertension (**4.3**) with bleeding taking place from miliary aneurysms on small perforating cerebral arteries (**4.46**). These aneurysms are usually multiple, tend to occur on blood vessels less than 250μm in diameter, and can measure about 2mm wide. They occur mainly in hypertensive subjects over the age of 50, but are also seen in normotensive subjects over 65 years of age.

Other causes of spontaneous intracerebral haemorrhage (**4.3**) include vasculitis, particularly in patients with collagen diseases, rupture of a mycotic or a saccular aneurysm, or a vascular malformation (**4.47**). Haemorrhage may occasionally occur in primary brain tumours, such as glioblastoma, or in secondary brain tumours, most often into deposits from primary carcinoma of the bronchus, malignant melanoma and chorion carcinoma. Multiple haemorrhages are often seen in the white matter of patients with thrombocytopenia. Patients on anticoagulant therapy and haemophiliacs are also at risk, although bleeding into the subdural space is more common than into brain substance.

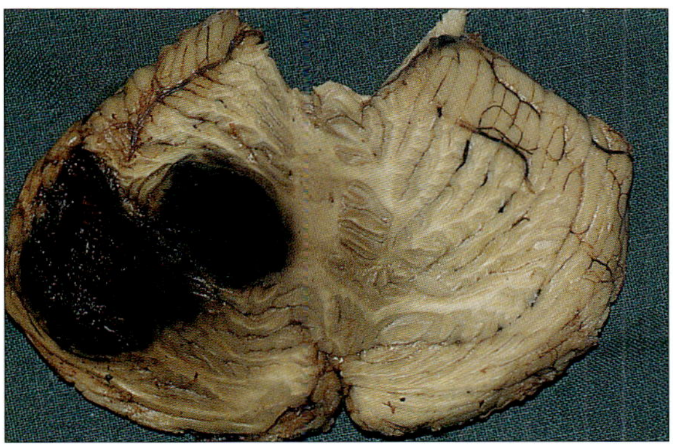

4.44 Spontaneous cerebellar haematoma: five days' survival. The haematoma was sufficiently large to distort CSF pathways and cause obstructive hydrocephalus.

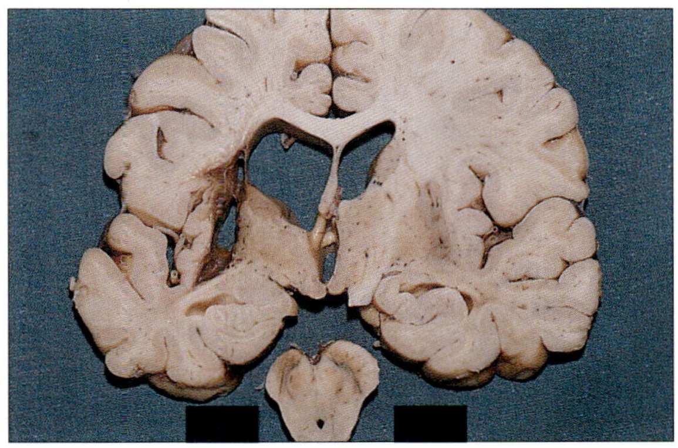

4.45 'Apoplectic cyst': three years' survival. There is an old cavity with orange-brown walls immediately deep to one insula: the lesion has crossed the internal capsule. Sequelae include un lateral hydrocephalus and descending long tract degeneration. The cyst represents residual haematoma cavity.

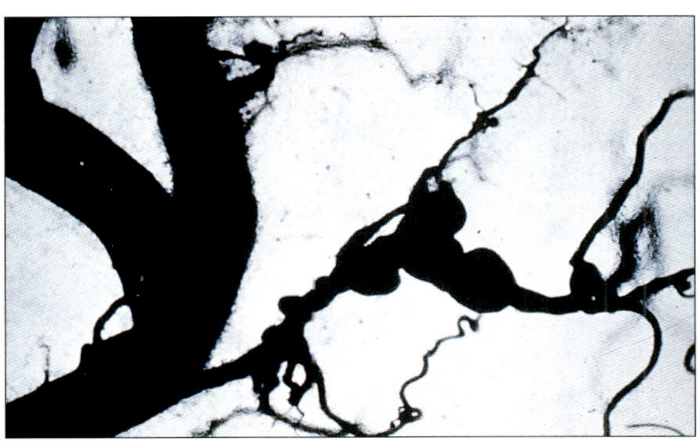

4.46 Miliary aneurysm. Cleared thick section of basal ganglia showing multiple aneurysms on lenticulostriate artery. (Injected specimen.)

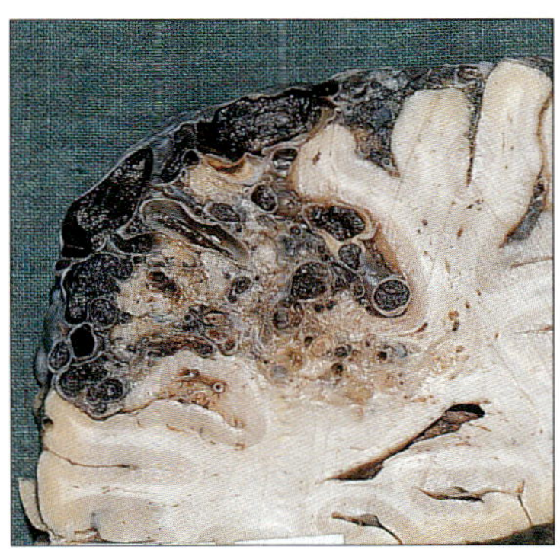

4.47 Arteriovenous malformation: incidental finding at autopsy. There is a tangle of abnormal vessels in the grey and white matter of one parietal lobe.

Haematomas occurring in atypical sites ('lobar haematomas') in normal individuals are increasingly thought to be due to cerebral amyloid (congophilic) angiopathy (**4.48**). Beta amyloid infiltrates the media and adventitia of blood vessels resulting in the formation of microaneurysms. There is an association with Alzheimer's disease. The haematoma may rupture into the ventricular system, and secondary brainstem haemorrhage is common. When fixed in formalin, the hardened clot may be difficult to cut with a brain knife.

Haemorrhage into the spinal cord

Spontaneous bleeding is rare but may occur with thrombocytopenia or a spinal vascular malformation (**4.49**).

Subarachnoid haemorrhage

There are several causes, the commonest of which is probably acute head injury (**4.50**). Non-traumatic subarachnoid haemorrhage is commonly due to rupture of a saccular aneurysm.

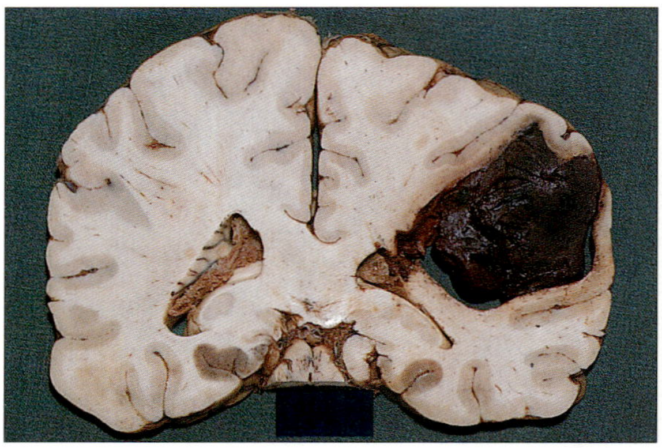

4.48 Lobar haematoma: three days' survival. There is a large haematoma in the white matter of one parietal lobe of an elderly demented patient. Histologically, there was evidence of amyloid angiopathy. There are bilateral tentorial herniae.

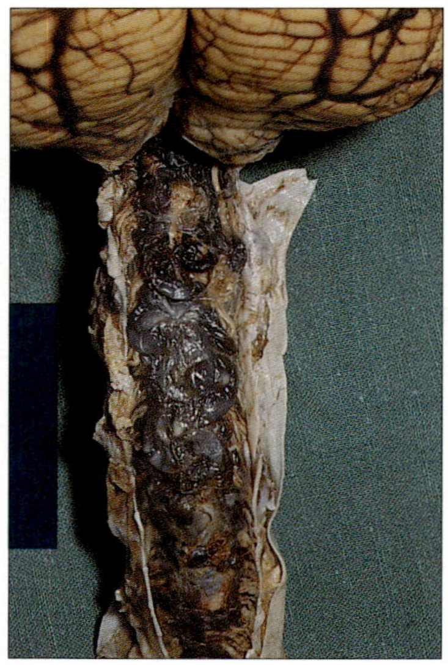

4.49 Spinal vascular malformation: two years' intermittent history. Variously diagnosed as multiple sclerosis and poliomyelitis, this female patient presented with quadriparesis. At post mortem there was a tangle of abnormal blood vessels over the dorsal aspect of the cervical cord. On section the malformation had ruptured to form a haematomyelia.

Causes	Frequency (%)
Traumatic	
Contusions and lacerations	100
Part of severe or diffuse injury	80
Spontaneous (non-traumatic)	
Rupture of saccular aneurysm	65
Arteriovenous malformation	5
Extension of intracerebral haematoma usually into ventricles and then into subarachnoid space	5–10
Idiopathic	5–10

4.50 Causes and frequency of bleeding into the subarachnoid space.

Saccular aneurysms

These occur in about 1–2% of the adult population and are found more commonly in women than in men. For a long time, they have been considered as congenital abnormalities because histologically there is often a defect of media and elastica in the structure of the aneurysmal wall. However, since the incidence of saccular aneurysms in childhood is low, it has been suggested that many saccular aneurysms are degenerative, resulting from an interaction of atheroma and hypertension at naturally weak points (bifurcations) in the walls of cerebral arteries. Support for the role of haemodynamic stress in the formation of saccular aneurysms is provided by their development on vessels supplying arteriovenous malformations.

Most saccular aneurysms are thin-walled, measuring between 2mm and 8mm in diameter (**4.51**). However, others are several centimetres across. They are usually thick-walled and often contain laminated thrombus (**4.52**).

About 90% of saccular aneurysms are located in the distributions of the internal carotid arteries; the remaining 10% are located on the vertebrobasilar arterial tree. Multiple aneurysms are found in 10–15% of patients with subarachnoid haemorrhage(**4.54**); these are said to be associated with coarctation of the

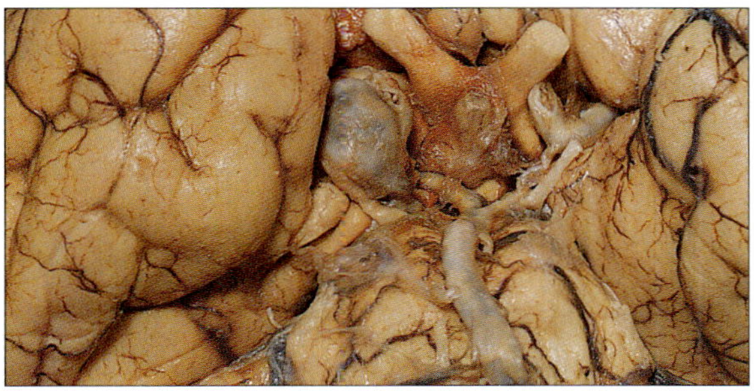

4.51 Saccular aneurysm: incidental finding. There is an aneurysm arising from the upper end of one of the internal carotid arteries. The lesion has compressed the ipsilateral IIIrd cranial nerve.

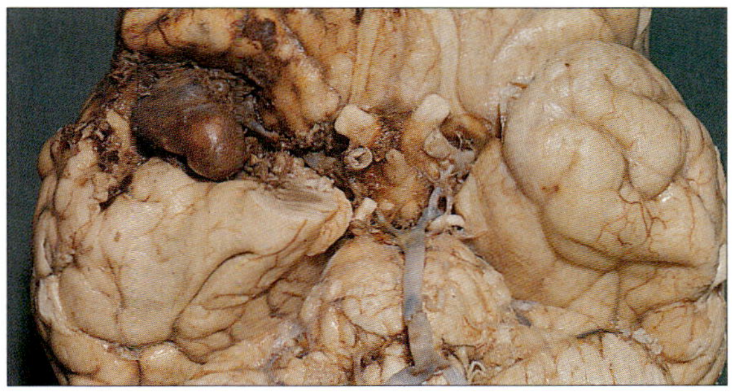

4.52 Giant saccular aneurysm: three days' survival following ligation of ipsilateral internal carotid artery. There is a 27mm aneurysm arising from one of the middle cerebral arteries which had ruptured to present with subarachnoid haemorrhage four weeks previously.

Location	Frequency (%)
Upper end of internal carotid artery	40
Anterior communicating artery	30
Middle cerebral artery	20
Basilar and vertebral arteries	5–10
Other arteries	5–10

4.53 Location and frequency of saccular aneurysms.

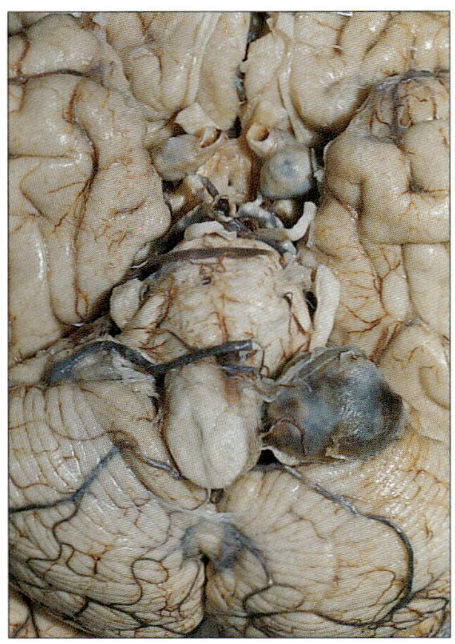

4.54 Multiple saccular aneurysms: incidental finding. There are unruptured aneurysms at the upper ends of each internal carotid artery and at the junction between one posterior inferior cerebellar and vertebral arteries.

aorta, adult type-3 polycystic disease of the kidney and renal artery stenosis, the possible common denominator being hypertension. However, in at least some instances, it is thought that there may be a developmental abnormality in the form of a collagen type-3 deficiency.

Rupture

Rupture of a saccular aneurysm may be associated with early (within three weeks) and late (after three weeks) intracranial complications (**4.55**).

Early intracranial complications

These are common, with about 10% of patients dying during the first bleed and a further 30% from its after-effects within the next few days. A further 35% of patients rebleed and die within the first year, mostly within the first two weeks. The causes include severe recurrent subarachnoid haemorrhage, intracerebral haematoma, subdural haematoma and a caroticocavernous fistula.

Subarachnoid haemorrhage usually accompanies rupture of a saccular aneurysm. This may be limited to the immediate vicinity of the aneurysm, but often there is extensive haemorrhage throughout the subarachnoid space (**4.56**). When fatal, the basal cisterns are filled with a recent blood clot. Sometimes, quite a large haematoma may develop in the subarachnoid space, usually within the Sylvian fissure in association with an aneurysm on the middle cerebral artery, or between the medial surfaces of the frontal lobe in association with an aneurysm on the anterior communicating artery. At post-mortem in such cases, it is important to try to identify the aneurysm before fixing the brain, since fixed blood clot is difficult to remove without destroying the aneurysm.

The formation of an **intracerebral haematoma** is a common sequel to rupture of a saccular aneurysm. The haematomas lie adjacent to the aneurysms, and occur in the inframedial part of the frontal lobes in association with anterior communicating artery aneurysms (**4.57**), and in the temporal lobe in association

Complications following rupture of intracranial saccular aneurysm	
Early	Subarachnoid haemorrhage Intracranial haematoma with or without extension into the ventricular system Subdural haematoma Caroticocavernous fistula Acute hydrocephalus
Late	Cerebral infarction Hydrocephalus Haemosiderosis of meninges

4.55 Complications following rupture of intracranial saccular aneurysm.

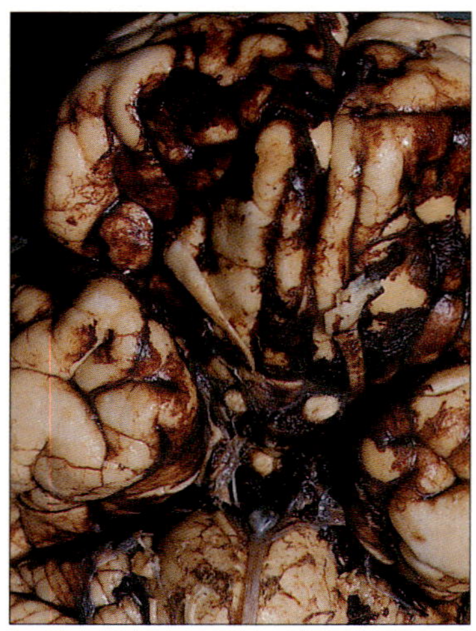

4.56 Subarachnoid haemorrhage arising from a saccular aneurysm: five days' survival. There are large amounts of fresh haemorrhage in the basal cisterns and over the base of the brain. Dissection showed an aneurysm arising from the upper end of the basilar artery.

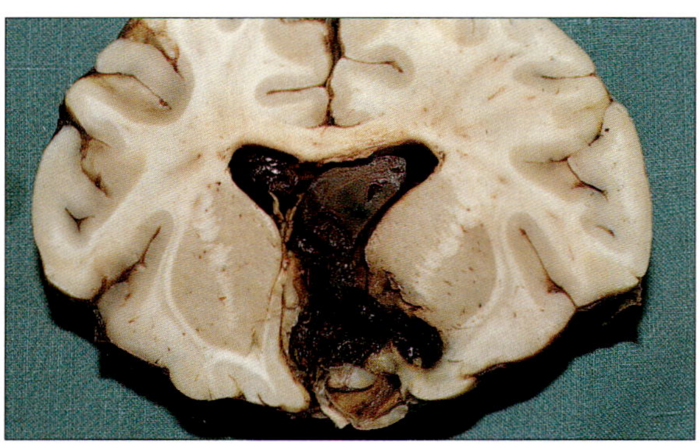

4.57 Intracerebral haematoma arising from a saccular aneurysm: two days' survival. There is a recently formed haematoma centred on the inferomedial aspects of each frontal lobe, which has extended into the ventricular system. The origin of the haematoma is an aneurysm arising from the anterior communicating artery.

with an aneurysm on a middle cerebral artery (**4.58**) or on a posterior communicating artery (**4.59**). Rupture of an aneurysm on the middle cerebral artery may occasionally produce an acute subdural haematoma while an aneurysm on the internal carotid artery may rupture into the cavernous sinus causing a caroticocavernous fistula.

Late intracranial complications

These include cerebral infarction, which occurs most commonly in the region of the brain supplied by the artery on which the aneurysm is situated. The infarct is probably partly attributable to arterial vasospasm. The situation, however, is complex and the infarct is often due to a combination of factors, including vasospasm, mass effects of intracerebral haematoma and raised intracranial pressure.

Acute **hydrocephalus** occurs within the first few days and a chronic type at about the second week. Both types are probably due to obstruction to the flow of CSF by blood in the subarachnoid space. Recurrent episodes of subarachnoid haemorrhage may cause haemosiderosis, in which the outer cortical layers become pigmented due to the presence of subpial haemosiderin-containing macrophages (**4.60**).

PETECHIAL HAEMORRHAGES

This is a non-specific term applicable to any condition of the brain characterised by the occurrence of multiple small haemorrhages (brain purpura). These vary in number but are usually confined to the white matter. There are many causes (**4.61**).

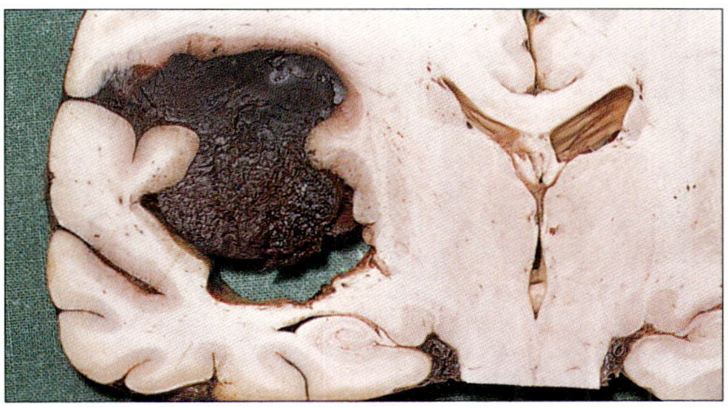

4.58 Intracerebral haematoma arising from a saccular aneurysm: 18 hours' survival. A recently formed haematoma lies partly in the subarchnoid space and partly intracerebrally. There was an aneurysm arising from the middle cerebral artery. Compare with **4.42** in which the haematoma is intracerebral.

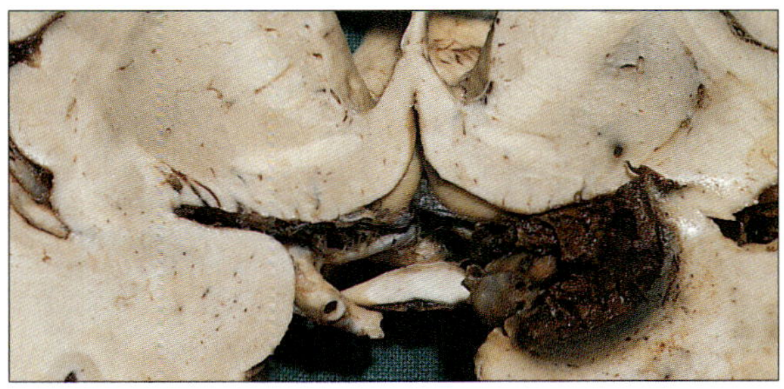

4.59 Intracerebral haematoma arising from a saccular aneurysm: two days' survival. An aneurysm arising from the upper end of the carotid artery has ruptured into the medial part of the temporal lobe.

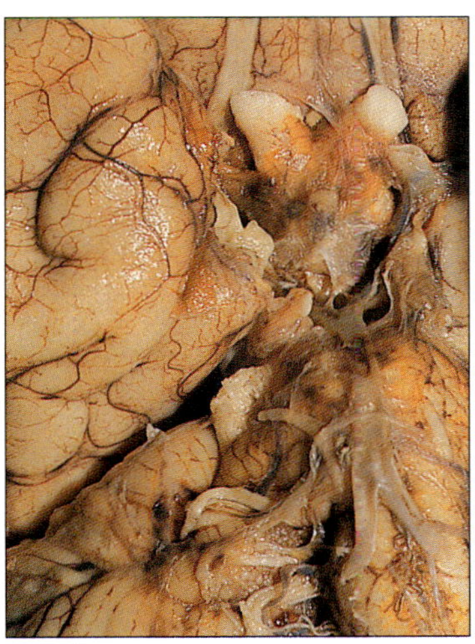

4.60 Meningeal haemosiderosis from a saccular aneurysm: three months' survival. There is a marked orange–brown discoloration of the meninges following earlier rupture of an aneurysm arising from the upper end of an internal carotid artery.

Causes of petechial haemorrhages	
Associated with trauma	Diffuse brain injury (including acute vascular injury) Fat embolism
Not associated with trauma	Asphyxia Thrombocytopenia Disseminated intravascular coagulation Hypertensive encephalopathy Acute haemorrhagic leucoencephalitis Cerebral malaria Endotoxic shock Allergic sensitivity to drugs

4.61 Causes of petechial haemorrhages.

HYPOXIC BRAIN DAMAGE

Irreversible hypoxic brain damage may occur whenever there is insufficient oxygen in the blood or a reduced blood flow to the brain, or both. Cerebral blood flow depends in turn on the cerebral perfusion pressure, which is the pressure difference between arteries and veins and the cerebrovascular resistance of the intervening vessels. The latter is determined by the intracranial pressure, the viscosity of the blood and the tone of the smooth muscle in vessel walls. Since blood flow is the most important factor for maintaining an adequate supply of oxygen to the brain, various protective mechanisms have evolved to preserve it. When these mechanisms fail or the insult is overwhelming, irreversible hypoxic brain damage is likely. Irreversible hypoxic damage may occur as a consequence of such diverse conditions as respiratory obstruction, lung and heart disease, shock, epilepsy, carbon monoxide poisoning, cardiac arrest, an episode of severe hypotension or a variety of anaesthetic accidents.

BRAIN DAMAGE DUE TO CARDIAC ARREST

At normal body temperature, if cardiac arrest of abrupt onset exceeds 5–7 minutes, complete clinical recovery is unlikely. If death occurs within 24–36 hours of cardiac arrest, the brain may appear normal externally and on section. By 36–48 hours, however, it is sometimes possible to identify patchy discoloration in the depths of the sulci, particularly in the posterior halves of the cerebral hemispheres (**4.62**) and selective necrosis in CA1 sector of the Ammon's horn (**4.63, 4.64**).

In patients who survive for several months or longer, there is a reduction in the weight of the brain and evidence of atrophy of both the cortical gyri (**4.65**) and the cerebellar folia (**4.66**). The cortex is reduced to a thin band of discoloured tissue in which it may be possible to discern laminar necrosis. There may be considerable ventricular enlargement and sclerosis of Ammon's horn is frequently seen (**4.67**). The thalami may appear normal but eventually retrograde degeneration is seen in the thalamic

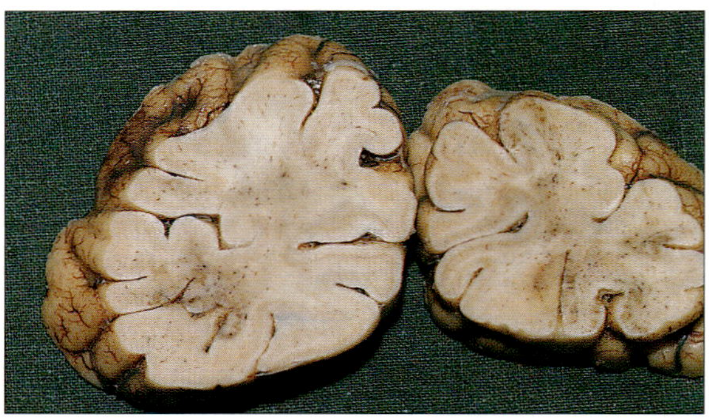

4.62 Sulcal necrosis: 48 hours' survival. There is discoloration of the cortex in the sides and depths of sulci. Histologically there was necrosis of neurons.

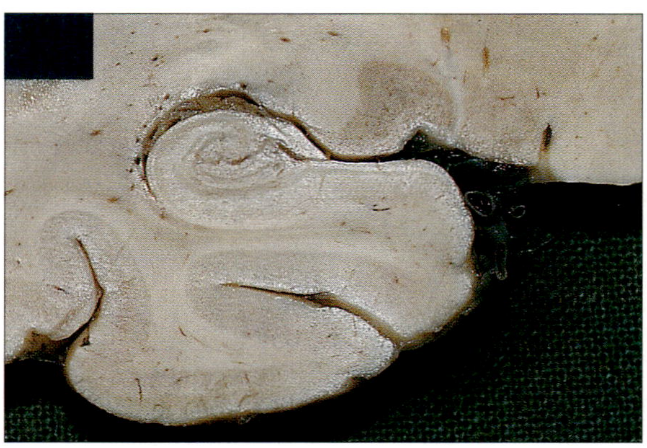

4.63 Normal hippocampus.

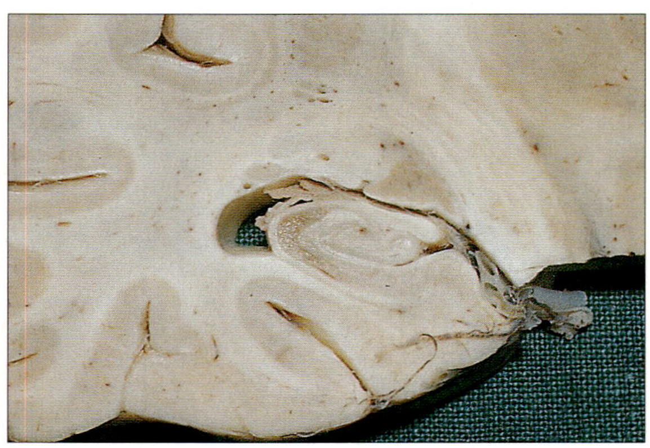

4.64 Hypoxic necrosis of hippocampus: 48 hours' survival. There is a band of slightly haemorrhagic necrosis limited to the CAI sector (Sommer sector). Compare with normal hippocampus in **4.63**.

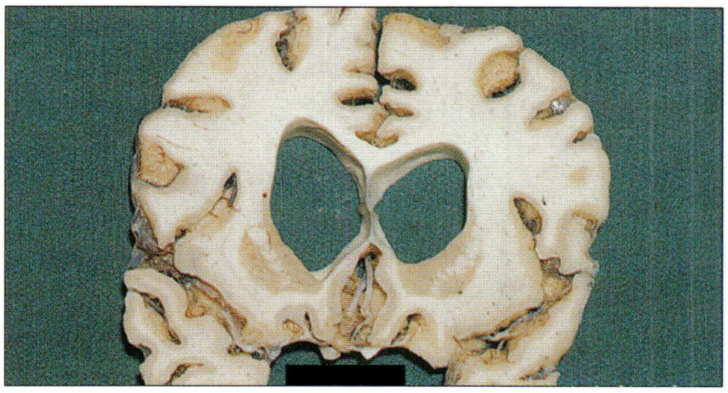

4.65 Cardiac arrest: five months' survival. Brain of patient who, following cardiorespiratory arrest, remained vegetative until death. Grey matter is discoloured and reduced in bulk. There is considerable symmetrical enlargement of the ventricles.

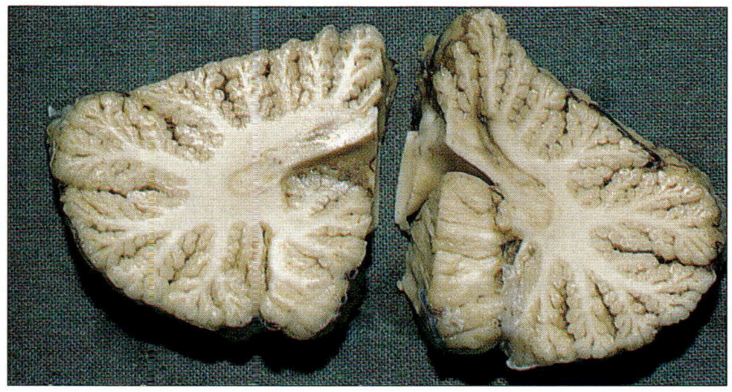

4.66 Cardiac arrest: five months' survival. This is the same case as in **4.65**. Note the diffuse atrophy of the cerebellar cortex.

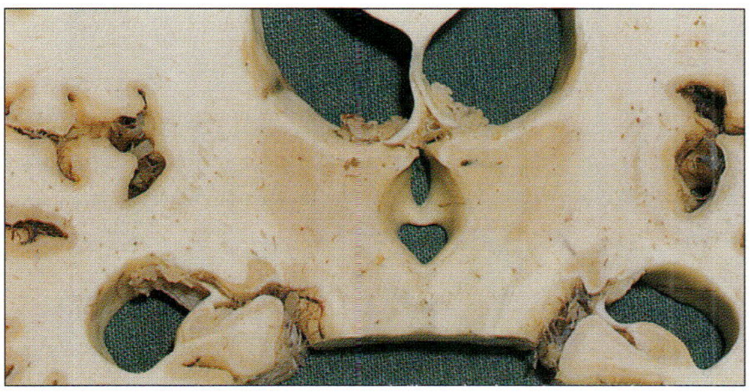

4.67 Cardiac arrest: five months' survival. This is the same case as in **4.65** and **4.66**. Note the bilateral sclerosis of Ammon's horn and marked symmetrical enlargement of ventricles.

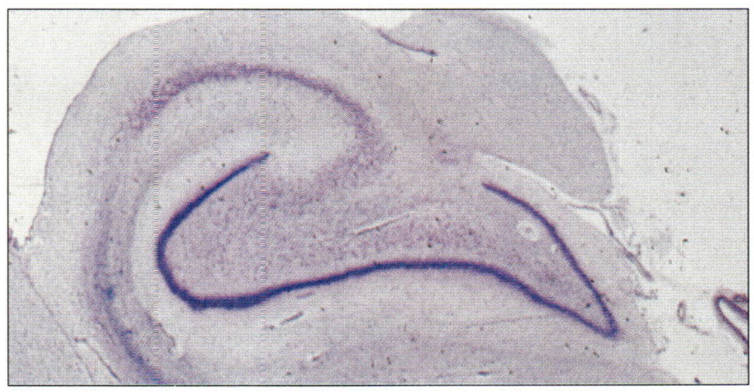

4.68 Cardiac arrest: five months' survival. This is the same case as in **4.65–4.67**. There is complete loss of neurons in CAI and a gliosis. (Celloidin: cresyl violet.)

Region	Histological appearance
Neocortex	Laminar necrosis in layers 3, 5 and 6, that is greatest in depths and sides of sulci than at crests of gyri, and maximal posteriorly
Hippocampus	Greatest in CAI and CA4 with least involvement of CA2 (so-called resistant sector)
Basal ganglia and thalamus	Variable involvement
Cerebellum	Diffuse necrosis of Purkinje cells
Brainstem	Sensory nuclei More severe in young children than adults

4.69 Histological patterns of selective vulnerability in hypoxia. CA1, CA2 and CA4 refer to the various subfields of the cornu ammonis (Ammon's horn) projection nuclei. Microscopy reveals a pattern of selective vulnerability (**4.68, 4.69–4.73**).

BRAIN DAMAGE DUE TO HYPOTENSION

In its most common form, damage is concentrated in the arterial boundary zones (watershed areas), which lie between the main cerebral and cerebellar arterial territories (**4.75**). This pattern of damage has been described:

- in neurosurgical patients operated on in a sitting position;
- following a sudden decrease in arterial pressure;
- after occlusion of one carotid artery;
- after the overzealous treatment of malignant hypertension;
- in fatal head injury.

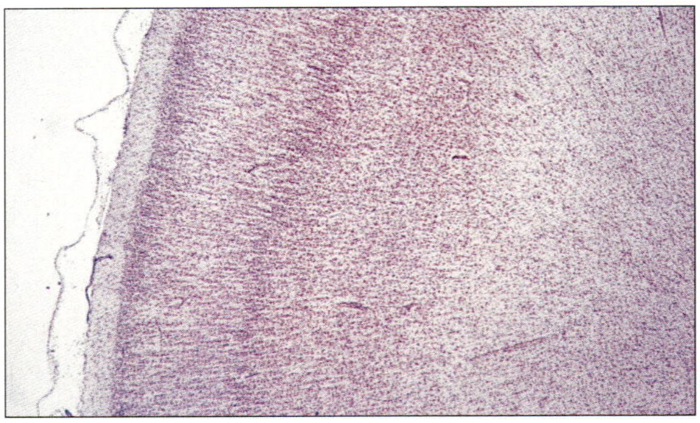

4.70 Selective vulnerability in the neocortex: 36 hours' survival. Normal temporal cortex showing six layers. (Celloidin: cresyl violet.)

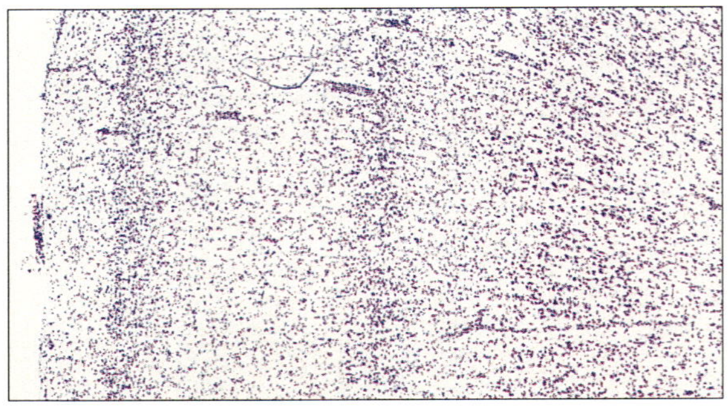

4.71 Selective vulnerability in the neocortex: 36 hours' survival. There is laminar necrosis of layers 3, 5 and 6 with relative preservation of layers 1, 2 and 4. (Celloidin: cresyl violet.)

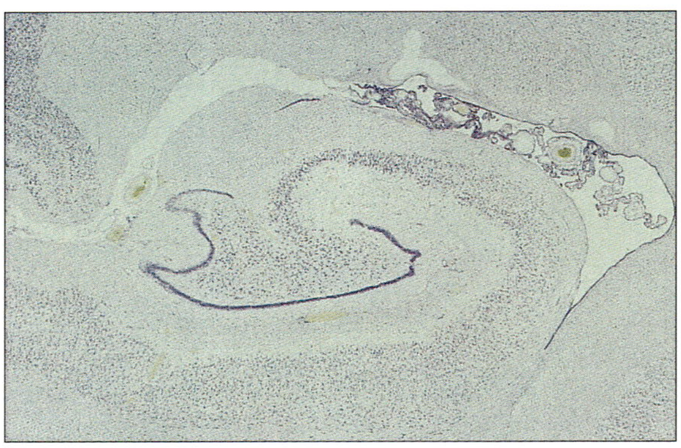

4.72 Normal hippocampus. (Celloidin: cresyl violet.)

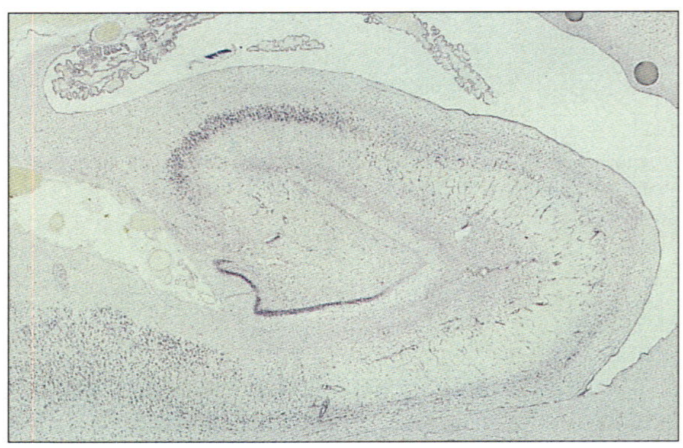

4.73 Selective vulnerability in the hippocampus: 36 hours' survival. There is selective necrosis of both CAI and CA4 with relative preservation of dentate fascia, CA3 and CA2. (Celloidin: cresyl violet.)

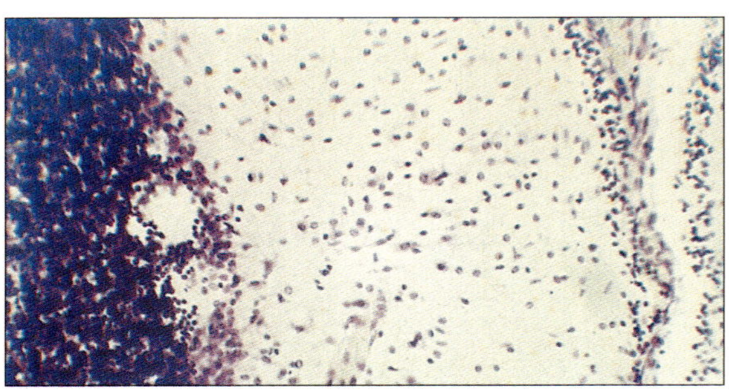

4.74 Selective vulnerability in the cerebellar cortex: 36 hours' survival. There is diffuse necrosis of Purkinje cells, which now appear as empty spaces surrounded by enlarged Bergmann astrocytes. There is also an early astrocytosis and microglial response in the molecular layer. (Celloidin: cresyl violet.)

If the lesions are several days old, they may be seen macroscopically. They vary in size from small foci of necrosis in the cortex to large wedge-shaped lesions, extending from the cortex almost to the angles of the lateral ventricles. Cortical damage is most frequent and most severe in the parieto-occipital regions, i.e. in the common boundary zones between the territories of the anterior, middle and posterior cerebral arteries. The lesions are usually asymmetrical (**4.76**), and may be unilateral. In the cerebellum, the boundary zones between the territories of the superior and posterior inferior cerebellar arteries lie just below the dorsal angle of each hemisphere (**4.77**).

BRAIN DAMAGE DUE TO CARBON MONOXIDE FOISONING

Carbon monoxide may give rise to structural brain damage because its affinity for haemoglobin is about 250 times that for oxygen. If the blood level of

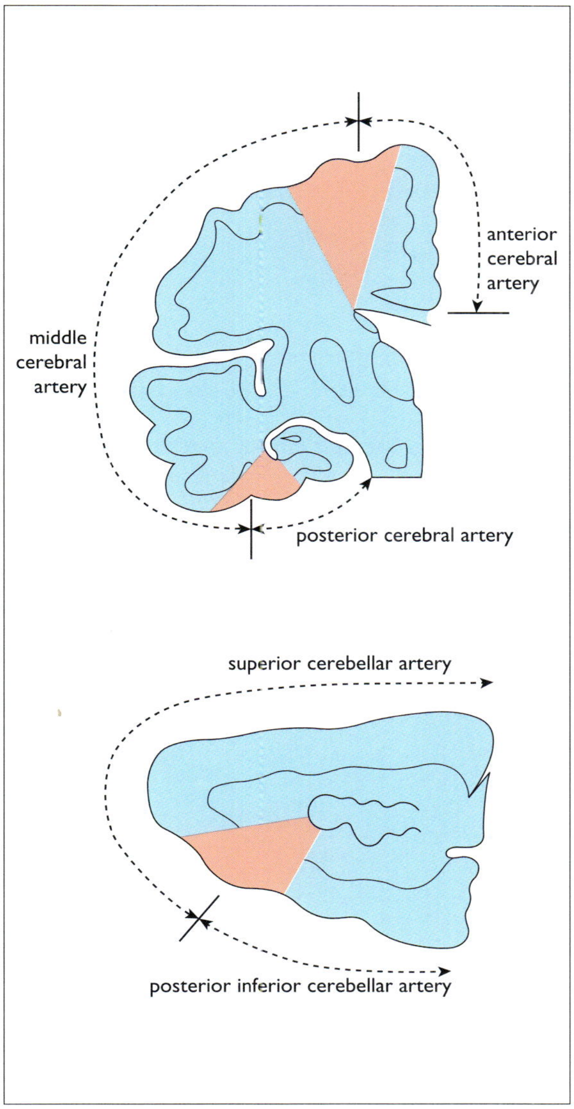

4.75 Arterial boundary zones in cerebral and cerebellar hemispheres. Each boundary zone is coloured red.

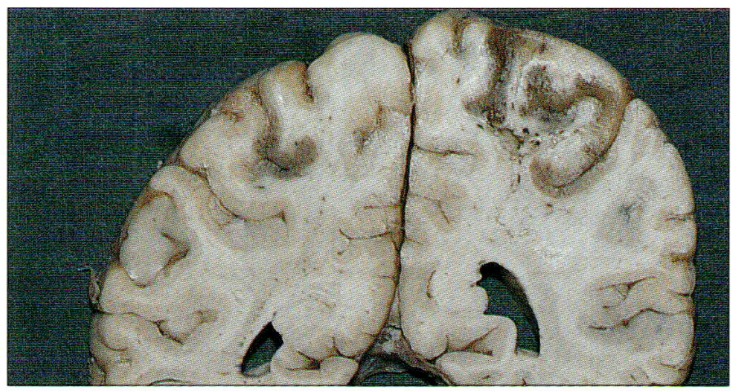

4.76 Infarction in arterial boundary zones: five days' survival. There is focally haemorrhagic infarction in the sides and depths of each parieto-occipital sulcus, i.e. in the boundary zones between the distributions of the anterior and middle cerebral arteries.

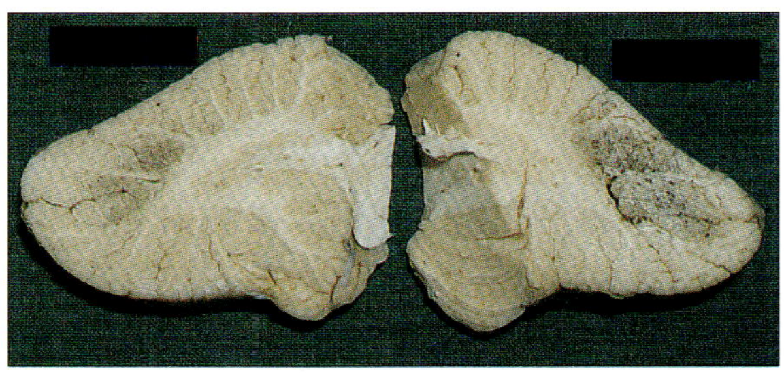

4.77 Infarction in arterial boundary zones: five days' survival. There is focally haemorrhagic infarction in the cortex of each cerebellar hemisphere just above the dorsal angles, i.e in the arterial boundary zones between the superior cerebellar and posterior inferior cerebral arteries.

carboxyhaemoglobin rises to about 60–70%, consciousness is lost, while above 70% concentration, death is rapid. Although there is a particular predilection for selectively severe structural damage in the globus pallidus, there is also widespread neuronal necrosis in other vulnerable areas, such as the hippocampi and the cerebellar cortex. In some cases of carbon monoxide poisoning, abnormalities are more conspicuous in white matter than in grey matter.

BRAIN DAMAGE DUE TO EPILEPSY

It is useful to distinguish between primary or idiopathic epilepsy for which there is no obvious cause, and secondary or symptomatic epilepsy for which the underlying cause of the seizures may vary, e.g. trauma, tumour or an infection. Discrete seizures are unlikely to produce irreversible brain damage, whereas status epilepticus has long been recognised as a serious danger to life at any age, particularly during childhood. The basic neuropathological changes are widespread necrosis of the cortex, hippocampus, basal ganglia, thalamus, cerebellum, and parts of the brainstem. In long-term survivors, damage may be limited to unilateral sclerosis of Ammon's horn.

HYPOGLYCAEMIC BRAIN DAMAGE

The respiratory quotient (CO_2/O_2) of the brain is almost one, indicating that the oxidation of glucose is the principal source of energy. Structural brain damage is unlikely unless there is a prolonged fall in the level of glucose below 1.1mmol/l, as in patients who die after insulin shock therapy, diabetic patients treated with insulin, and in infants with idiopathic hypoglycaemia. The pattern of damage is similar to that found in other categories of hypoxia, except that unlike in other types, there is preservation of Purkinje cells.

FURTHER READING

Allen CMC, Harrison, MJE., Wade, DT. *The Management Of Acute Stroke*. Colchester, Castle House Publications, 1988.

Barnett HJM, Mohr JP, Stein BM, Yatsu F (eds). *Stroke: Pathophysiology, Diagnosis and Management*, Vols 1 and 2. Edinburgh, Churchill–Livingstone, 1986.

Graham DI. Vascular Disease and Hypoxic Brain Damage. In: Weller RO (ed). *Systemic Pathology*. 3rd edn.Vol. 4. Edinburgh, Churchill–Livingstone, 1990, pp 89–124.

Hachinski VC, Norris JW. *The Acute Stroke*. Philadelphia, FA Davis, 1985.

Stroke Octet. *The Lancet*, 1992.

5. Trauma

Either as a cause of death or of persisting disability, trauma remains a major health problem facing society. Thus, in the UK, trauma is responsible for more deaths in all age groups under 45 than any other single cause, and head injury is the single most important factor in death due to trauma. In the UK, with a population of about 55 million, there are about 10 deaths from head injury per 100,000 of the population, between 200 and 300 people per 100,000 are admitted to hospital because of head injury, and probably about 1500 others per 100,000 report to Accident and Emergency departments. Furthermore, morbidity is high: some 10% of severe head injuries remaining vegetative or severely disabled six months after injury and only some 22% make a good recovery. Spinal injury is a smaller problem: published reports suggest that in the UK some 1.3–2.7 patients per 100,000 of the population sustain severe paralysis as a result of such an injury, and that in some 50% of patients hospitalized for paraplegia or quadriplegia trauma has been the cause. In non-military practice about 45% of all new cases of spinal injury result from road accidents, 30% are due to falls and the remainder are due to sporting injuries and occasionally to gunshot wounds.

Classification and frequency of principal types of lesions in fatal non-missile head injury

Primary damage	
Fracture of the skull	75%
Surface contusions and lacerations	95%
Diffuse axonal injury (DAI) as diagnosed by silver impregnation	30%
Secondary damage	
Intracranial haematoma	60%
Brain swelling	53%
Ischaemic brain damage	55%
Infection	4%
Due to raised intracranial pressure	75%

5.1 Classification and frequency of principal types of lesions.

TRAUMA TO THE HEAD

These are of two types: non-missile and missile. The mechanisms of brain damage are different in the two types. In non-missile head injury there is sudden acceleration/deceleration of the head, as a result of which the brain moves within the cranial cavity causing it to come in contact with bony protuberances within the skull resulting in contusions and lacerations and engendering various shear strains within the brain. These strains are particularly severe when there is a rotational element, and lead to subdural haematoma and diffuse axonal injury (DAI). In missile injuries brain damage is inflicted by various types of objects which fall, or are propelled, through the air.

BRAIN DAMAGE DUE TO NON-MISSILE HEAD INJURY

This is by far the most common type encountered in civilian practice and is most frequently due to road traffic accidents, falls, and assaults. The principal types of damage to the skull and brain and their frequency are shown in **5.1**. In the account that follows brain damage is classified as primary and secondary with the aim of helping pathologists reconstruct the sequence of events leading to the fatal outcome. Such clinicopathological classification helps to identify preventable complications in patients with a head injury who 'talk and die' or 'deteriorate and die'.

Primary damage

Principal amongst types of primary damage are: lesions of the scalp, fractures of the skull, surface contusions and DAI.

Lesions of the scalp

The scalp may be lacerated or bruised and such injuries may bleed profusely: they may also be a potential route for later infection.

Fracture of the skull

Most fractures are fissure fractures (**5.2**) and they often extend into the base of the skull. The more localised fracture is often depressed: such a fracture is said to be compound if there is an associated laceration of the scalp. Fractures of the base of the skull may pass through the middle ear or the anterior cranial fossa producing CSF otorrhoea or rhinorrhea, and they are potential sources for later infection. Patients with a fracture of the skull have a much higher incidence of intracranial haematoma than patients who do not have a fracture. Occasionally, there may be fractures in the roofs of the orbits in association with a fall on the occiput: these are referred to as contrecoup fractures. Growing fractures occur in infancy when brain tissue or meninges protrude through the fracture, preventing it from healing.

Surface contusions and lacerations

These are the hallmark of brain damage due to a head injury (**5.3**). They vary in amount and may extend into subcortical white matter: they are usually asymmetrical. Most contusions are found over the lateral surfaces of the hemispheres (**5.4, 5.5**), on the undersurfaces of the frontal and temporal lobes (**5.6**), in the cortex above and below the Sylvian fissures

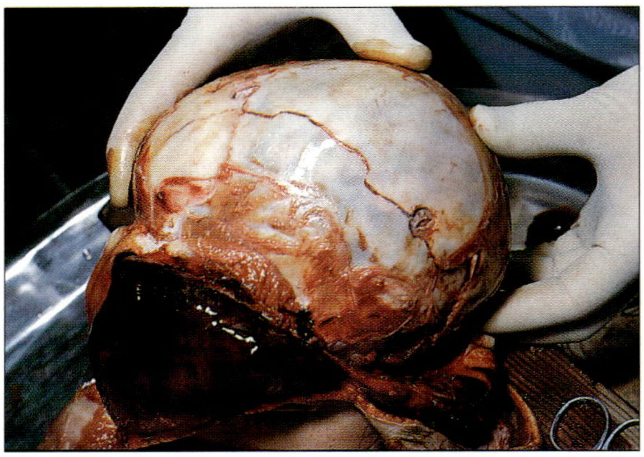

5.2 Fissure fracture of skull (44-hour survival). There is a linear fracture of the vault that extends from the occiput, across the coronal suture, to the frontal region. Note the extensive bleeding into the deeper layers of the scalp overlying the fracture.

Surface contusions and lacerations

Pia-arachnoid intact with contusions, but torn with lacerations

Affect crests of gyri

At vertex related to fractures, and inferiorly correspond to irregular bony contours of base of skull

Healed contusions are found incidentally in 4% of adult autopsies *post mortem*

5.3 Surface contusions and lacerations.

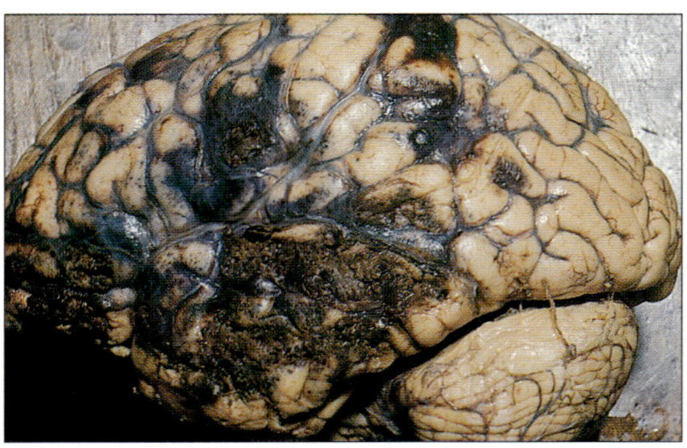

5.4 Surface contusions (eight day survival). There are extensive haemorrhagic defects over the lateral aspects of the temporal lobe and to a lesser extent those of the frontal and parietal lobes.

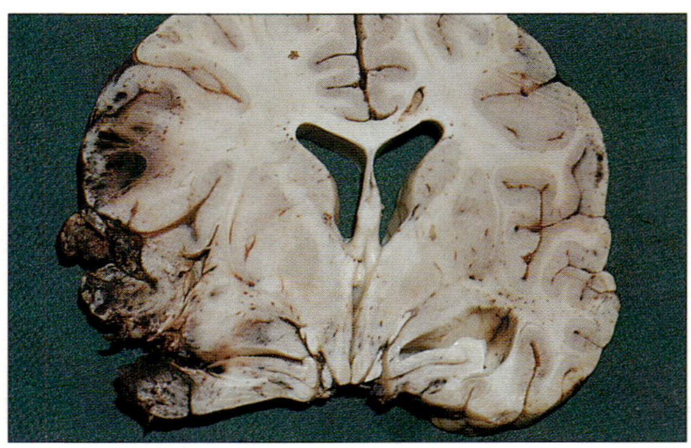

5.5 Surface contusions and lacerations. Coronal section to show extent and depth of haemorrhagic defects over lateral aspect of temporal and frontal lobes.

(**5.7**), and less commonly on the undersurface of the cerebellar hemispheres.

With the passage of time, the contusions come to be represented as brownish shrunken scars which are characteristic in appearance and distribution (**5.8**). Various names have been applied to surface contusions (**5.9**); contrecoup contusions are considered to be more severe than coup contusions. This is not always so: frontal injury is rarely associated with occipital contusions although occipital contusions are usually associated with severe contusions of the orbital surfaces of the frontal lobes.

Contusions of the types described earlier occur at all ages apart from infancy: non-missile head injury in this age group produces tears at the junction between the cortex and the white matter, particularly in the frontal and the temporal lobes.

Diffuse axonal injury (DAI)

This is one of the most important types of brain damage resulting from a non-missile head injury. It occurs at the moment of injury and is the commonest cause of coma in the absence of an intracranial haematoma. Using classical silver impregnation

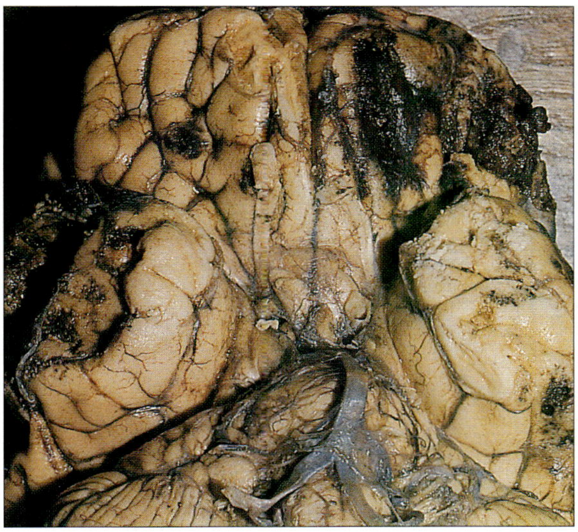

5.6 Surface contusions (eight day survival – same case as **5.4**). Asymmetrical haemorrhagic defects are present on the under aspects of the frontal and temporal lobes.

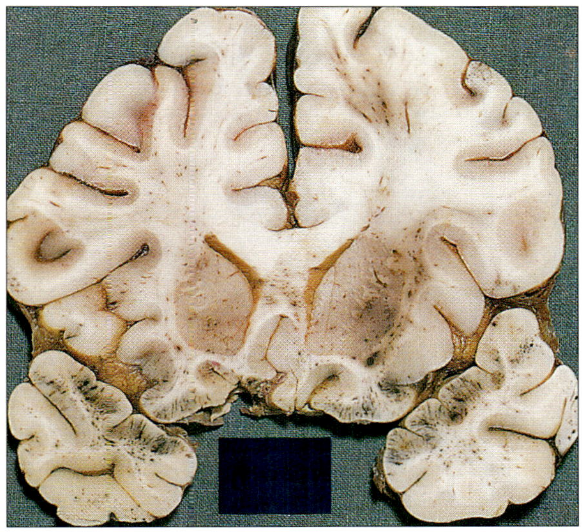

5.7 Surface contusions (4-hour survival). Haemorrhagic defects are seen in relation to the operculum of each Sylvian fissure.

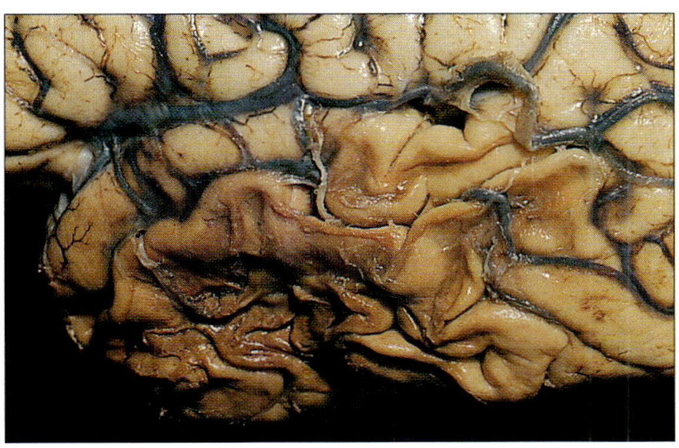

Fig. 5.8 Surface contusions (old). There are orange-brown defects on the lateral aspect of the temporal lobe.

Various types of surface contusions and lacerations

Coup (at point of impact)

Contrecoup (diametrically opposite point of impact)

Herniation (at point of impact between hernia – tentorial, cingulate and free edge of tentorium or the falx, respectively)

Fracture (related to fracture of skull)

5.9 Various types of surface contusions and lacerations.

techniques, DAI as shown by the presence of axonal bulbs is present in some 30% of fatal head injuries. However, immunohistochemistry using an antibody to β-amyloid precursor protein has suggested that axonal injury may be much more common after head injury than has been appreciated previously. Also it seems likely that milder degrees of this type of brain damage are responsible for concussion and less severe degrees of permanent disability. It is the commonest cause of the vegetative state after head injury.

In DAI there is widespread disruption of axons attributable to shear and tensile strains affecting axons at the time of an acceleration/deceleration injury. In these patients there is a remarkably uniform pattern of brain damage (**5.10**). In patients surviving for only a few days the lesions are usually haemorrhagic and often apparent macroscopically. They consist of discrete lesions in the corpus callosum (**5.11**) and in the dorsolateral quadrant(s) of the rostral brainstem (**5.12**). Gliding contusions refer to haemorrhage into the parasagittal white matter (**5.11**): they are often bilateral. Histological evidence of diffuse axonal damage depends on the length of survival after injury: if this is short (days)

Diffuse axonal injury (DAI): frequency of principal macroscopic lesions and their anatomical distribution

Site	Frequency
Rostral upper brainstem	95%
Corpus callosum	92%
Parasagittal (gliding contusions)	88%
Hippocampal formation	88%
Interventricular septum	80%
Thalamus	56%
Caudate nucleus and putamen	17%

5.10 Diffuse axonal injury – sites of lesions.

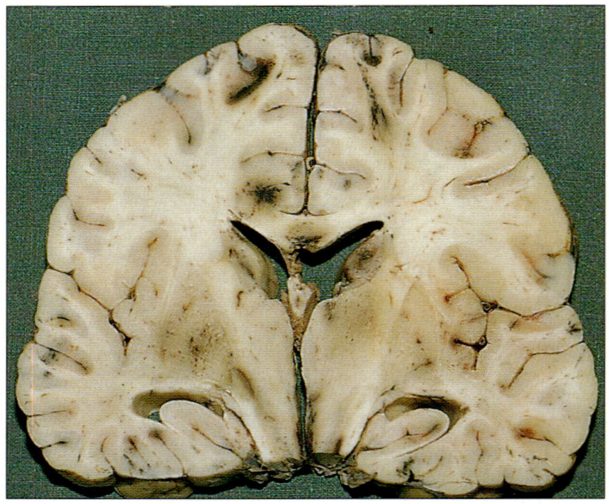

5.11 DAI (six day survival). Coronal slice that shows haemorrhagic lesions concentrated in midline structures viz. corpus callosum, interventricular septum, parasagittal white matter and basal ganglia. Note absence of surface contusions.

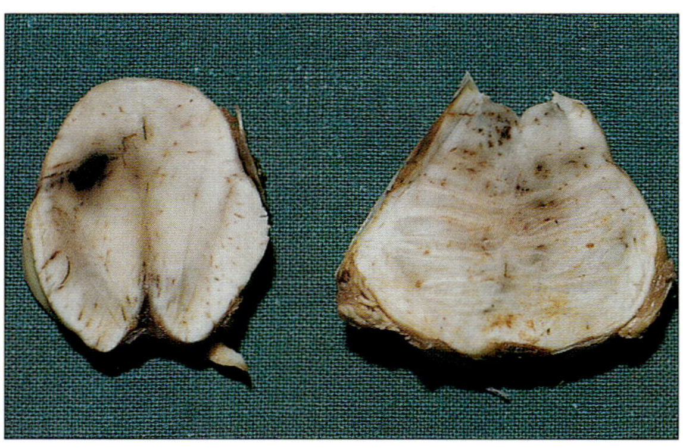

5.12 DAI (32-hour survival). Upper brain stem to show concentration of haemorrhagic lesions in dorso-lateral quadrants of rostral midbrain and pons. Compare with centrally placed haemorrhages (Duret) that are normally a feature of vascular damage secondary to raised intracranial pressure (*see Chapter 2*).

there are numerous axonal bulbs throughout the brain, particularly in the parasagittal white matter of the cerebral hemispheres, and in midline structures that include the corpus callosum, the midbrain and rostral pons (**5.13, 5.14**). If the patient survives some weeks, a striking histological finding is the presence of multiple clusters of microglia throughout the white matter of the brain (**5.15**). If the patient survives for two to three months there is established Wallerian degeneration in the white matter in the cerebral hemispheres, cerebellum, ascending and descending tracts of the brainstem (**5.16**) and the descending tracts of the spinal cord.

In patients who have survived for months or years, external abnormalities post mortem may be limited to small healed surface contusions.

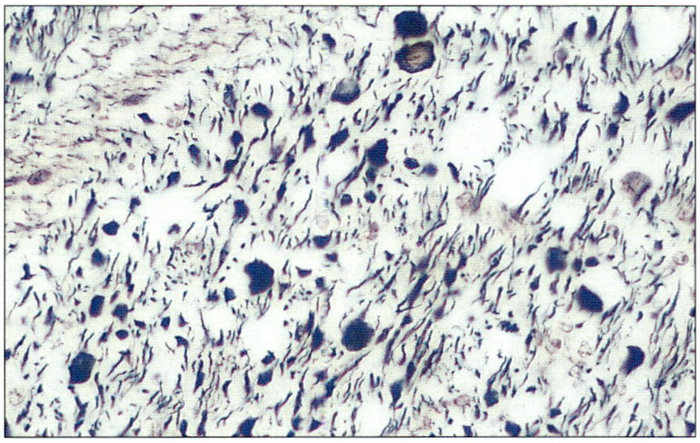

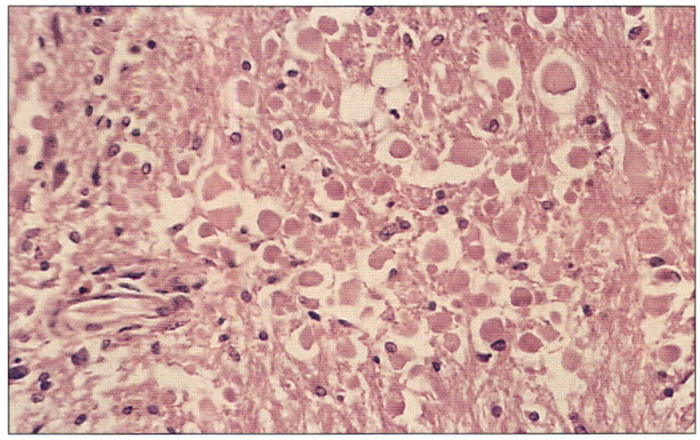

5.13, 5.14 DAI (ten day survival). Superior cerebellar peduncle to show many axonal bulbs stained by (**5.13**, left – silver impregnation (Palmgren), and (**5.14**, right) H & E.

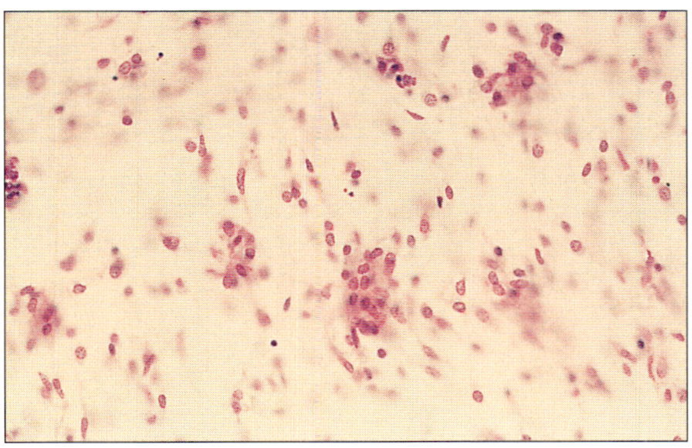

5.15 DAI (six week survival). There are multiple clusters of microglia throughout the white matter. (Cresyl violet)

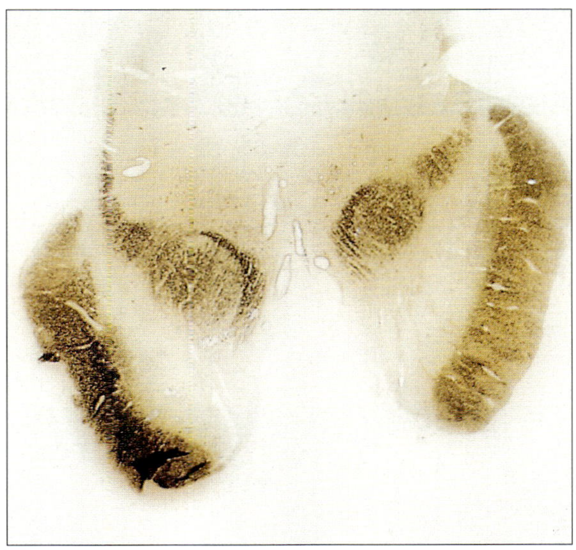

5.16 DAI (21-month survival). There is both ascending (medial lemnisci) and descending (cerebral peduncles) long tract degeneration in a patient who was vegetative from the time of injury until death. The appearances are similar to those described by Dr S. Strich as diffuse degeneration of white matter. (Marchi)

In coronal sections the ventricles are enlarged (**5.17**) because of a reduction in the white matter, and there are characteristically small shrunken lesions in the corpus callosum (**5.18**) in one or both superior cerebellar peduncles (**5.19**). Three grades of DAI are recognized (**5.20**). There is a good correlation between these grades and the patient's clinical state; patients with grade 3 DAI always remain unconscious or in a vegetative state until death.

Other types of primary damage

In patients who die within minutes of a head injury, there are often multiple petechial haemorrhages throughout the cerebral hemispheres, particularly the white matter of the frontal and temporal lobes (**5.21**), and in the brainstem (**5.22**): this is known as diffuse vascular injury. Occasionally there is a tear at the pontomedullary junction (**5.23**). Other structures may be torn at the time of injury, such as cranial nerves; the cavernous part of the internal carotid artery, leading to a caroticocavernous fistula; and the pituitary stalk, leading to infarction of the anterior lobe of the pituitary gland due to disruption of the long portal hypothalamohypophyseal blood vessels. Blows to the upper part of the neck just below the ear may cause rupture of a vertebral artery: this is usually rapidly fatal and the principal finding at autopsy is massive traumatic subarachnoid haemorrhage within the posterior fossa. Injuries to the neck may also cause dissection (see **4.40**) of the internal carotid artery, and subsequent thrombosis leading to cerebral infarction.

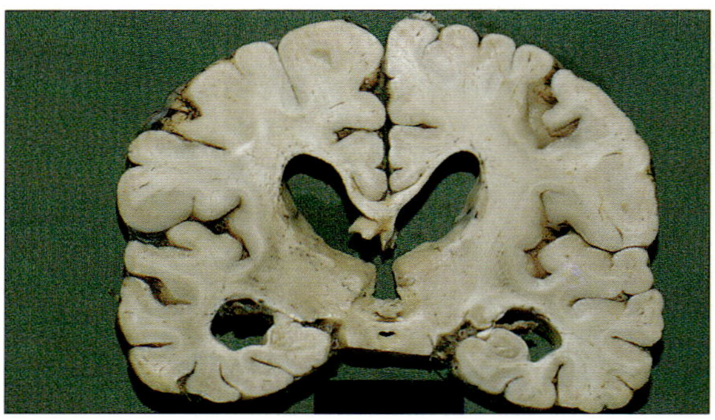

5.17 DAI (17-month survival). Coronal slice showing symmetrical enlargement of the ventricles, thinning of the corpus callosum and a reduction in the bulk of the centrum semiovale, absence of surface contusions and near-normal thickness of the cortex. Patient in vegetative state.

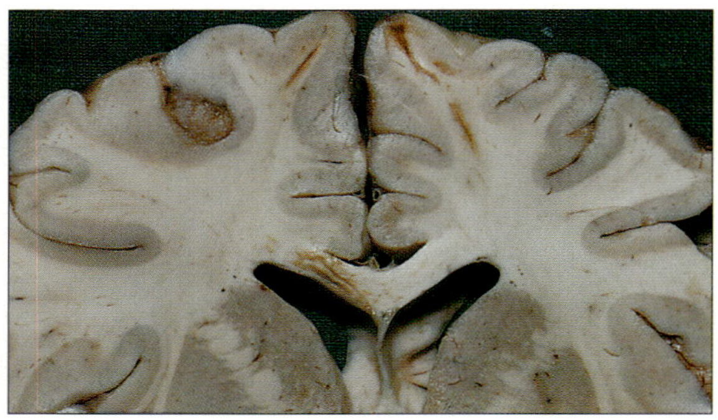

5.18 DAI (three-month survival). Coronal slice showing orange-brown lesion in (a) corpus callosum to one side of midline, and (b) parasagittal white matter (gliding contusion). Patient in vegetative state.

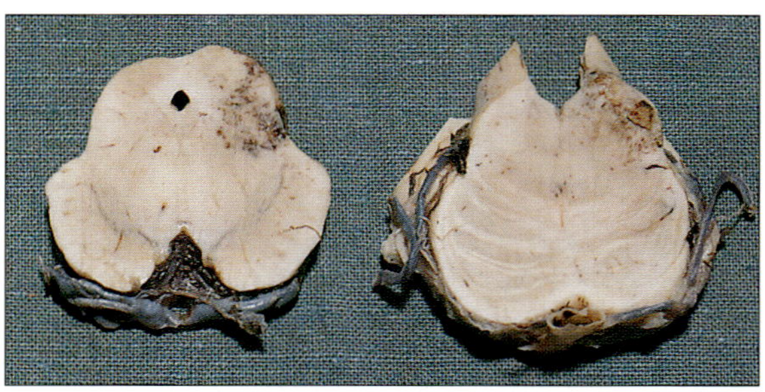

5.19 DAI (12-day survival). Upper brain stem showing orange-brown lesions in dorsolateral quadrant of midbrain and upper pons.

Diffuse axonal injury (DAI): grading

1. Scattered axonal bulbs throughout white matter
2. Also a focal lesion (usually haemorrhagic) in the corpus callosum
3. In addition there is a lesion in the rostral brainstem

5.20 Diffuse axonal injury – grading.

Secondary damage

The main types are: intracranial haematoma; brain swelling; ischaemic brain damage; infection, and brain damage secondary to raised intracranial pressure.

Intracranial haematoma

This is a frequent complication (about 66%) of a non-missile head injury and is the most common cause of deterioration and death in patients who have experienced a lucid interval after their injury; most are evacuated surgically. The incidence of haematoma is much higher in patients with a fracture of the skull than in those who do not have a fracture. The increasing use of CT scanning has established that the haematoma may be present very soon after the injury and before it produces clinical deterioration. However, serial scans have also shown that some haematomas do not develop until two or three days after the injury: these are referred to as delayed haematomas.

There are several types of traumatic intracranial haematoma (**5.24**).

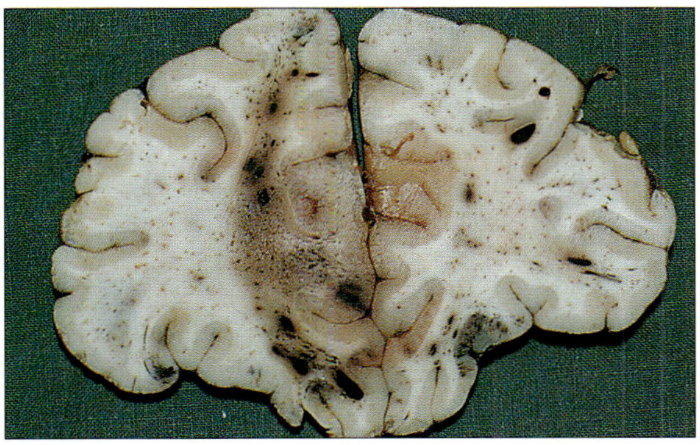

5.21 Diffuse vascular injury (10-minute survival). Coronal section showing multiple small haemorrhages in white matter of each frontal lobe. Note relative absence of surface contusions.

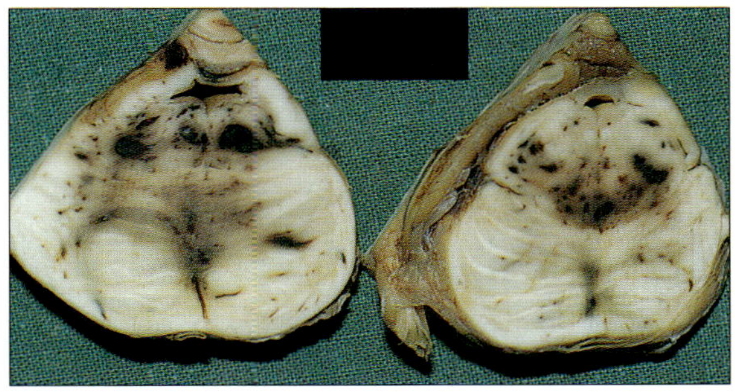

5.22 Diffuse vascular injury (10-minute survival). There are multiple haemorrhages throughout the pons.

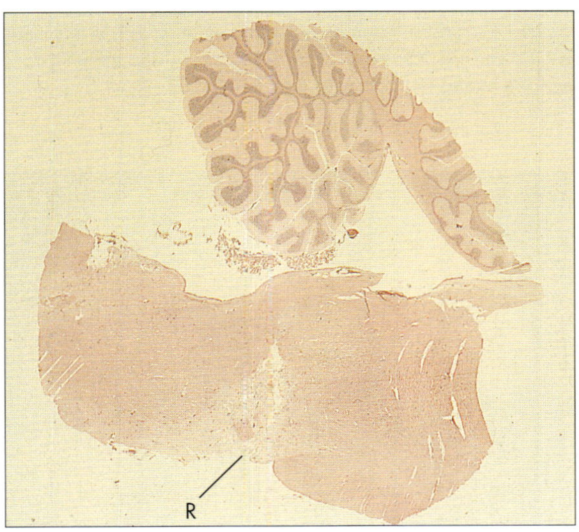

5.23 Pontomedullary rent (22-day survival). In severe cases there is avulsion and death is immediate. In other cases the patient survives with a wedge-shaped rent in the brainstem at the junction between the pons and medulla (R).

Intracranial haematoma is a complication of 66% of cases of non-missile head injury

Extradural	10%
Intradural	**56%**
Subdural	13%
Subarachnoid	3%
Discrete intracerebral or intracerebellar haematomas not in continuity with the surface of the brain	15%
'Burst lobe': an intracranial or intracerebellar haematoma in continuity with a related subdural haematoma	25%

5.24 Large intracranial haematomas in fatal head injury

Extradural haematoma is present in about 10% of fatal cases. It is usually a complication of a fracture in the temporoparietal region that involves the middle meningeal artery; it may also develop in other sites and may be bilateral. In children the haematoma may develop in the absence of a skull fracture. As it strips the dura from the skull it forms a large ovoid circumscribed mass that indents the adjacent brain (**5.25**). Often there is only a small amount of underlying brain damage. If untreated, there is midline shift leading to the formation of internal herniae and compression of the midbrain. Associated brain damage is often minimal (**5.26**).

Intradural haematoma is subdivided into subdural haematoma, intracerebral and intracerebellar haematoma, and a 'burst' lobe. Subdural haemorrhage is present in about 13% of fatal cases; it tends to spread diffusely over the cerebral hemispheres: thin bilateral haematomas are common. Usually, they are unilateral and large enough to act as expanding lesions (**5.27**) and they are associated with contusions of the underlying brain which may be sufficiently extensive to constitute a 'burst' lobe (**5.28**). As the haematoma expands there is progressive shift of the midline structures, internal herniae and compression of the brainstem. Diffuse swelling of the underlying hemisphere is common and not infrequently when the haematoma is evacuated there is little or no reduction in the midline shift. Subdural haematomas are attributed to rupture of bridging veins.

Subdural haematomas are usually defined as acute, subacute or chronic (**5.29**). Chronic subdural haem-

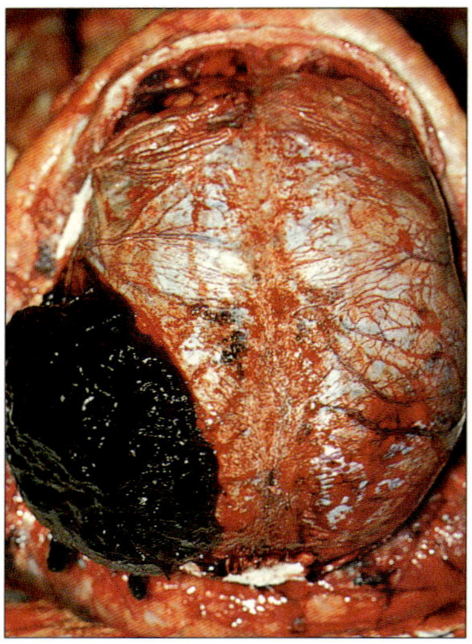

5.25 Extradural haematoma (24-hour survival). There is an ovoid circumscribed mass of blood clot external to the dura.

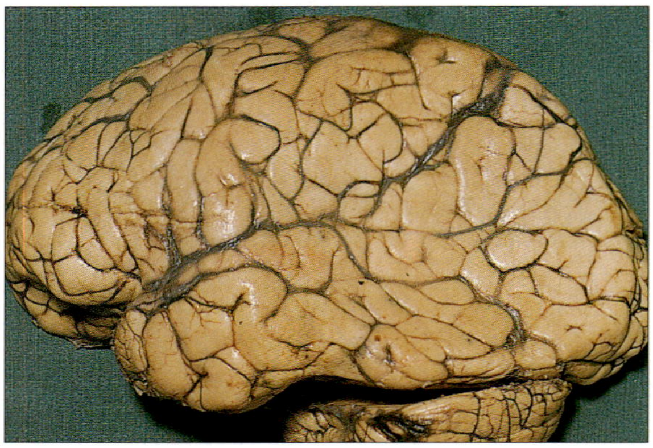

5.26 Extradural haematoma (24-hour survival). Same case as shown in **5.25**. Note distortion of brain and minimal surface contusion (compare with **5.28**).

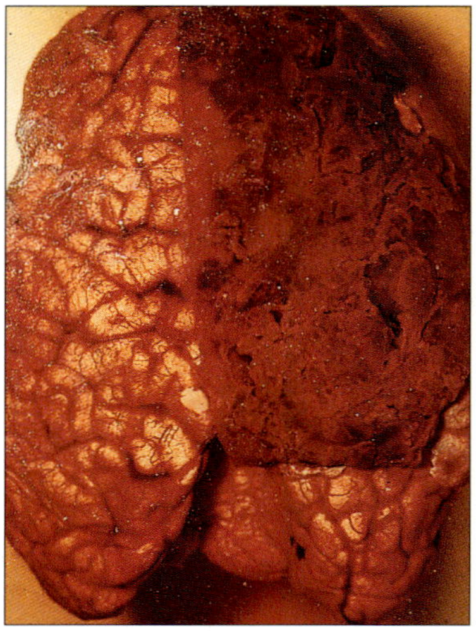

5.27 Acute subdural haematoma (three day survival). There is a large recently formed blood clot in the subdural space overlying one cerebral hemisphere.

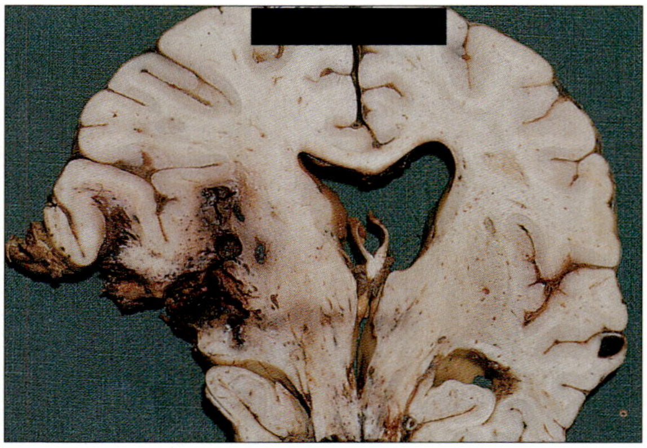

5.28 'Burst' temporal lobe (24-hour survival). The haematoma in the temporal lobe was in continuity with an overlying acutely formed subdural haematoma.

atoma presents weeks or months after what may have appeared to have been a trivial head injury. The precise aetiology is not clear but there is an association with long-term anticoagulant therapy, and patients with coagulation defects such as haemophilia. The haematoma increases in size slowly, probably as a result of repeated small haemorrhages. Eventually, it becomes large enough to produce the effects of raised intracranial pressure (**5.30**).

Subdural haematoma is found in a proportion of victims of child abuse (*see Chapter 9*) in the battered baby syndrome. Diagnosis is confirmed by needling the fontanelle, which yields yellow fluid with a high protein content (subdural hygroma).

Intracerebral or intracerebellar haematoma is present in some 15% of fatal cases. It may be single or multiple and is usually related to surface contusions of the brain, and occurs principally in the sub-frontal (**5.31**) and temporal regions, or less commonly in the cerebellum (**5.32**) Some deeply seated haematomas are not related to contusions: these are often referred to as basal ganglia haematomas and are usually indicative of a severe head injury. They are often found in association with DAI.

A 'burst' lobe is a combination of an intracerebral (or intracerebellar) haematoma in continuity through contusions with a subdural haematoma, and is present in some 25% of fatal cases. If a solitary haematoma is found in the brain of a patient who has had a head injury, the possibility that it is due to hypertension or to a ruptured saccular aneurysm, and hence precipitating the injury, has to be borne in mind.

Subdural haematoma: classification

48–72 hours	Acute: composed of clotted blood
3–20 days	Subacute: mixture of clotted and fluid blood
3 weeks plus	Chronic: encapsulated haematoma is fluid

5.29 Subdural haematoma.

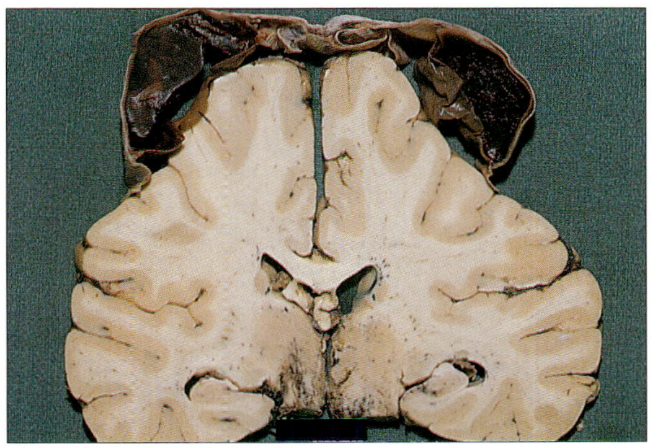

5.30 Bilateral chronic subdural haematomas (three month survival). There is symmetrical distortion of both cerebral hemispheres by masses of encapsulated haematoma lying in the subdural space. Haemorrhagic infarction of the thalami and upper brain are secondary to raised intracranial pressure.

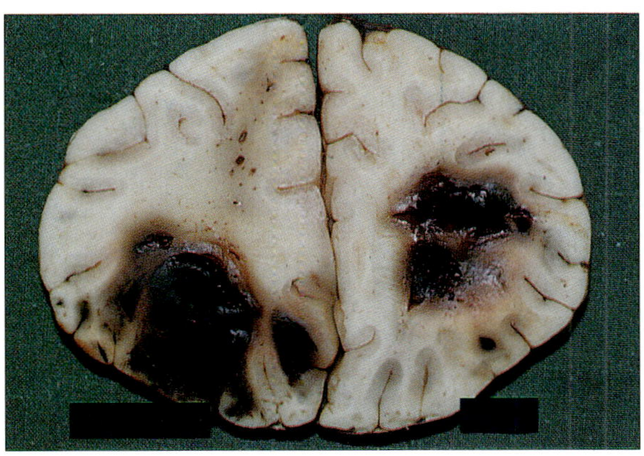

5.31 Intracerebral haematomas (15-hour survival). There are bilateral frontal haematomas.

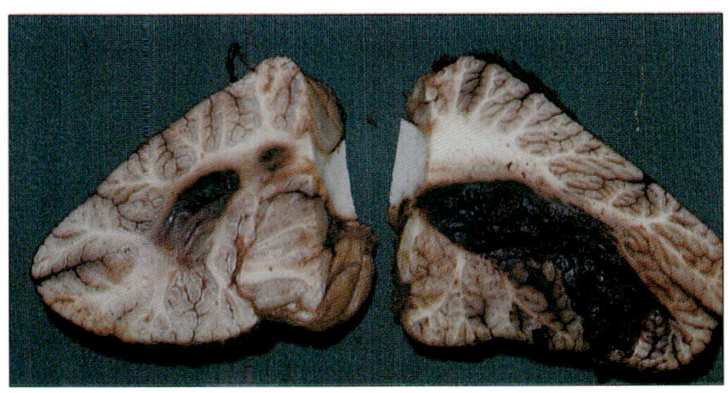

5.32 Intracerebellar haematomas (15-hour survival). There are bilateral haematomas.

Brain swelling
Swelling due to vasogenic oedema is found frequently adjacent to contusions (**5.33**), and around haematomas. Diffuse swelling of the entire cerebral hemisphere occurs in about 33% of patients with an acute traumatic intracranial haematoma, but is particularly common in an acute subdural haematoma (**5.34**). Diffuse swelling of both hemispheres occurs in young children (**5.35**), and the original injury may have been apparently trivial or severe.

Ischaemic brain damage
Much of this occurs adjacent to contusions and haematomas or is secondary to raised intracranial pressure, shift and distortion of the brainstem. Although some of this damage may be identifiable to the naked eye, much can only be identified microscopically. It is found most often in the hippocampus (81%) and in the basal ganglia (79%); within the cortex the damage may be diffuse, in arterial boundary zones or lie within arterial territories (**5.36, 5.37**). The pathogenesis of ischaemic damage resulting from a head injury is not yet established: available evidence suggests that it occurs soon after injury, and is present in some 90% of patients who die as a result of a non-missile head injury. Singly or in combination there are many factors that contribute to ischaemic brain damage (**5.38**). Extensive ischaemic brain damage may be a cause of both severe disability and the vegetative state. If an infarct is found in the brain of a patient who has suffered a head injury the possibility of it being primary, and hence precipitating injury, has to be considered.

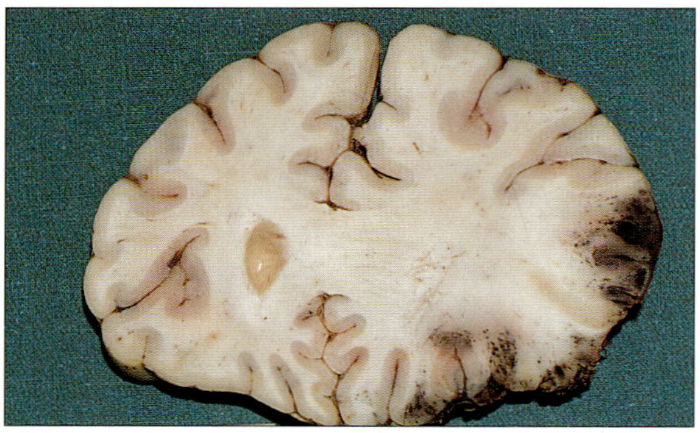

5.33 Swelling in relation to contusions (five day survival). The swelling is ipsilateral to the surface contusions.

Infection
Meningitis is a well recognized complication after head injury, and is invariably associated with a fracture of the base of the skull. If there is also a tear of the dura the latter may be associated with CSF rhinorrhoea or otorrhoea. Subdural or intracerebral abscesses are uncommon complications of non-missile head injuries but are not uncommon after penetrating injuries.

Brain damage secondary to raised intracranial pressure
Brain damage, usually haemorrhage or infarction in the brainstem, secondary to a high intracranial pressure and shift and herniation of the brain, is the most common important factor contributing to death.

Other abnormalities
The possibility of massive cerebral fat embolism should always be considered in patients with fractures of the long bones.

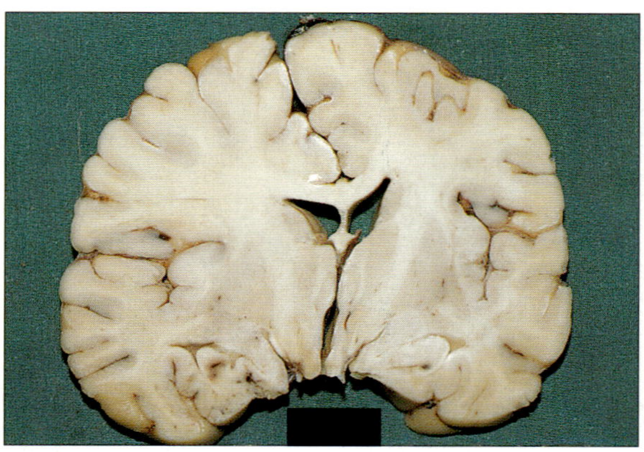

5.34 Swelling (36-hour survival). Swelling on same side as an acute subdural haematoma had been evacuated.

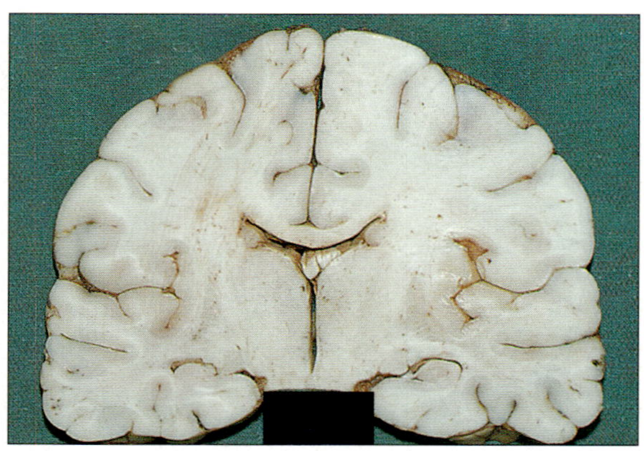

5.35 Bilateral swelling (18-hour survival). There is diffuse swelling of both cerebral hemispheres and symmetrical reduction in size of ventricles in a 16-year-old who died from raised intracranial pressure. Note absence of other traumatic pathologies.

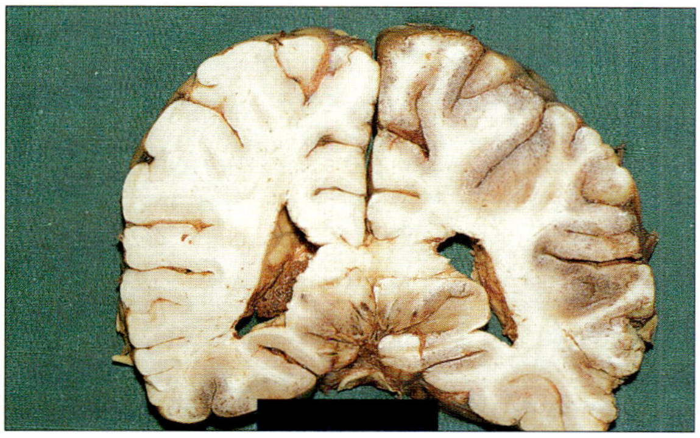

5.36 Ischaemic brain damage (32-hour survival). There is recent infarction in distributions of one middle and both posterior cerebral arteries following surgical evacuation of an acute subdural haematoma.

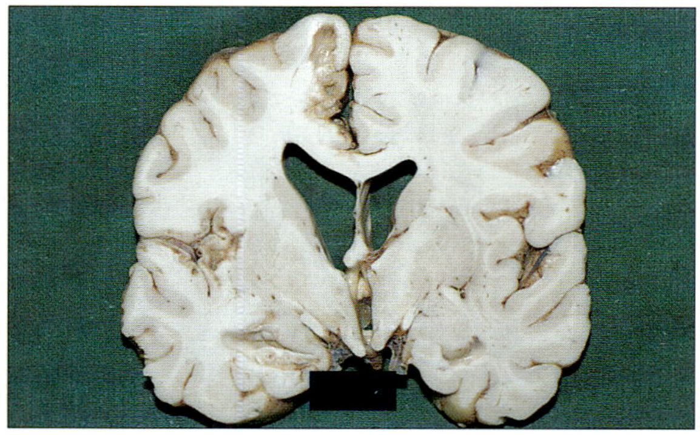

5.37 Ischaemic brain damage (28-day survival). There is subtotal infarction in distribution of one anterior and middle cerebral artery. Note absence of raised intracranial pressure and asymmetry of ventricular system due to loss of tissue in the distribution of the internal carotid artery.

LATE COMPLICATIONS

In adults, early onset post-traumatic epilepsy is unusual except in association with prolonged post-traumatic amnesia, depressed fracture of the skull or intracranial haematoma. In contrast, it is more common in children even after trivial injuries. Late onset epilepsy complicates some 40% of missile head injuries compared with 5% of non-missile head injuries.

There are many causes of residual neurological deficit after head injury, many of which result in asymmetrical enlargement of the ventricular system – hydrocephalus *ex vacuo*. In other cases there is symmetrical enlargement of the entire ventricular system due to obstruction at the exit foramina of the fourth ventricle: this may be due to haemosiderosis of the meninges.

There is a group of patients who make a reasonably good recovery from a head injury but who subsequently develop a progressive neurological illness with the features of organic dementia. Thus, examples of Alzheimer's disease and Pick's disease have been reported. Many of these cannot be substantiated but occasionally the temporal relationship between the head injury and the appearance of a progressive organic dementia is such that it is difficult to believe that they are purely coincidental.

It is now generally accepted there is an organic basis for dementia pugilistica – 'punch drunk' syndrome – since a recurring pattern of damage has been found in the brains of ex-boxers (**5.39**). Features include a large and fenestrated septal cavum, scarring of the folia around the groove formed by the sloping edge of the foramen magnum on the undersurface of the cerebellum, degeneration of the substantia nigra, the presence of numerous neurofibrillary tangles and β-amyloid deposits, diffusely through the cerebral cortex.

Ischaemic brain damage: patterns and causes

Diffuse	Cardio-respiratory arrest
Focal	Raised intracranial pressure, shift, distortion and internal herniae
	Vasospasm
	Hypotension
	Embolism
	Penetrating injuries

(Patterns in part determined by congenital and acquired vascular disease; influence of stage of development; blood gases; haematocrit and temperature)

5.38 Ischaemic brain damage.

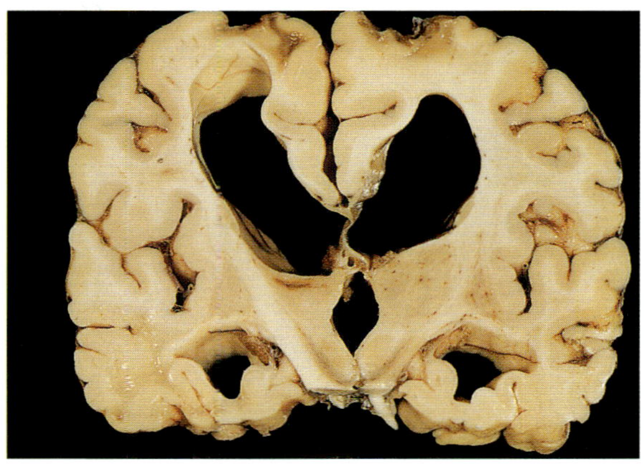

5.39 Dementia pugilistica (many years survival). Ex-professional boxer with ventricular enlargement, thinning of the corpus callosum and interventricular septum, and healed pigmented scars in each parasagittal region and the thalamus. There is also some pallor of the substantia nigra.

MISSILE HEAD INJURY

Typically, there is focal damage to the brain in the form of lacerations, haemorrhage into the region of the brain destroyed by penetration of the object, and varying degrees of associated swelling (**5.40, 5.41**). However, brain damage is not restricted to the region of injuries since multiple contusions may be produced by high-velocity missiles. These are attributed to contact of the surface of the brain against the skull as a result of radial displacement forces from the missile.

HEAD INJURY IN CHILD ABUSE

Intracranial damage with or without a fracture of the skull is the most common cause of death in abused children. Subdural haemorrhage is usual and may result from a blow or fall. Vigorous shaking can also rupture blood vessels in the subdural space to cause a haematoma. Associated brain damage may be of any type and there may be associated injuries to the skeleton, to viscera, and to the eyes, ears and mouth.

MECHANICAL BIRTH INJURY

In 2.5% of all births there is a cephalohaematoma. Fractures of the skull are unusual and are found only in association with prolonged labour and forceps deliveries. Subdural haemorrhage at full term is usually due to either a tear in the falx cerebri or in the tentorium cerebelli during a precipitate or breech delivery. In premature babies bleeding is likely to occur during breech presentation, high forceps delivery or excessive distortion of skull bones during birth. Subarachnoid haemorrhage is common and may be due to rupture of vessels within the subarachnoid space or in the cerebral hemispheres, to direct extension from the ventricles, or to a tear in the falx or the tentorium.

TRAUMA TO THE SPINAL CORD

The lumbar spine is damaged most commonly in crush injuries of the type seen in mining accidents, and the cervical and thoracic spine are injured most commonly in road accidents. Trauma to the spinal cord may be non-missile or missile in type. The mechanisms are various and include a combination of flexion, rotation, extension and compression, and injuries occurring in association with cervical spondylosis or ankylosing spondylitis may cause severe damage to the cord. The spinal canal may be narrowed by fracture dislocation or compressive fractures. Missile injuries are caused by bullets, and the cord may be injured by a stab wound, especially if the knife enters the spinal canal anterolaterally.

The outcome depends on the severity of irreversible damage and the level of injury where there are varying degrees of haemorrhagic necrosis. The affected cord is soft to touch and swollen and there is often a traumatic haematomyelia (**5.42**). This often extends as a fusiform mass for some distance above and below the level of injury, usually in the posterior columns immediately dorsal to the central canal. With survival the dead tissue is removed, and Wallerian degeneration occurs in ascending tracts

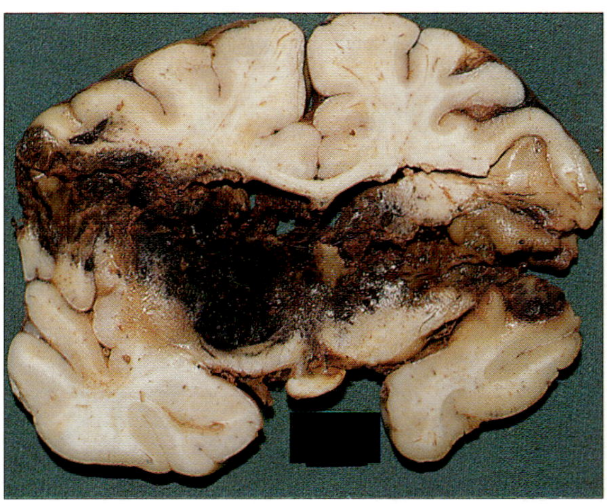

5.40 Missile injury (immediate death). There is an obliquely running haemorrhagic bullet tract through the brain in a patient who died quickly.

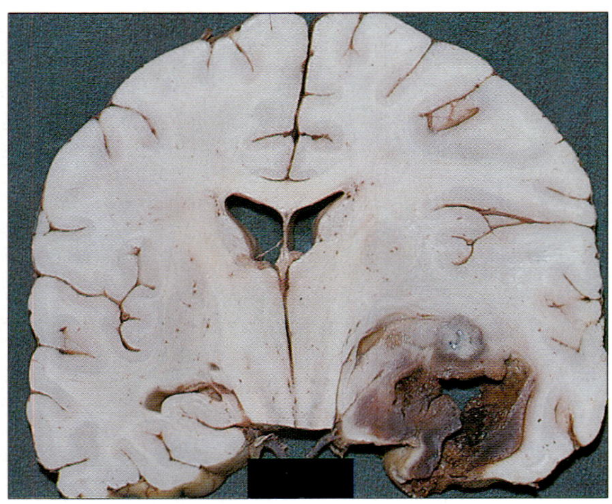

5.41 Missile injury (21-month survival). There is an abscess due to an air gun pellet that had become lodged in the medial part of the temporal lobe. Note associated swelling.

above (**5.43**), and in descending tracts below (**5.44**), the level of injury.

Histological examination of the spinal cord at the level of the injury in longstanding paraplegia often shows regenerative features in the form of proliferating Schwann cells and axons in the region of the posterior nerve roots.

A delayed result of traumatic paraplegia is the development of post-traumatic syringomyelia (**5.45**). This takes the form of a centrally situated cystic cavity which may extend upwards or downwards from the damaged segment (*see Chapter 9*).

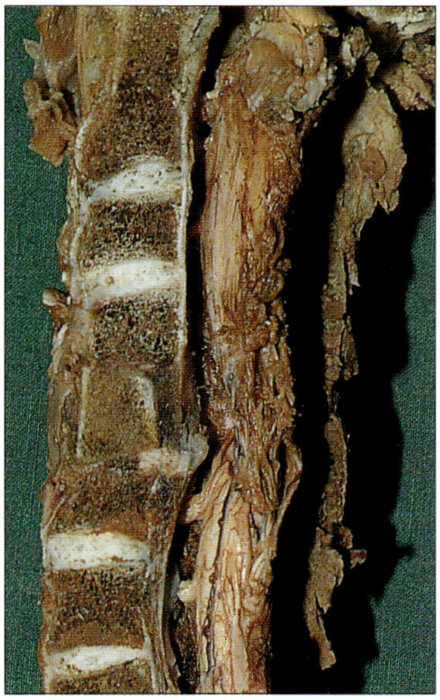

5.42 Fracture/dislocation of spine (eight week survival). There was a crush fracture of vertebral body C5 with compression of the spinal cord in a patient who sustained a fall. Note haemorrhagic discoloration of the spinal cord.

Injury to the spinal cord during forcible breech extraction or mid and high forceps extraction with cephalic delivery may result in damage to the cervical segments of the cord and the spinal nerve roots.

COMPRESSION OF THE SPINAL CORD

The causes of spinal compression are many and varied (**5.46**) and there are different causes in the young, middle-aged and elderly. The clinical effects depend to a considerable extent on the rate of development of the compressive lesion: these may extend over many months, whereas some of the more rapidly expanding lesions can produce paraplegia within days. Tumours that may cause spinal cord compression are discussed in Chapter 10.

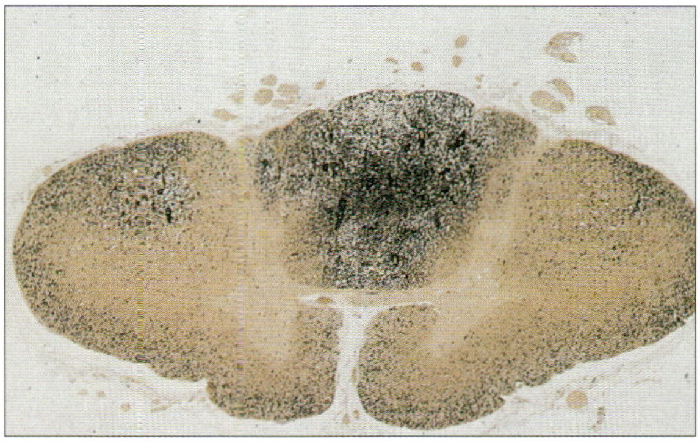

5.43 Ascending degeneration in thoracic cord (several weeks' survival). There is considerable osmophilia (dark area) of the posterior columns and to a lesser extent of the dorsal spinocerebellar tracts. (Marchi preparation)

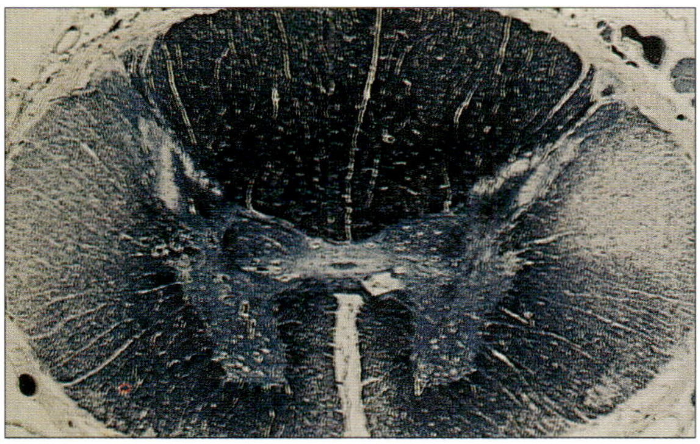

5.44 Descending degeneration in thoracic cord (several weeks' survival). There is pallor of staining in the lateral columns (crossed corticospinal tracts) and to a lesser extent in the anterior columns (uncrossed corticospinal tracts). (Myelin stain)

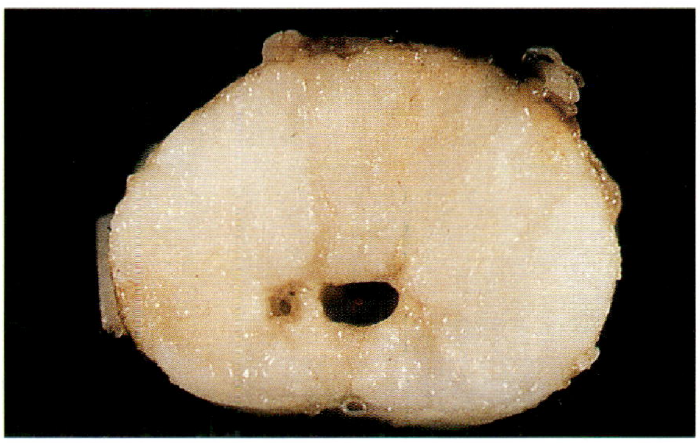

5.45 Post-traumatic syringomyelia (four month survival). There is a cavity close to the central canal at the base of the dorsal columns. There is also a small cavity to one side of the main lesion

Prolapsed intervertebral disc

The central part of an intervertebral disc consists of soft fibrocartilage (the nucleus pulposus) and this is surrounded by a ring of much firmer fibrocartilage (the annulus fibrosus). Most disc protusions occur posteriorly and are secondary to degenerative disease: the most commonly affected are L5/S1 and L4/5.

Cervical spondylosis

This results in degeneration of intervertebral discs in the cervical region. The disc spaces are narrowed and transverse bars develop in the vertebral canal as a result of posterior protrusion of the annulus fibrosus. There is a reactive osteophytosis and thickening of intervertebral ligaments leads to compression of nerve roots and fibrosis of the dural root sleeves. As the spondylosis progresses there may, in addition to compression of nerve roots, be interference with the blood supply to the spinal cord where the vertebral canal is most narrow. When this occurs cervical myelopathy develops and the structural changes in the spinal cord are a combination of focal infarction and subtotal degeneration of the lateral part of the posterior columns secondary to damage to axons in the cervical posterior nerve roots.

SELECTIVE LESIONS IN NEUROSURGERY

As a result of improved drug treatment these procedures have been used less than they were in the past. One of the first techniques to be introduced was prefrontal leucotomy for patients with severe schizophrenia. The original procedure cut most fibres to and from the frontal poles and caused considerable destruction of brain tissue (**5.47**). Thalamotomy or pallidotomy was sometimes undertaken for movement disorders including parkinsonism, while cordotomy is sometimes undertaken in patients with intractable pain.

Principal causes of compression of the spinal cord	
Lesions in vertebral column	Prolapsed intervertebral disc Cervical spondylosis Kyphoscoliosis Fracture dislocation Metastatic tumour
Spinal extradural lesions	Metastatic carcinoma Lymphoma Myeloma Abscess
Intradural extramedullary lesions	Meningioma Schwannoma
Intramedullary lesions	Astrocytoma Ependymoma Cyst formation

5.46 Principal causes of compression of the spinal cord.

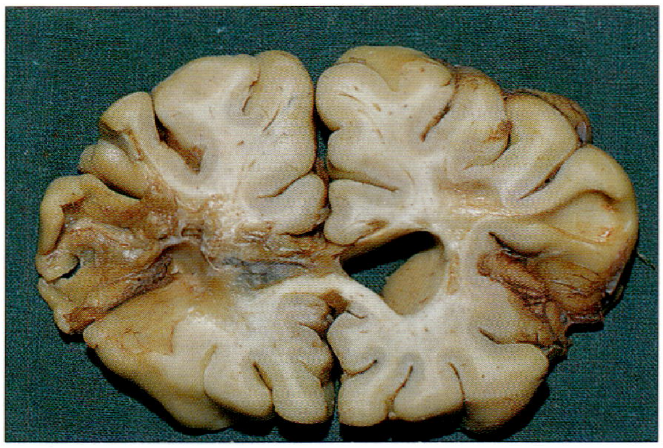

5.47 Prefrontal leucotomy (40-year survival). There is long-standing pigmented destruction of white matter in the frontal lobes.

FURTHER READING

Becker DP and Povlishock JT (eds) Central Nervous System Trauma Status Report 1985. Washington, USA, NINCDS.

Cooper PR (ed) *Head Injury* 3rd ed. Baltimore, Williams & Wilkins, 1993.

Graham DI. Trauma. In Weller RO (ed) *Systemic Pathology*, 3rd ed, vol. 4. Edinburgh, Churchil–Livingstone, 1990, pp125–150.

Jane JA, Anderson DK, Turner JC, Young W (eds) Central Nervous System Trauma Status Report 1991. Washington, USA, NINCDS.

6. Demyelinating Diseases

Demyelination in the CNS is the destruction of the myelin sheath around an intact axon. This may occur as an initial event in conditions such as multiple sclerosis which are considered primary demyelinating diseases. Secondary demyelination is used to describe the demyelination that occurs as part of a wide spectrum of pathological processes in the CNS (**6.1**). Secondary loss of myelin may also be a result of axonal damage, a common process which occurs in a wide variety of diseases, including neurodegenerative disorders and cerebrovascular disease. Staining reactions for myelin and the demonstration of demyelination are discussed in *Chapter 2*.

Myelin in the CNS is formed by oligodendrocyte cell membranes, with each oligodendrocyte believed to myelinate about 30–40 internodes. CNS myelination is incomplete at birth and continues for several years afterwards (*see Chapter 9*), and myelin development may be delayed or significantly impaired by malnutrition during this period in life. Disturbed myelin formation also occurs in a group of inherited metabolic disorders known as leucodystrophies (*see Chapter 8*). In some of these disorders, although myelination occurs, the myelin formed is both chemically and structurally abnormal; dysmyelination is the term used to describe this abnormality. Myelin formation may also be disturbed in generalised disorders of lipid metabolism, inluding low-density lipoprotein deficiency (abetalipoproteinaemia) and high-density lipoprotein deficiency (Tangier disease).

Demyelinating disorders of the CNS	
Primary demyelinating diseases	Multiple sclerosis and its variants Acute disseminated encephalomyelitis Acute haemorrhagic leucoencephalitis
Secondary demyelinating diseases	Miscellaneous disorders Central and extra pontine myelinolysis Progressive multifocal leucoencephalopathy Vacuolar myelopathy in AIDS Cerebral leucoencephalopathy in AIDS Subacute combined degeneration of the spinal cord (vitamin B_{12} deficiency) Marchiafava–Bignami disease Subacute sclerosing panencephalitis Cockayne's syndrome Low- and high-density lipoprotein deficiencies Prolonged cerebral oedema Demyelination following axonal degeneration
Leucodystrophies and metabolic disorders	Sudanophilic leucodystrophy Metachromatic leucodystrophy Adrenoleucodystrophy Krabbe's leucodystrophy Alexander's disease Canavan's spongiform leucodystrophy
Toxic demyelination	Hexachlorophane Cyanide Carbon monoxide Chronic solvent vapour abuse

6.1 Demyelinating disorders of the CNS.

PRIMARY DEMYELINATING DISORDERS

MULTIPLE SCLEROSIS

By far the commonest demyelinating disease in man is multiple sclerosis, which has a prevalence rate in northern Europe of around 50–100 per 100,000 population. The disease usually presents in early adult life with characteristic signs and symptoms (**6.2**) and pursues a relapsing and remitting course over a period of years. Most patients die from late complications of the disease, e.g. bronchopneumonia, urinary tract infections and chronic bedsores. The disease occurs more frequently in females than in males and genetic studies have shown an association

Feature	Frequency (%)
Limb weakness	50
Optic neuritis	20
Diplopia	10
Paraesthesiae	10
Bladder dysfunction	5
Vertigo and nystagmus	5

6.2 Presenting features of multiple sclerosis.

with HLA haplotypes, including HLA-A3, -B7, -DR2, -DW2 and -DQw1.

Multiple sclerosis also has a characteristic geographic distribution, being relatively uncommon in the tropics and subtropics (**6.3**).The cause of this disorder is unknown. A wide range of dietary, metabolic and infective disorders have been postulated to account for its characteristic epidemiology. The most popular current theory is that of an autoimmune process directed against myelin in the CNS, which occurs as a consequence of a viral infection in a genetically predisposed individual. Several viruses have been implicated in the pathogenesis of multiple sclerosis, particularly the measles virus although there is as yet no conclusive evidence.

Pathological features

The pathological features of this disease depend on the stage of evolution of lesions in the CNS. Demyelination in multiple sclerosis occurs in the form of plaques which appear as pale ill-defined pink-yellow lesions in the unfixed brain. Acute plaques (**6.4**) may occasionally present as space-occupying lesions and consequently have been biopsied. As the lesions evolve, myelin is broken down within the plaque and undergoes phagocytosis by macrophages. There is an accompanying astrocytosis, particularly in chronic or burnt-out plaques. These appear as sharply demarcated grey-white lesions which may be present on the surface of the brainstem or spinal cord on external examination (**6.2**). Optic nerve involvement is common, and one or both optic nerves may appear pale and shrunken. The cut surfaces of the brain show demyelinated plaques characteristically present around the lateral ventricles in the central white matter, corpus callosum (**6.6**) and temporal and occipital lobes. Plaques may also occur in the white matter regions of the basal ganglia, thalamus, hypothalamus (**6.7**) and around the fourth ventricle in the brainstem. Multiple brainstem lesions are common (**6.8**), particularly in the pons and region of the middle cerebellar peduncle, but the cerebellar white matter is less commonly involved. Spinal cord involvement is common, particularly in the cervical region (**6.9**).

Demyelination occurs without a direct relationship to anatomical tracts, though Wallerian degeneration may sometimes be present in ascending or descending tracts in longstanding cases. Both acute and chronic plaques may be present at different anatomical locations in individual cases. Demyelination in the CNS is usually most extensive in patients with longstanding disease, but it is not always easy to establish a direct relationship between the distribution of demyelinated plaques in the CNS and documented neurological abnormalities in individual patients. Solitary demyelinated plaques have been reported as incidental findings in the brains of individuals with no clinical history to suggest multiple sclerosis; these are sometimes referred to as 'silent' plaques.

The demyelinated plaques in multiple sclerosis are usually detectable in MRI scans of the brain and spinal cord. CSF examination in an active phase of multiple sclerosis shows evidence of a chronic inflammatory reaction (see **3.5**) with increased numbers of lymphocytes and macrophages (usually up to 30 cells/mm^3). The protein level in the CSF is elevated, with oligoclonal bands of IgG; some of the latter show an antimeasles specificity.

Histological features

Histological examination of multiple sclerosis plaques shows a variety of appearances which relate to the stage of evolution of the lesions. In the early or acute phase, the lesions are markedly hypercellular, with widespread perivascular lymphocytic cuffing and oedema in the surrounding tissues (**6.10**). Astrocytosis can usually be seen at this stage, and there is evidence of widespread macrophage infiltration with phagocytosis of myelin breakdown products (**6.11**). Oligodendrocyte nuclei can still be identified, and evidence of oligodendrocyte proliferation may be seen, particularly at the edges of the lesions.

In chronic plaques, there is a widespread loss of myelin and oligodendrocyte nuclei with relatively good axonal preservation, though axonal loss has been demonstrated in very longstanding chronic plaques. Astrocytosis is common throughout these lesions and at their edges. Perivascular lymphocytic cuffing is usually not a prominent feature unless there

Area	Crude prevalence/100,000 of the population
Northeast Scotland	144
England	50
Italy	20
Syria	12
Malta	4
Mexico	1.5

6.3 Geographical prevalence of multiple sclerosis.

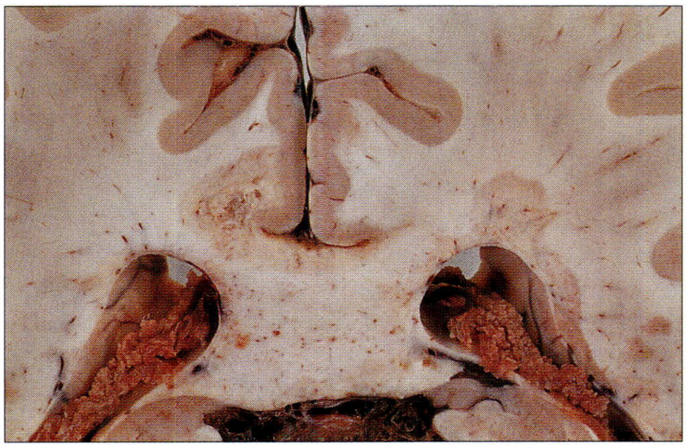

6.4 In acute multiple sclerosis, the demyelinated plaques are yellow-brown in colour, with an ill-defined edge which blends in places into the adjacent white matter. Small foci of cavitation are evident in the large plaque on the left.

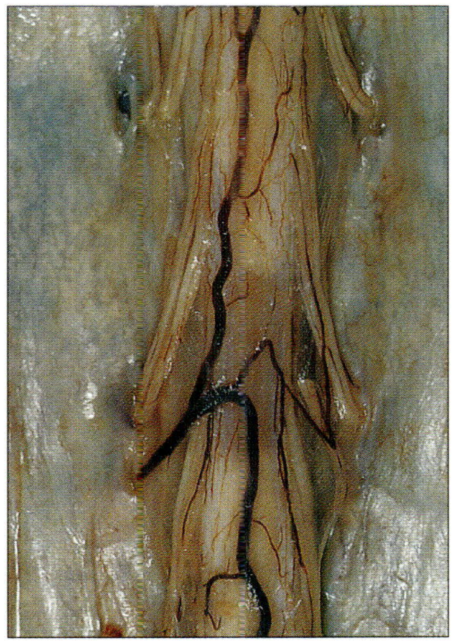

6.5 A chronic multiple sclerosis plaque on the posterior surface of the thoracic spinal cord appears as a grey-brown shrunken lesion.

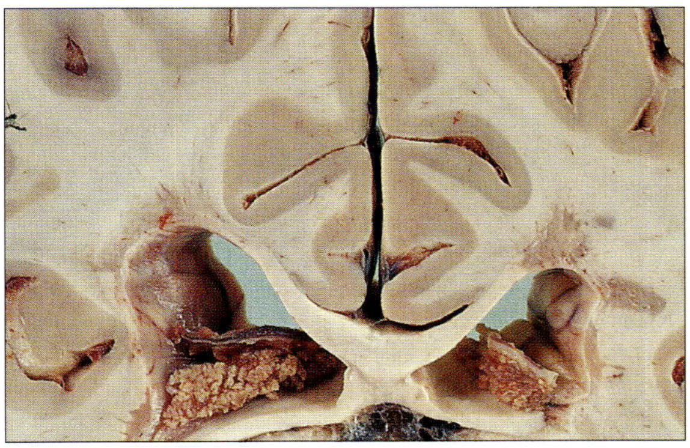

6.6 Chronic multiple sclerosis plaques (in contrast to those in **6.4**) appear as well-demarcated grey-brown lesions in the white matter, in this example classically situated around the lateral ventricles.

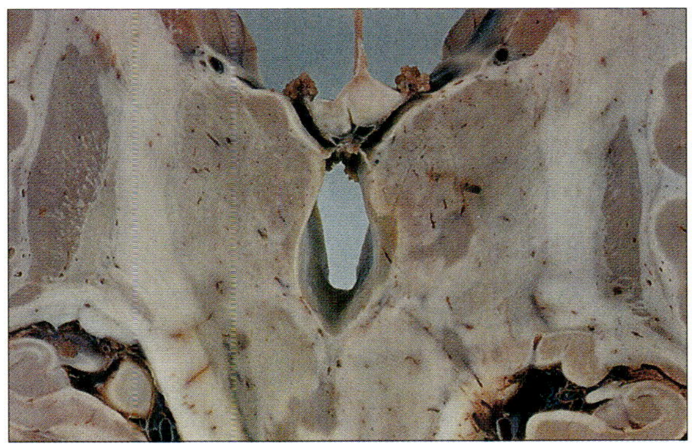

6.7 Chronic multiple sclerosis plaques can be identified as sharply demarcated lesions occurring in the thalamus, particularly around the third ventricle.

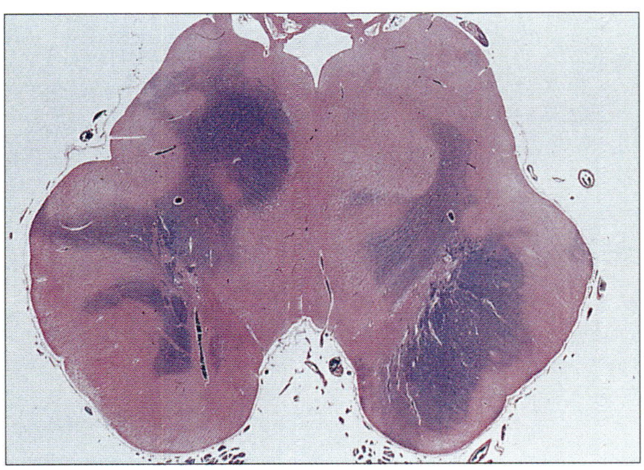

6.8 Multiple areas of demyelination are present in the mid-brain in this case of chronic multiple sclerosis. (Luxol fast blue/H & E stain: myelin is blue.)

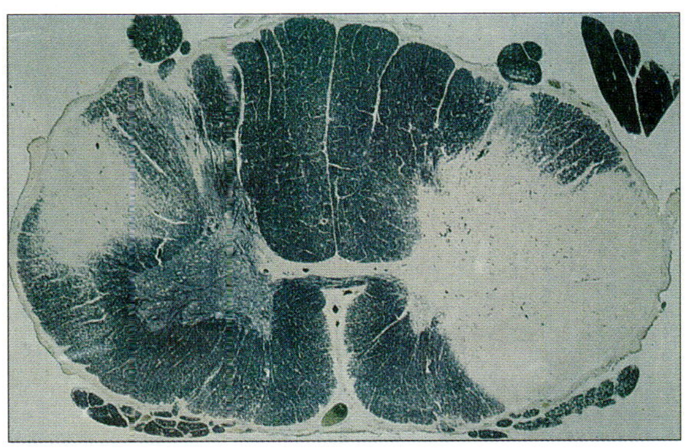

6.9 Chronic multiple sclerosis plaques in the spinal cord show a non-anatomical distribution, involving both ascending and descending fibre pathways. (Loyez stain: myelin is black.)

is other evidence of continuing disease activity (**6.12**). The surrounding tissues are usually not oedematous, and once myelin breakdown is complete there is little evidence of residual macrophage infiltration. Towards the edges of some chronic plaques, there may be hypercellular areas of remyelination ('shadow' plaques) in which oligodendrocyte proliferation may be identified (**6.13**). Oligodendrocytes have a limited capacity for remyelination, which does not occur to a significant degree either in multiple sclerosis or any other demyelinating disorder.

Demyelinating plaques often appear to be centred around small veins or venules (**6.14**), and these vessels may occasionally show evidence of vessel damage, with signs of previous haemorrhage or thrombosis and scarring of the wall, particularly in chronic plaques.

Perivascular lymphocytic cuffing is a hallmark of disease activity in multiple sclerosis, and the

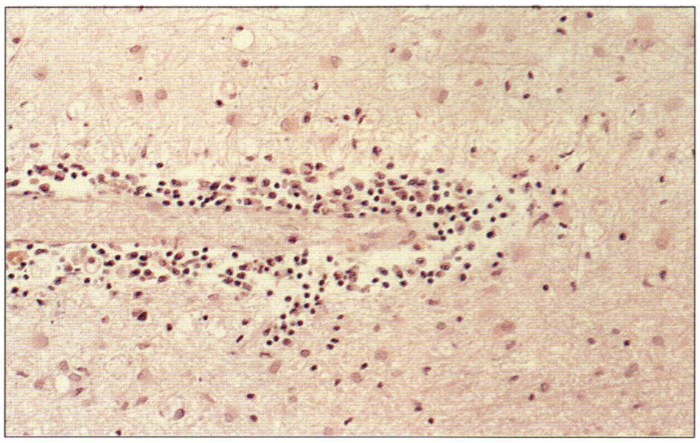

6.10 In acute multiple sclerosis, perivascular lymphocytic cuffing is a common feature with numerous plasma cells also present in this case. The adjacent white matter is oedematous and exhibits astrocytosis.

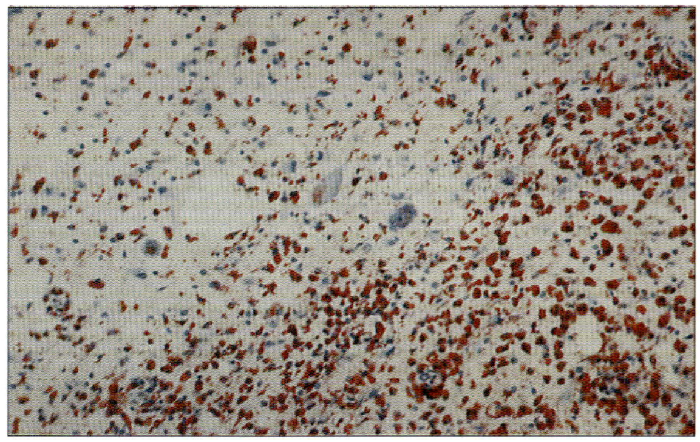

6.11 Myelin breakdown in acute multiple sclerosis is demonstrated in this cryostat section stained with Oil Red O, in which numerous droplets of myelin breakdown products are present within macrophages.

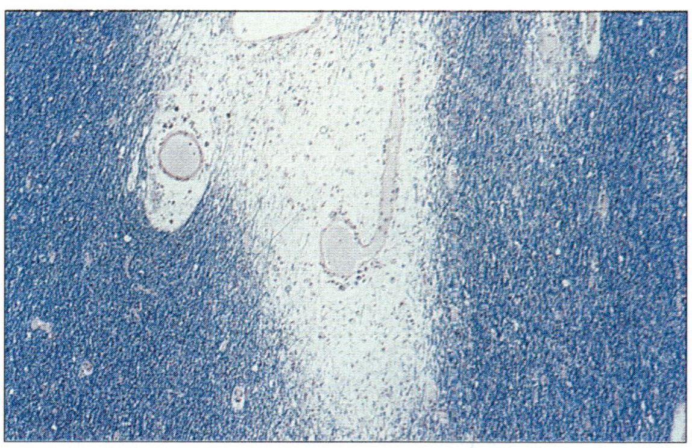

6.12 In chronic active multiple sclerosis, perivascular cuffing with lymphocytes and macrophages is present around blood vessels at the edge of the demyelinating lesion. (Luxol fast blue/H & E stain: myelin is blue.) (Reproduced from Underwood JCE (ed.) *General and Systematic Pathology*, with permission from Churchill Livingstone, Edinburgh.)

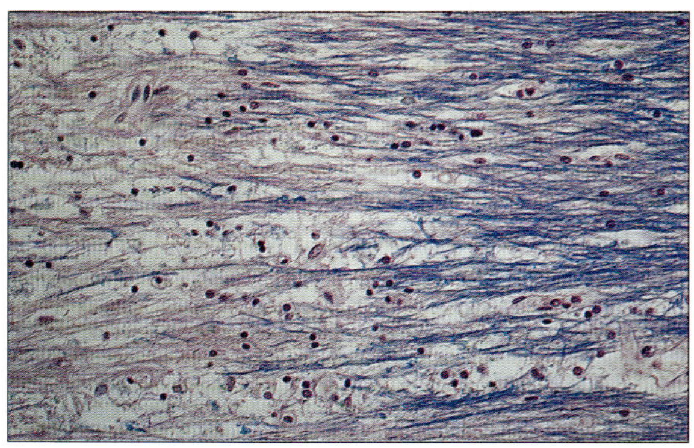

6.13 Irregular collections of oligodendrocyte nuclei are present in this 'shadow' multiple sclerosis plaque towards the centre and right of the picture. The myelinated fibres in this region appear abnormally thin; towards the left of the picture there is total myelin loss. (Luxol fast blue/H & E stain: myelin is blue.)

perivascular lymphocytes comprise both T and B cells. Plasma cells which usually contain cytoplasmic IgG may also be identified around blood vessels. However, T lymphocytes and macrophages comprise most cells at sites of active demyelination. Both CD4 and CD8 T cells are present, but CD4 T cells are most numerous at the edge of a demyelinating lesion. These cells are functionally activated and express HLA class II molecules (**6.15**) and interleukin-2 (IL-2) receptors.

MULTIPLE SCLEROSIS VARIANTS

Schilder's disease

Schilder's disease or diffuse sclerosis (**6.16**) is often regarded as a variant of multiple sclerosis, although some cases exhibit similarities to sudanophilic leucodystrophy (**6.17**).

Schilder's disease is an uncommon disorder that usually affects younger patients and is rapidly progressive, often with a monophasic clinical course.

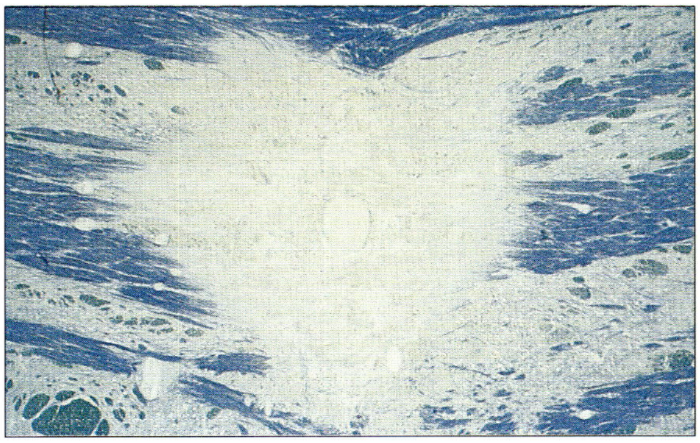

6.14 Demyelination in this chronic active multiple sclerosis plaque is centred around a central venule. (Luxol fast blue: myelin is blue.)

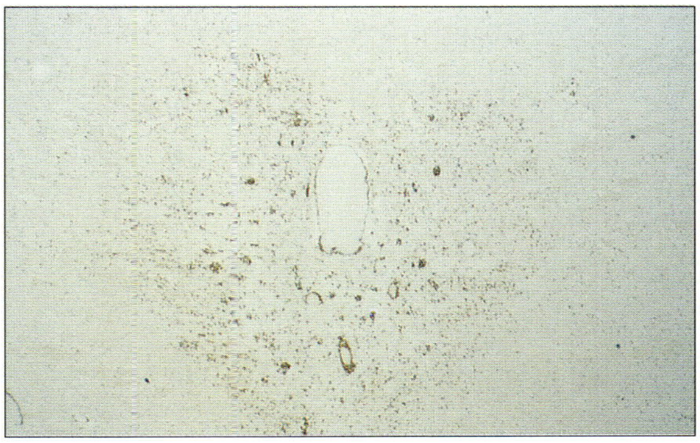

6.15 In an adjacent section to that shown in **6.14**, large numbers of reactive T lymphocytes can be seen stained by immunocytochemistry for HLA class II molecules. (Brown stain is positive.)

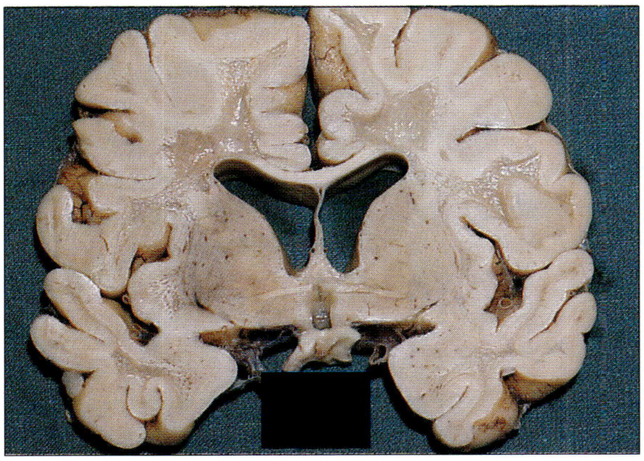

6.16 A female aged 38 years with Schilder's disease, showing extensive myelin loss throughout the cerebral hemispheres.

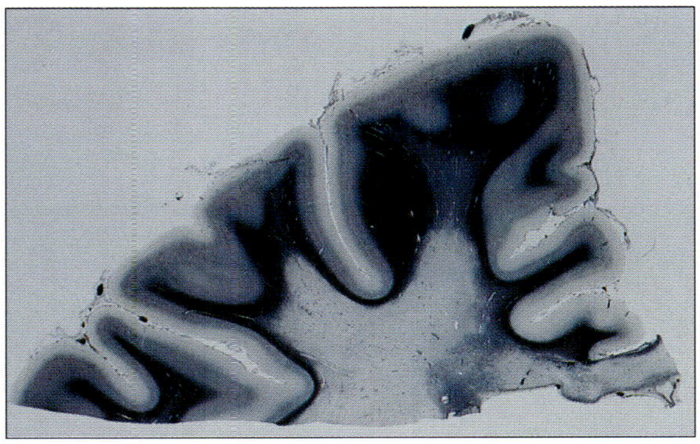

6.17 Schilder's disease. In this condition, the myelinated subcortical U fibres are usually preserved, in contrast to the central white matter where there is extensive myelin loss. (Loyez stain: myelin is black.)

Devic's disease

Devic's disease (neuromyelitis optica) is an uncommon disorder, in which a single focus of demyelination with inflammation is present within the spinal cord, often in the cervical region (**6.18**). This lesion may become frankly necrotic (**6.19**) and is usually accompanied by evidence of demyelination in the optic pathway (**6.20**).

Baló's disease

Baló's disease is a rare and unusual disorder. It is characterised by concentric rings of demyelination in the cerebral white matter in association with a rapid clinical disease progression. The unusual pattern of these lesions may indicate areas of remyelination.

ACUTE HAEMORRHAGIC LEUCOENCEPHALITIS

This extremely uncommon disorder is characterised by a sudden clinical onset with profound neurological disturbances, a rapid clinical course and death in most cases.

Many cases occur as an apparent complication in a range of other disorders (**6.21**), several of which are thought to be autoimmune in nature. There is evidence for immune complex deposition and complement activation around blood vessels in the CNS and other organs in these conditions.

In this disorder, the brain is swollen with multiple petechial haemorrhages within the white matter

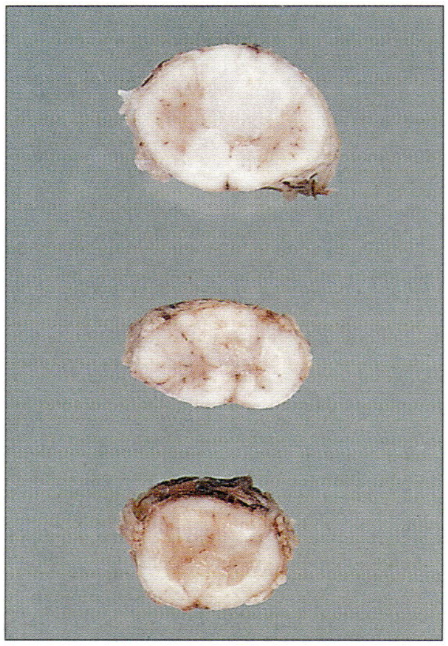

6.18 Devic's disease. A solitary focus of demyelination is present within the spinal cord, accompanied by necrosis (macroscopic view).

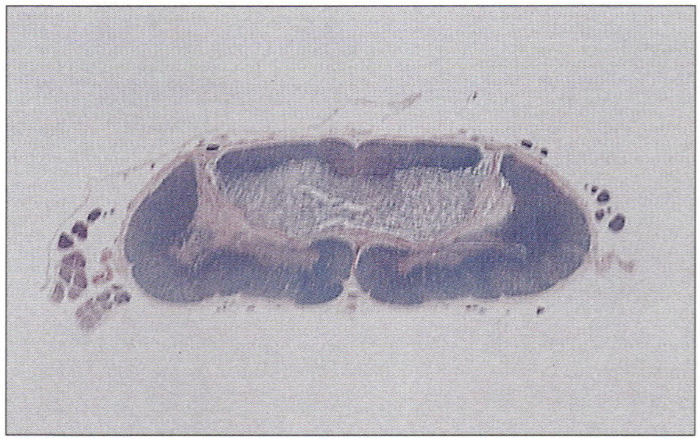

6.19 Devic's disease. A section is stained with Luxol fast blue/H & E (myelin stains blue) to show extensive central necrosis and myelin loss (same case as **6.18**).

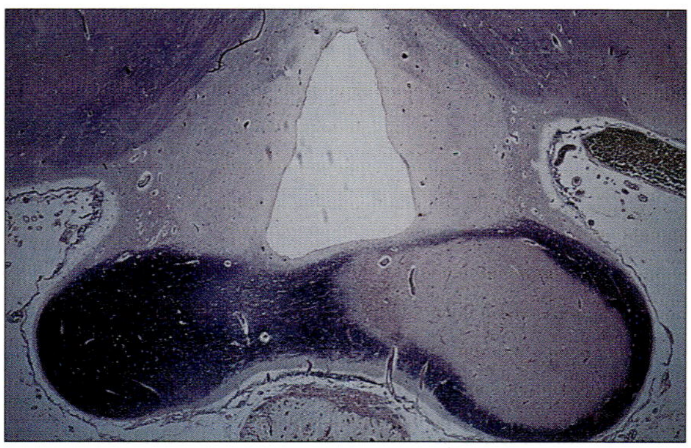

6.20 Devic's disease. An extensive focus of demyelination is present in the optic chiasm (same case as **6.18** and **6.19**). (Phosphotungstic acid haematoxylin: myelin is dark purple.)

Antecedent disorders associated with acute haemorrhagic leucoencephalitis
Upper respiratory tract viral infections
Septicaemia
Ulcerative colitis
Rheumatoid arthritis
Acute glomerulonephritis
Asthma
Drug reactions

6.21 Antecedent disorders associated with acute haemorrhagic leucoencephalitis.

(**6.22**). These may occasionally become confluent and can involve deep grey matter structures, particularly the basal ganglia. The subcortical white matter is most commonly involved but the cerebellum and brainstem may also be affected.

Histological examination shows fibrinoid necrosis of venules with inflammatory cell infiltration and oedema within the surrounding tissue. The cellular infiltrate is initially composed of neutrophil polymorphs, which are eventually followed by lymphocytes and macrophages. There is widespread haemorrhage into the surrounding tissues, often with a 'ball-and-ring' pattern. Ischaemic damage is common in this disease, and multiple small areas of infarction may be seen around the affected blood vessels.

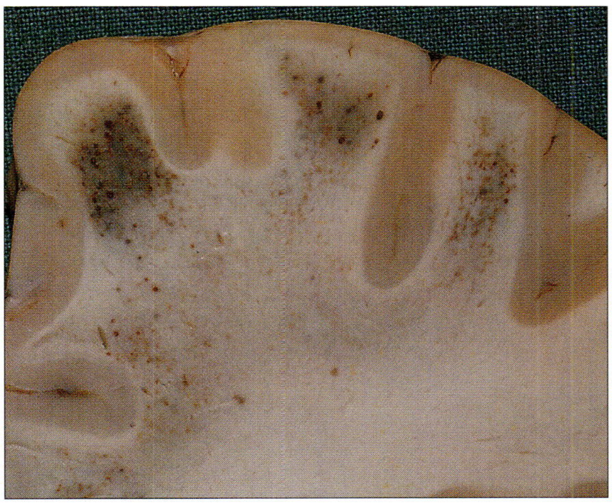

6.22 A male aged 30 years with a two-week history of a flu-like illness. Sections of the cerebral hemispheres show acute haemorrhagic leucoencephalitis, with multiple small confluent haemorrhages in the subcortical white matter.

ACUTE DISSEMINATED ENCEPHALOMYELITIS

This disease is uncommon, but occurs at an increased frequency in relation to acute haemorrhagic leucoencephalitis. Many cases of acute disseminated encephalomyelitis are self-limiting monophasic illnesses.

Disease onset is usually rapid, often occurring about 6–14 days following the onset of a viral infection in children and young adults (when the term postinfectious encephalitis is sometimes used). It occurs most commonly after upper respiratory tract infections, but also after other viral infections such as measles, mumps, rubella or chickenpox.

A mortality rate of 10–20% has been reported, particularly after measles infections. A similar disorder has been described following primary vaccination against smallpox and antirabies inoculations (sometimes referred to as postvaccinial encephalitis). The disease has been claimed to occur following inoculation with pertussis vaccine, but this remains unproven.

External inspection of the brain may show a mild degree of swelling and oedema. Histological examination shows widespread perivascular cuffing with lymphocytes and macrophages, which extend into the surrounding white matter (**6.23**). Most of the involved vessels are venules and there is variable patchy perivascular demyelination (**6.24**). These patches of demyelination may become confluent and are associated with astrocytosis in later stages.

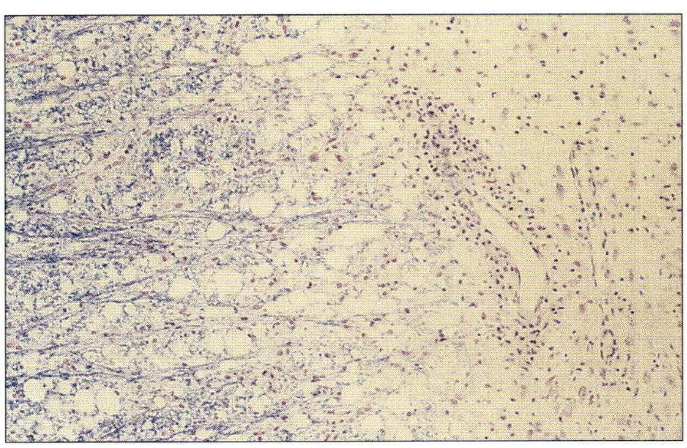

6.23 The same case as in **6.24**, showing perivascular lymphocytic cuffing and myelin breakdown around a small venule. (Luxol fast blue/cresyl violet: myelin is blue.)

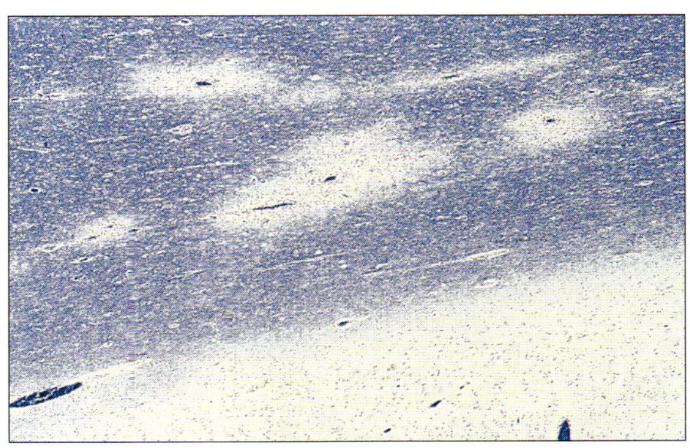

6.24 A female aged eight years with acute disseminated encephalomyelitis following a measles infection. Multiple small areas of demyelination are present around venules in the white matter. (Luxol fast blue/cresyl violet: myelin is blue.)

SECONDARY DEMYELINATION

CENTRAL PONTINE MYELINOLYSIS

This unusual disorder occurs most often in middle-aged or elderly patients who are malnourished and chronically debilitated. It is associated with fluid–electrolyte imbalance, particularly when a hyponatraemic patient has been rapidly treated with hyperosmolar saline. The mechanism of demyelination is unknown, but may possibly relate to impaired vascular perfusion during the episode of rapid electrolyte flux.

As its name suggests, demyelination in this disorder occurs in the central pons, often involving the tegmentum but not extending into the subpial or periventricular regions (**6.25**). Myelin loss is usually sharply defined (**6.26**) with axonal preservation and no evidence of perivascular lymphocytic cuffing. Astrocytosis is noted in established lesions.

Occasional patients may also exhibit similar small foci of demyelination in other regions of the CNS, including the subcortical white matter, cerebellum and spinal cord. This is often referred to as extrapontine myelinolysis.

PROGRESSIVE MULTIFOCAL LEUCOENCEPHALOPATHY

Demyelination in this disorder results from a lytic infection of oligodendrocytes by the JC papovavirus. This virus is widespread in the community, and can be detected in other organs of the body including the kidney. Demyelination as a consequence of oligodendrocyte infection is most common in debilitated or immunosuppressed individuals. The disease was first described in patients with systemic lymphoma and is now a well-recognised complication of AIDS.

As its name implies, demyelination in this disease is multicentric, often around small venules. In the fixed brain, this results in a number of small, sometimes cavitated lesions which are usually sharply defined and may become confluent (**6.27**). Virtually any region of white matter in the CNS may be involved, but the subcortical white matter (**6.28**) and cerebellum are commonly affected.

Histological examination of the lesions shows demyelination with axonal preservation and oligodendrocyte loss. Surviving oligodendrocytes may contain eosinophilic intranuclear inclusions (**6.29**) which on electron microscopy can be seen to represent viral nucleic acid. The demyelinated lesions are commonly infiltrated by macrophages, with associated myelin breakdown and phagocytosis. Astrocytosis is common, with many of the astrocytic cells having bizarre nuclear morphology suggestive of neoplastic change (**6.29**). Astrocytic gliomas have occasionally been described in patients with this unusual disorder, but this appears to be an exceptional event. Viral DNA is demonstrable in the nuclei of oligodendrocytes and enlarged bizarre astrocytes using an *in situ* hybridisation technique for JC papovavirus DNA (**6.30**). This investigation is of diagnostic value, particularly in small biopsy specimens.

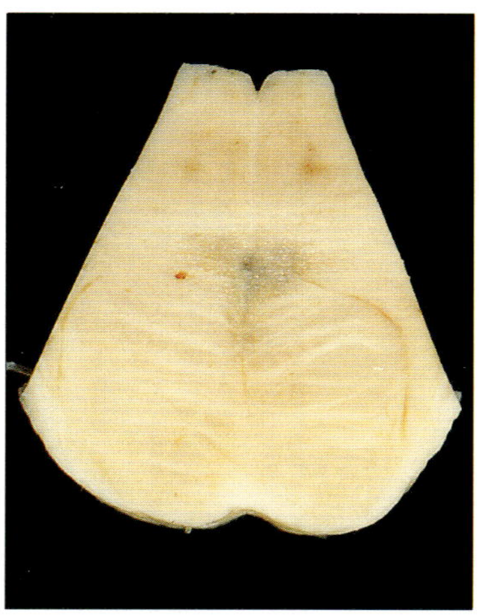

6.25 A section of the pons of a chronic alcoholic male, aged 58, found unconscious in the street. There is an ill-defined central grey-brown lesion, characteristic of central pontine myelinolysis.

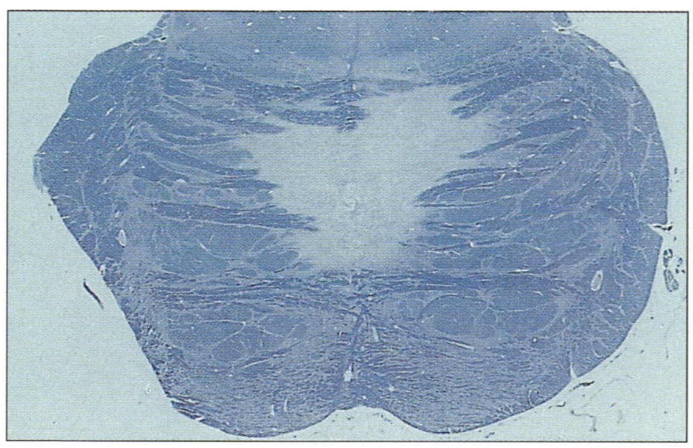

6.26 The zone of demyelination in central pontine myelinolysis is sharply defined. (Solochrome cyanin: myelin is blue.) (*Acknowledgement in the Preface.*)

OTHER CAUSES

Demyelination may occur following a wide range of toxic conditions, deficiency states and metabolic disorders, as listed in **6.1** and further discussed in *Chapter 8*.

It may also occur as a consequence of axonal loss within the CNS, in a manner analogous to Wallerian degeneration in the peripheral nervous system. This form of demyelination is found most often in the corticospinal pathway in patients, who have survived for several months or years, following an ischaemic stroke in which the internal capsule region was damaged. In these patients, the corresponding cerebral peduncle often appears shrunken, gliotic and discoloured in the region of the corticospinal pathway, as distal axonal degeneration is accompanied by myelin loss (*see Chapter 4*). Similar changes may be

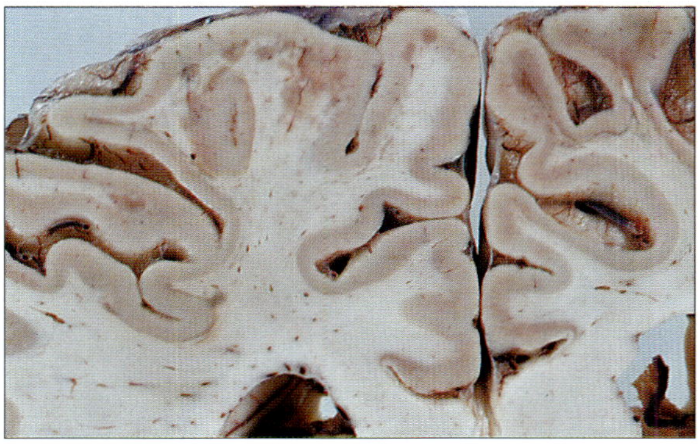

6.27 A female aged 58 years with a history of chronic rheumatoid arthritis treated with steroids. Multiple cavitated lesions are present in the subcortical white matter, several of which are confluent. This appearance is characteristic of progressive multifocal leucoencephalopathy.

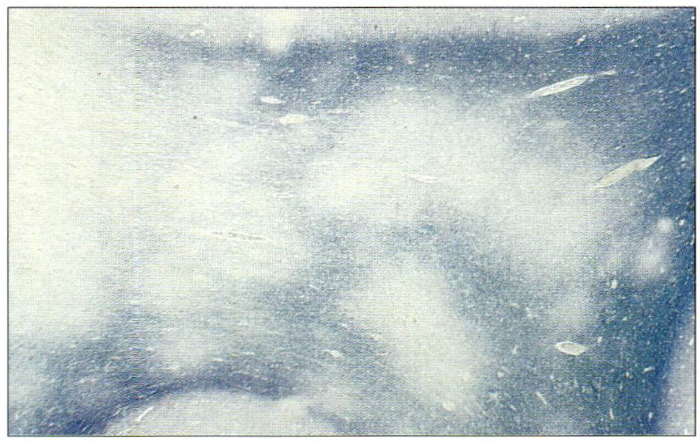

6.28 A male aged 53 years with AIDS and a sudden onset of visual disturbances. A section of the right optic radiation shows multiple confluent areas of demyelination, which extend up to the cortical margin. This pattern of demyelination is typical of progressive multifocal leucoencephalopathy. (Luxol fast blue/cresyl violet: myelin is blue.)

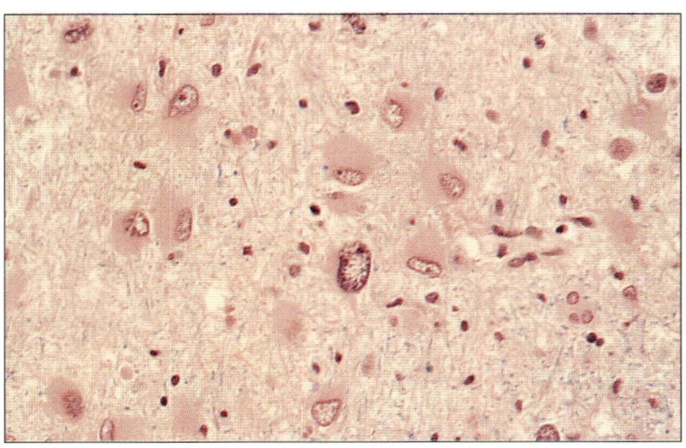

6.29 Histology of the demyelinated lesions shown in **6.28** shows oligodendrocytes with large homogenous nuclei containing viral inclusions (centre) and hyperplastic astrocytes with bizarre nuclei.

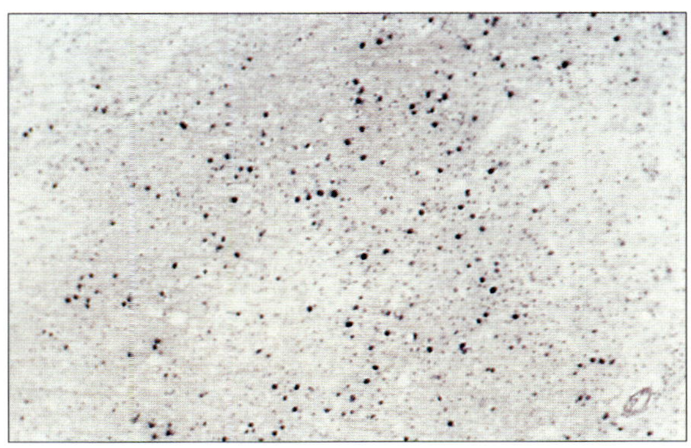

6.30 *In situ* hybridisation for the JC papovavirus using a biotinylated DNA probe shows a positive blue-black reaction in oligodendrocyte nuclei (in the same case as **6.28** and **6.29**). This confirms the diagnosis of progressive multifocal leucoencephalopathy.

seen in the ipsilateral medullary pyramid and in the corresponding descending corticospinal fibres in the cord. Ascending sensory tract degeneration may also be accompanied by myelin loss, for example, in subacute combined degeneration of the spinal cord (*see Chapter 8*), Friedreich's ataxia (*see Chapter 7*) and tabes dorsalis (*see Chapter 3*) within defined neuro-anatomical pathways

FURTHER READING

Adams CWM. *A Color Atlas of Multiple Sclerosis and Other Myelin Disorders.* London, Wolfe Medical, 1989.

Allen IV, Kirk J. Demyelinating Diseases. In: Adams JH, Duchen LW (eds). Greenfield's *Neuropathology.* 5th edn. London, Edward Arnold, 1992, pp 447–520.

Mathews WB (ed). McAlpine's *Multiple Sclerosis*. Edinburgh, Churchill–Livingstone, 1991.

Raine CS. Demyelinating Diseases. In: Davis RL, Robertson DM (eds). *Textbook of Neuropathology.* 2nd edn. Baltimore, Williams and Wilkins, 1990, pp 535–620.

Weller RO. Demyelinating Disease: Multiple Sclerosis. In: Weller RO (ed). *Systemic Pathology.* Vol 4. 3rd edn. Edinburgh, Churchill–Livingstone, 1990, pp 224–243.

7. Degenerative Diseases

Most degenerative disorders of the CNS occur in elderly patients, and many of these disorders show some histological features which also occur as a result of normal ageing in the CNS. Familiarity with these age-related changes is therefore essential if one is to make an appropriate neuropathological assessment of degenerative CNS disorders in elderly patients (**7.1, 7.2**). The extent and severity of age-related changes in the CNS is enormously variable, particularly in patients over the age of 60 years. However, characteristic progressive features can be identified (**7.3, 7.4**).

Primary degenerative diseases of the CNS are an important large group of disorders. They occur most often in elderly patients, and their prevalence is increasing in industrialised societies as the average age of the population continues to rise. They are usually confined to the CNS and comprise a diverse group of disorders characterised by neuronal cell death and gliosis. There is increasing evidence to suggest that these disorders may be influenced by both environmental and genetic factors. Some occur as familial disorders, but in many cases the aetiology is poorly understood.

Recent advances in clinical investigative techniques, particularly neuroradiology, have enabled some neurodegenerative disorders to be more accurately diagnosed during life. Nevertheless, neuropathological examination of the CNS after autopsy still remains the most accurate method for diagnosis. The importance of a thorough neuropathological examination in this group of disorders is paramount. Such an examination often requires specialised histological techniques including histochemistry and immunocytochemistry for diagnosis. Brain banks have been established for many neurodegenerative

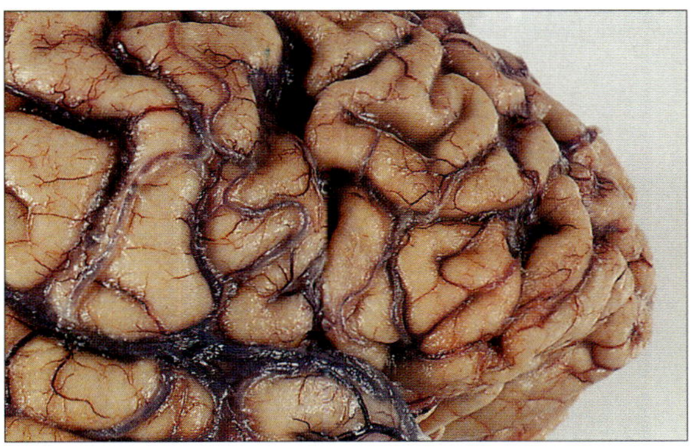

7.1 A normal male aged 75 years, with age-related atrophy of the cerebral cortex resulting in narrowing of the gyri and widening of the sulci. The meninges are thickened, particularly over the widened sulci.

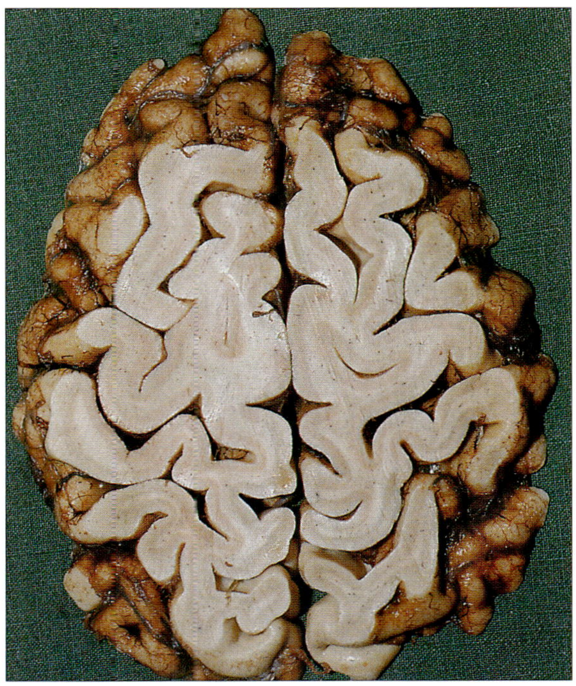

7.2 Horizontal section of the cerebral hemispheres from the case shown in **7.1**. This shows generalised cortical atrophy with sulcal widening.

Age-related changes in the CNS	
Thickening and fibrosis of the leptomeninges with prominent arachnoidal granulations	
Reduction in the weight of the brain with a fall in the ratio of brain to skull volume, narrowing of gyri and widening of sulci and compensatory dilatation of the ventricular system	
Variable neuronal loss which is most conspicuous in the hippocampus and cerebral cortex, resulting in cerebral cortical atrophy and sulcal widening	
Neuronal changes	Lipofuscin accumulation in cytoplasm Altered dendritic pattern Loss of neuromelanin in pigmented cells
Changes in neurotransmitter activity (e.g. reduced acetylcholine (ACh) activity in the cerebral cortex, some of which is related to neuronal loss)	
Neuronal inclusions	Neurofibrillary tangles Hirano bodies Granulovacuolar degeneration } in hippocampal neurons
Lewy bodies in pigmented neurons	
Neuritic plaques in the hippocampus and in relatively sparse numbers elsewhere in the cerebral cortex	
Glial changes	Astrocytosis Corpora amylacea
Vascular changes	Arteriosclerosis Atheroma Calcification of blood vessel walls (particularly in the basal ganglia – pallidal siderosis) Enlarged perivascular spaces in deep grey matter Perivascular Aß amyloid deposition Microaneurysms on intracerebral arterioles

7.3 Age-related changes in the CNS.

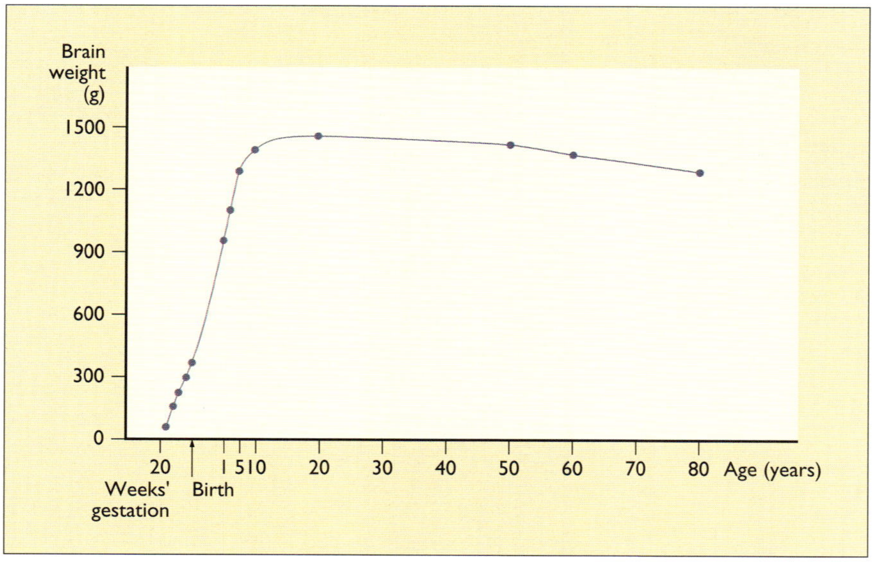

7.4 Graph of normal brain weight in relation to age. The most rapid phases of brain growth occur prenatally and from birth to five years. A slowly progressive decline in brain weight occurs from the fifth decade onwards.

disorders. These are important resources of frozen unfixed tissues allowing neurochemical and molecular biological investigations which cannot be performed on fixed tissues.

Primary neurodegenerative disorders can conveniently be considered in two main groups based on both clinical and neuropathological features:

- system degenerations;
- dementias.

Although there is considerable overlap, this subcategorisation provides a useful framework for investigation and differential diagnosis.

SYSTEM DEGENERATIONS

Neuronal loss in this group of disorders characteristically occurs within regions of the brain which are functionally and structurally related. Many of these diseases spare the cerebral cortex and patients often present with signs and symptoms of dysfunction in clearly defined neuroanatomical pathways, e.g. the motor or sensory systems. Classification is based mainly on clinical signs and symptoms. It should be remembered that a wide variety of disease processes within the CNS may result in similar clinical features of varying severity.

MOTOR SYSTEM DISORDERS

Motor neuron disease

This condition has an incidence of about 4–5 per 100,000 of the population in Western countries. Some cases occur as familial disorders, but most are sporadic and progressive, usually resulting in death from respiratory failure in about 4–5 years after diagnosis. The disease usually occurs in middle-aged or elderly individuals and affects males more often than females. The cause of the disorder is unknown, though genetic studies have implicated abnormalities of the superoxide dismutase gene in familial cases.

Both upper and lower motor neurons may be involved, resulting in a range of clinical features in which three main variants are recognised (**7.5**). Macroscopic examination of the CNS occasionally reveals selective atrophy of the motor cortex (**7.6**). More commonly, the anterior spinal nerve roots are shrunken and grey in appearance in comparison with the sensory nerve roots (**7.7**), particularly in the cervical region and in the cauda equina where axonal loss and degeneration can be identified (**7.8, 7.9**).

On histological examination, there is loss of anterior horn cells in the spinal cord, with accompanying gliosis. Occasional surviving nerve cells show chromatolysis (**7.10, 7.11**), or neuronophagia may be observed. Other surviving nerve cells may contain filamentous inclusions which are most easily identified using immunocytochemical techniques for ubiquitin (**7.10, 7.11**). In the white matter of the spinal cord, there is usually extensive degeneration of the corticospinal tracts, particularly in the lateral columns which exhibit marked pallor of myelin staining as a consequence of axonal (Wallerian) degeneration (*see Chapter 2*) and secondary demyelination. In cases with bulbar involvement, there is usually extensive loss of nerve cells in the hypoglossal nucleus and in the motor nucleus of the vagus nerve.

Nerve cell loss in the motor cortex of the cerebrum is more difficult to identify, but can be marked in cases with predominant upper motor neuron features. As in the spinal cord, immunocytochemistry for ubiquitin can reveal the presence of small filamentous inclusions within nerve cells in the motor cortex.

In some cases of motor neuron disease, there is evidence of nerve cell loss elsewhere in the cerebral cortex, particularly in the frontal lobes with characteristic inclusions present in nerve cells. Occasionally this is accompanied by clinical features of dementia of frontal lobe type (*see below*).

In the peripheral nervous system, there may also be atrophy and loss of motor fibres. Skeletal muscle exhibits the features of neurogenic atrophy, with evidence of continuing denervation (**7.12**) and ultimately extensive atrophy of muscle fibres with replacement by fibroadipose connective tissue.

Clinical subgroups of motor neuron disease	
Progressive muscular atrophy	Predominant lower motor neuron involvement Flaccid weakness Muscle fasciculation Absent tendon reflexes
Amyotophic lateral sclerosis	Both upper and lower motor neuron involvement Spasticity Exaggerated reflexes Weakness Fasciculation
Progressive bulbar palsy	Involvement of motor nuclei of lower cranial nerves in brainstem Wasting Fasciculation of tongue Dysarthria Dysphagia

7.5 Clinical subgroups of motor neuron disease.

Spinal muscular atrophy

This term encompasses a group of disorders which are inherited as autosomal-recessive conditions. The gene for this group of disorders has been identified on chromosome 5q and all disease subtypes appear to be allelic variants. Clinically, four main categories

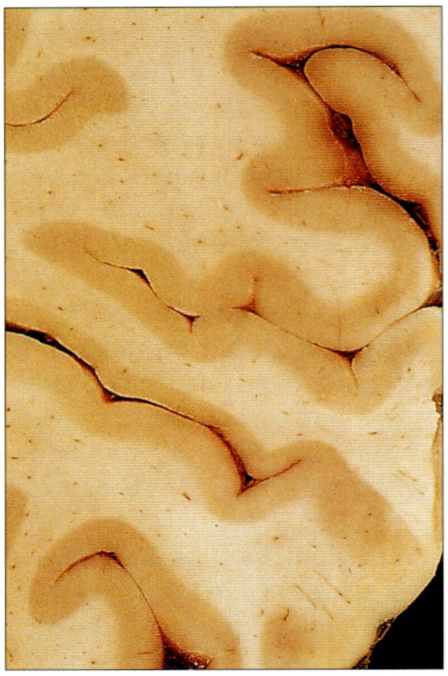

7.6 The motor cortex in this case of motor neuron disease exhibits irregular thinning (centre) as a consequence of neuronal loss.

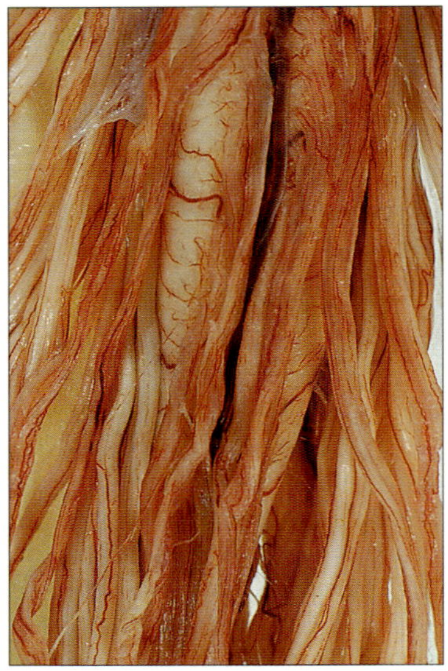

7.7 In motor neuron disease, the anterior spinal nerve roots (centre) appear thinned and grey-brown in colour, in contrast to the posterior sensory nerve roots (left and right) which are normal.

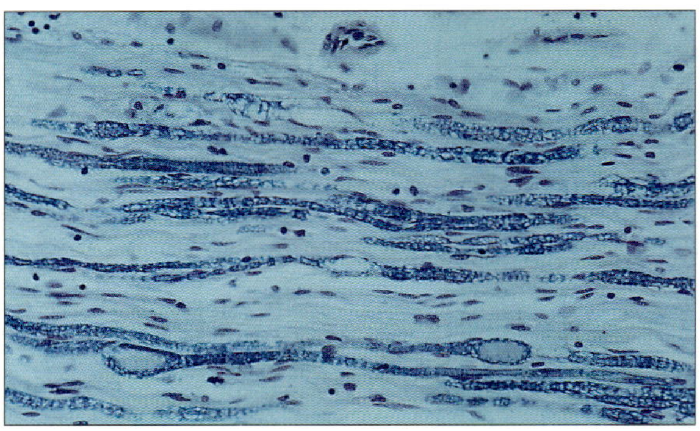

7.8 Histology of the anterior spinal nerves in motor neuron disease shows extensive axonal loss with Wallerian degeneration of surviving nerves, which appear swollen and fragmented. (Luxol fast blue/cresyl violet: myelin is blue.)

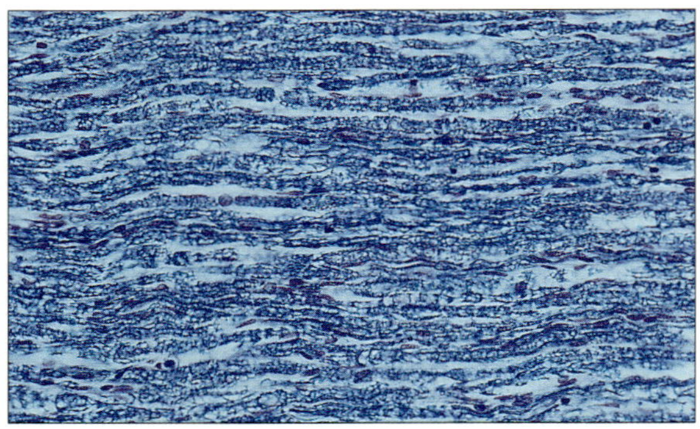

7.9 Normal age-matched comparison to the case shown in **7.8**. (Luxol fast blue/cresyl violet: myelin is blue.)

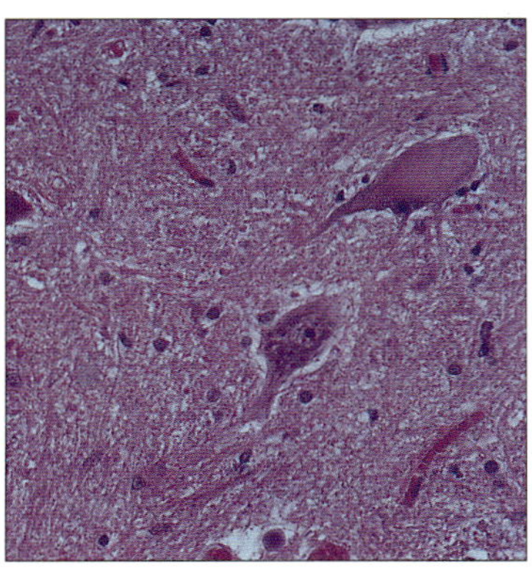

7.10 Surviving anterior horn cells in motor neuron disease exhibit chromatolysis, with cytoplasmic swelling.

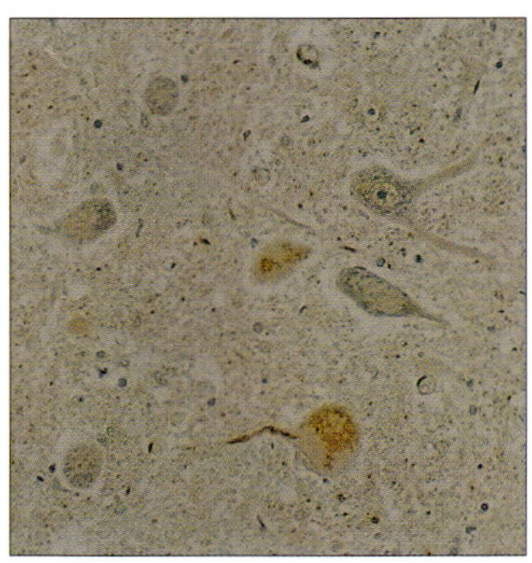

7.11 Immunocytochemistry for ubiquitin shows irregular filamentous inclusions within surviving anterior horn cells.

are recognised (**7.13**). In this group of disorders, there is progressive degeneration of the anterior horn cells (**7.14**) of the spinal cord with accompanying atrophy of spinal nerve roots and motor nerve fibres and neurogenic muscular atrophy (**7.15**). These features are most striking in spinal muscular atrophy type 1 (SMA1), while the diagnosis in SMA4 may be more difficult to establish at initial presentation. It is anticipated that molecular genetic investigations will be of primary diagnostic value in this group of disorders.

A similar X-linked disorder has been identified, referred to as bulbospinal muscular atrophy. The onset of this extremely rare disorder is in adult life, with progressive facial and bulbar weakness and proximal limb weakness. The disease is slowly progressive and associated with a good prognosis.

SPINOCEREBELLAR DISORDERS

This group of disorders includes numerous rare conditions, many of which are of unknown aetiology. The neurological features overlap extensively in this group of diseases, making precise clinical diagnosis difficult, particularly on initial presentation.

Friedreich's ataxia

This is the most common spinocerebellar disorder, occurring as an autosomal dominant condition and

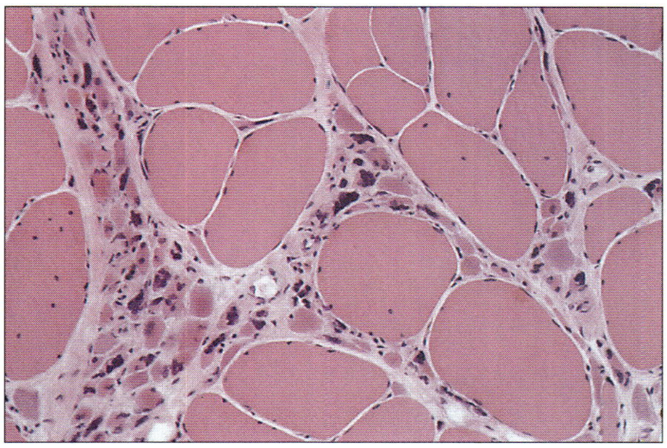

7.12 Skeletal muscle in advanced motor neuron disease shows denervation atrophy in many fibres. Surviving innervated fibres are enlarged and contain internal nuclei.

Subtypes of spinal muscular atrophy (SMA)	
SMA1 (Werdnig–Hoffmann disease)	Severe weakness and hypotonia present at or shortly after birth Rapid progressive course
SMA2	Juvenile onset Slow progressive course
SMA3 (Kugelberg–Welander disease)	Onset in late childhood or early adult life Very slow progressive course
SMA4	Onset in adult life and a benign clinical course which may include a normal life expectancy Previously, some patients with this disorder were diagnosed as having a slowly progressive form of motor neuron disease

7.13 Subtypes of spinal muscular atrophy.

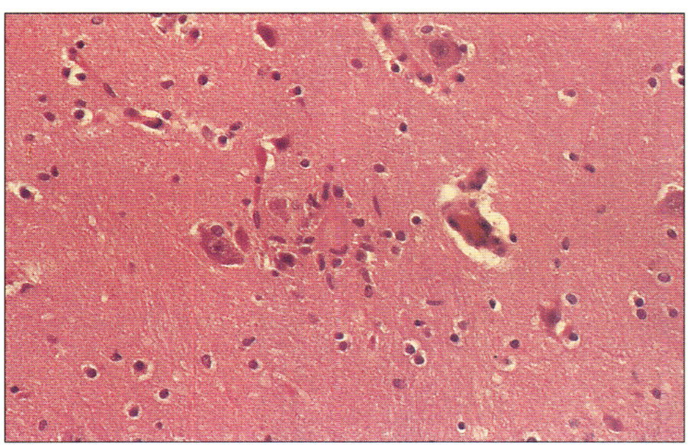

7.14 In spinal muscular atrophy type 1, loss of anterior horn cells is accompanied by neuronophagia with a prominent microglial reaction (centre).

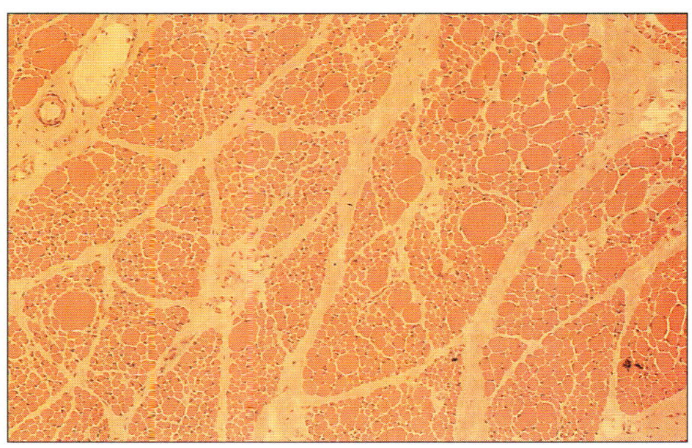

7.15 Skeletal muscle in spinal muscular atrophy type 1 shows characteristic widespread denervation atrophy, with surviving innervated fibres appearing massively enlarged. There is an excess of fibrous connective tissue around the muscle fibre bundles.

affecting around two per 100,000 of the population. The gene for this disorder is located on chromosome 9, but the precise genetic defect has not yet been identified. The disease usually presents in early adult life with progressive sensory abnormalities, ataxia and dysarthria, which may be accompanied by a number of systemic disorders (**7.16**).

Macroscopic examination of the CNS in this disorder may not reveal any striking abnormality in the cerebral hemispheres. The spinal cord often appears atrophied and on cross-section there is atrophy and discoloration in the posterior columns (particularly the gracile tracts) and in the spinocerebellar tracts (**7.17**). Histological examination confirms these abnormalities with extensive loss of axons and secondary myelin loss in these regions. The dorsal root ganglia often exhibit neuronal loss, which may also be identifed in Clarke's column in the spinal cord. The lateral corticospinal fibres may also show myelin pallor and a more subtle axonal loss. Neuronal loss is also usually evident in the dentate nucleus of the cerebellum and in some of the brainstem cranial nerve nuclei (usually of the VIIIth, IXth and XIIth cranial nerves). The visual pathway may also be involved with ganglion cell loss in the retina and degeneration of the optic nerves and tracts, and neuronal loss in the lateral geniculate nucleus. The heart is often abnormal with progressive cardiomyopathy in this disorder.

Cerebellar cortical atrophies

Atrophy of the cerebellar cortex can occur in a range of conditions (**7.18**). The commonest primary neurodegenerative disorder resulting in selective cerebellar cortical atrophy is the cerebello-olivary degeneration of Holmes. This is a rare familial disorder characterised by a progressive cerebellar ataxia, dysarthria and tremor, usually with onset in mid-adult life.

Systemic abnormalities in Friedreich's ataxia
Peripheral axonal neuropathy
Muscle weakness
Pes cavus and kyphoscoliosis
Diabetes mellitus
Hypertrophic cardiomyopathy

7.16 Systemic abnormalities in Friedreich's ataxia.

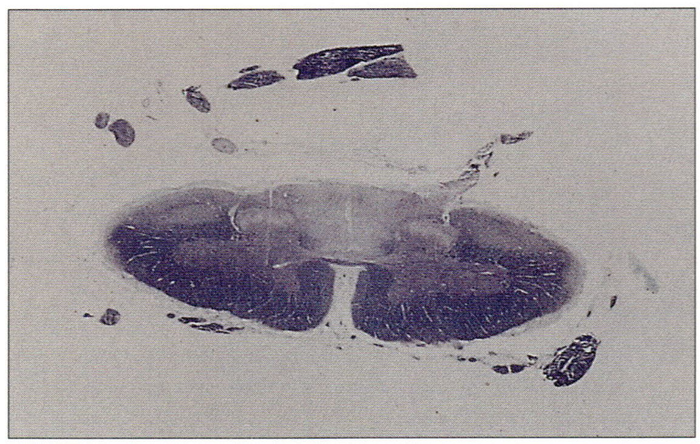

7.17 The spinal cord in Friedreich's ataxia shows myelin loss in the posterior columns and spinocerebellar tracts. (Luxol fast blue/cresyl violet: myelin is blue.)

Disorders associated with cerebellar cortical atrophy	
Cerebellar degenerations	Cerebellar cortical degeneration Olivopontocerebellar degeneration Friedreich's ataxia Ataxia – telangiectasia
Generalised neurodegenerative disorders	Huntington's disease Creutzfeldt–Jakob disease Gerstmann–Straussler–Scheinker syndrome Multiple system atrophy
Systemic disorders	Involving the vermis: Chronic alcoholism Involving the entire cerebellum: Irradiation Paraneoplastic subacute cerebellar degeneration Hypoxia (cardiac arrest, epilepsy)

7.18 Disorders associated with cerebellar cortical atrophy.

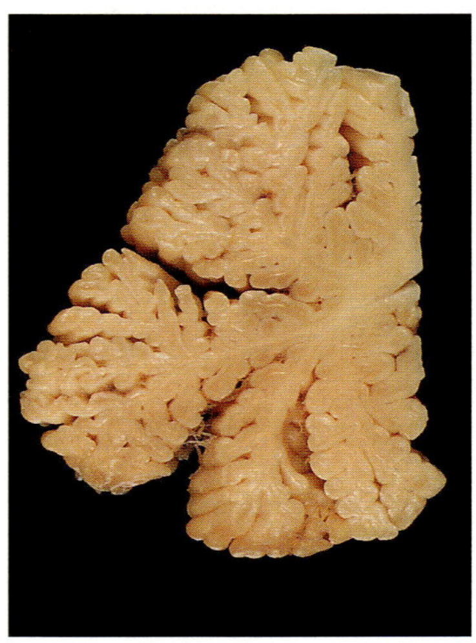

7.19 In Holmes' cerebellar degeneration, the cerebellar cortex appears shrunken with widening of the spaces between the folia and discoloration of the subcortical white matter.

Examination of the CNS shows marked atrophy of the cerebellum (**7.19**), with almost complete loss of Purkinje cells and extensive granular cell loss. This is accompanied by gliosis and loss of myelinated fibres in the white matter. Occasional surviving Purkinje cells may exhibit axonal torpedos. There is usually an accompanying atrophy with neuronal loss in the inferior and accessory olivary nuclei, as a result of retrograde trans-synaptic degeneration.

Olivopontocerebellar atrophy

This uncommon autosomal dominant condition has an onset in late middle-age and presents with slowly progressive cerebellar signs and symptoms. Macroscopic examination of the CNS characteristically shows atrophy of the ventral pons (**7.20**), the middle cerebellar peduncles, the olivary nuclei and the cerebellar cortex (**7.21**).

On histological examination, there is an extensive loss of neurons in the pontine nuclei and loss of transverse pontine fibres. The cerebellar atrophy is of mild to moderate severity, often being most marked in the hemispheres. In these atrophic areas there is a loss of Purkinje cells with relative sparing of the granular neurons, accompanied by gliosis. These changes are also present in the inferior olivary nuclei. Examination of the spinal cord usually shows degeneration of the spinocerebellar tracts and posterior columns, and loss of neurons in the thalamus and basal ganglia has also been described in the cerebral hemispheres.

Hereditary spastic paraplegia

This is an uncommon slowly progressive disorder which occurs most frequently in male patients. Onset of the disease usually occurs in early adult life with weakness of the lower limbs progressing to paraplegia. Histological examination of the CNS shows a distal axonopathy with degeneration of the lateral corticospinal tracts (particularly in the lower thoracic and lumbar segments) and degeneration of the dorsal columns and spinocerebellar tracts, particularly in the upper thoracic and cervical segments. The cerebrum and cerebellum are usually not involved.

MULTIPLE SYSTEM ATROPHY

In this uncommon group of disorders, patients present with a variety of signs and symptoms which indicate a degenerative disorder involving multiple systems in the CNS (**7.22**) Parkinsonian symptoms are particularly common and often accompanied by features of cerebellar and autonomic dysfunction (sometimes referred to as the Shy–Drager syndrome).

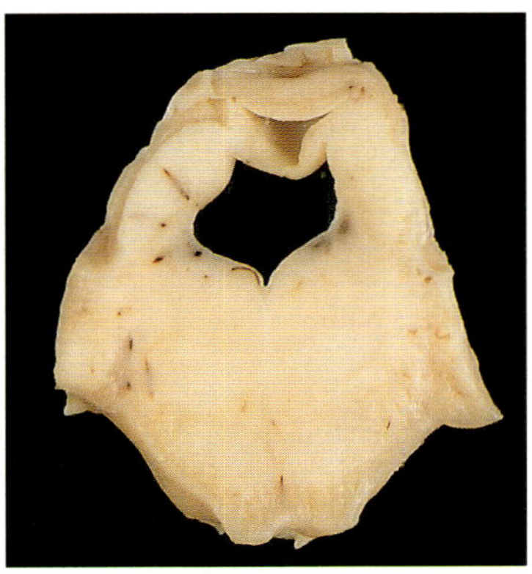

7.20 In olivopontocerebellar atrophy, the pons appears shrunken with marked loss of transverse pontine fibres and compensatory dilatation of the fourth ventricle.

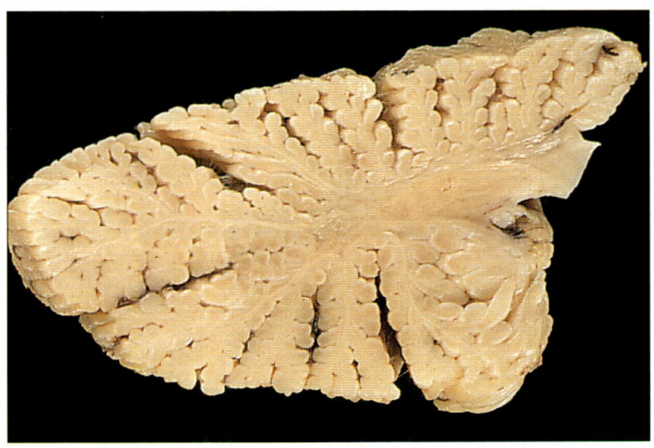

7.21 The cerebellar hemisphere in the same case as **7.20** shows marked cortical atrophy with discoloration of the subcortical white matter and atrophy of the dentate nucleus, which has an abnormal yellow-brown appearance.

Degenerations of multiple system atrophy
Striatonigral system (with or without Lewy body disease)
Pontocerebellar and spinocerebellar systems
Motor system
Autonomic system
Vestibular system

7.22 The degenerations of multiple system atrophy.

Macroscopic examination of the CNS may show atrophy of the cerebellum and basal ganglia (**7.23**), while histological examination usually shows features of striatonigral degeneration (sometimes with Lewy body disease), pontocerebellar atrophy and loss of autonomic neurons in the intermediolateral nucleus of the spinal cord, Onuf's nucleus, and in sensory and autonomic ganglia. Motor neuron loss may be identified in the cerebral cortex, brainstem and spinal cord. Immunocytochemical studies have revealed small cytoplasmic inclusions in glial cells (mainly in oligodendrocytes) on staining for ubiquitin (**7.24**). The nature and significance of these inclusions is uncertain, but they seem to be a characteristic feature of this group of disorders.

DISEASES OF THE BASAL GANGLIA

Parkinson's disease

This disorder is characterised by a clinical triad of tremor, bradykinesia and rigidity. The clinical features of Parkinson's disease result from a deficiency of dopamine in the projection sites of substantia nigra neurons in the corpus striatum, particularly the putamen. In this region, dopamine acts as an inhibitory neurotransmitter on cholinergic neurons. This relative deficiency can be replaced therapeutically, though the long-term results of oral therapy are sometimes disappointing. A considerable functional reserve appears to exist in the substantia nigra, as more than 50% of nerve cells need to be lost from this region before the characteristic clinical features of this disease emerge. Similar clinical features can result from other unrelated disorders which affect the function of the striatonigral system; such cases are referred to as Parkinson's syndrome or parkinsonism (**7.25**).

Idiopathic Parkinson's disease is a slowly progressive disorder that occurs most often in late middle-aged or elderly patients, with a prevalence of 1% in the general population over the age of 60 years. Macroscopic examination of the brain usually reveals no significant external abnormality.

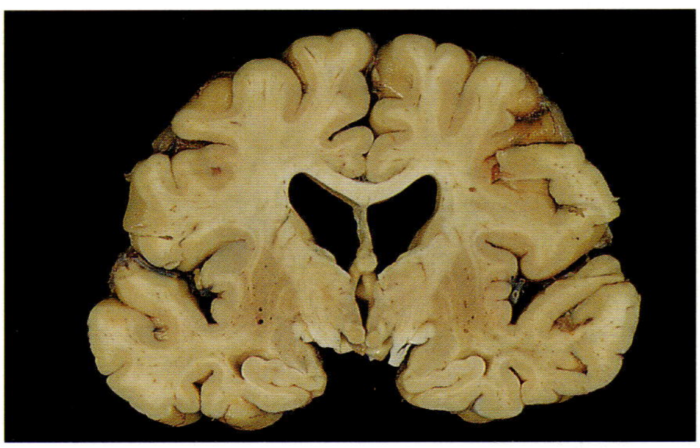

7.23 A male aged 54 years with multiple system atrophy, showing a mild degree of cortical atrophy and more severe atrophy of the basal ganglia and hypothalamus.

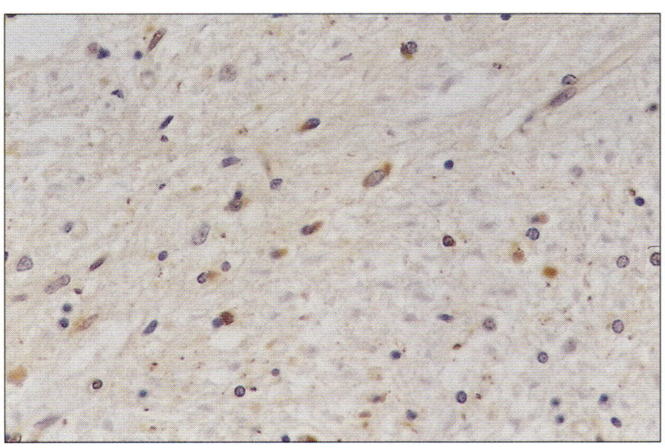

7.24 In the same case as **7.23**, immunocytochemical staining for ubiquitin in the medulla shows numerous small brown inclusions within the cytoplasm of glial cells, predominantly oligodendrocytes.

Disorders causing Parkinsonism	
Idiopathic neurodegeneration	Parkinson's disease
Drugs depleting dopamine reserves	Reserpine Tetrabenzene
Striatal dopaminergic receptor blockade	Phenothiazines
Toxic dopaminergic neuronal damage	Manganese Methyl-phenyl tetrahydropyrine (MPTP)
Viral infection of dopaminergic neurons	Encephalitis lethargica Japanese B encephalitis
Trauma	Dementia pugilistica
Striatal neuronal degeneration	Striatonigral degeneration Multiple system atrophy
Miscellaneous	Wilson's disease Neurosyphilis

7.25 Disorders causing Parkinsonism.

The most characteristic feature on cross-section of the brainstem is depigmentation of the substantia nigra (particularly in the zona compacta) and in the locus ceruleus (**7.26**). Histological examination shows evidence of neuronal loss at these sites accompanied by gliosis. Surviving neurons are usually depigmented and neuromelanin can be found lying free within the neuropil or within macrophages. Residual neurons contain Lewy bodies, which are rounded intracytoplasmic inclusions (**7.27**).

Lewy bodies are usually circular in outline, with a brightly eosinophilic hyaline core surrounded by a pale halo. Their precise chemical composition is unknown, but they are made up of filamentous structures and give a positive reaction for neurofilament protein and ubiquitin on immunocytochemistry. Ubiquitin immunostaining is also useful in demonstrating Lewy bodies in other sites within the CNS, including other brainstem nuclei, e.g. the dorsal nucleus of the vagus, and in diffuse Lewy body disease (**7.28, 7.29**),

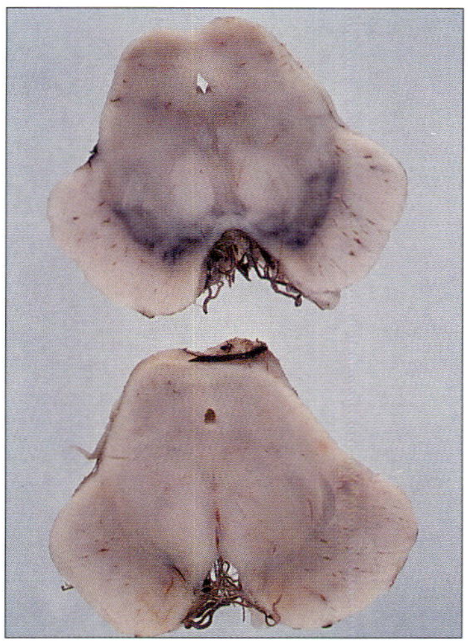

7.26 Parkinson's disease is characterised by shrinkage and discoloration of the substantia nigra (bottom) in contrast to a normal age-matched control (top).

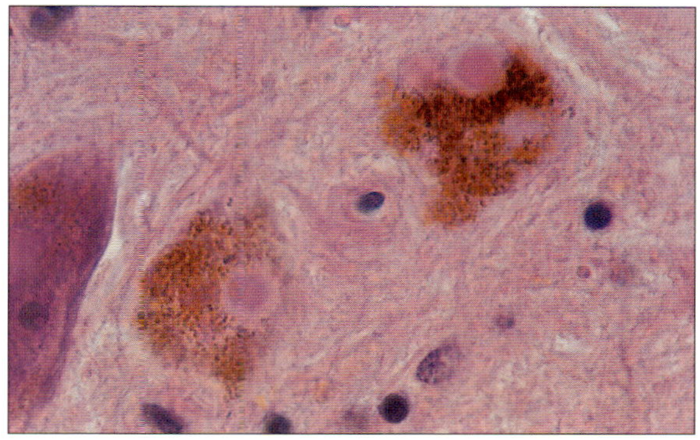

7.27 Surviving neurons in the substantia nigra in Parkinson's disease contain numerous rounded eosinophilic inclusions known as Lewy bodies, which classically comprise a dense core surrounded by a pale halo.

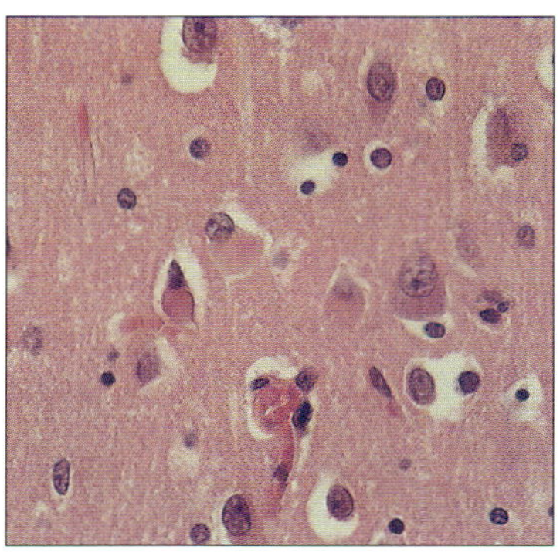

7.28 In cortical Lewy body disease, numerous ill-defined eosinophilic cytoplasmic inclusions are present within neurons (centre).

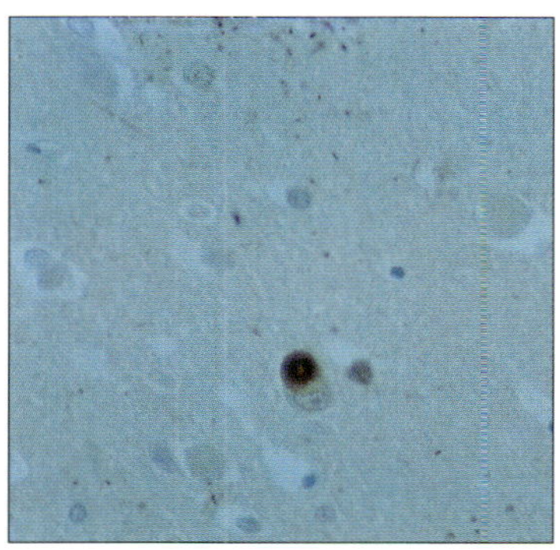

7.29 These inclusions give a strong positive reaction on immunocytochemistry for ubiquitin.

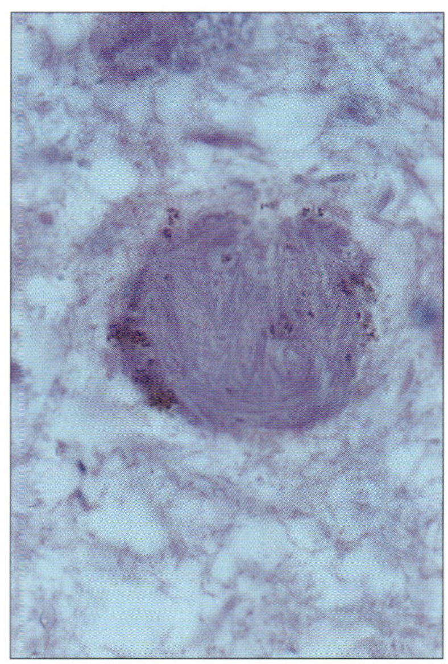

7.30 In postencephalitic parkinsonism, surviving pigmented neurons in the substantia nigra contain neurofibrillary tangles.

where Lewy body inclusions in the cerebral cortex are often accompanied by dementia (*see below*). Lewy bodies are occasionally found in the brainstem of otherwise normal individuals, but in Parkinson's disease, they are much more numerous and several inclusions may be present within a single neuron.

Postencephalitic parkinsonism

This clinical entity was described in survivors of the pandemic of encephalitis lethargica in the early 1920s. In affected individuals, parkinsonian symptoms are accompanied by loss of nerve cells in the substantia nigra with gliosis. Lewy bodies are not present, but many surviving neurons contain neurofibrillary tangles composed of paired helical filaments (**7.30**).

Striatonigral degeneration

The clinical features of this disorder are very similar to those of idiopathic Parkinson's disease. Unlike Parkinson's disease, neuronal loss and gliosis occur in the putamen in areas of dopaminergic projection sites from neurons in the substantia nigra. No intraneuronal inclusions are usually visible. This disorder has been associated with other system diseases, particularly pontocerebellar atrophy.

Progressive supranuclear palsy

Like Parkinson's disease, this uncommon condition occurs in late middle-aged and elderly patients. Of unknown aetiology, the disease is characterised clinically by the features of parkinsonism with supranuclear ophthalmoplegia.

Neuronal loss and gliosis are present in the substantia nigra in adjacent nuclei, including the red nucleus of the thalamus, the subthalamic nucleus and the periaqueductal grey matter. Lewy bodies are not present in excess numbers, but neurons in affected sites usually contain characteristic globose neurofibrillary tangles (**7.31**). On electron microscopy, these are composed of straight filaments approximately 15nm in diameter. The lesions are occasionally most widespread in the basal ganglia and cerebral cortex, resulting in dementia.

Neuroaxonal dystrophy

This uncommon group of inherited disorders affects not only the basal ganglia but other regions of the CNS, including particularly the brainstem and subcortical white matter. The aetiology of this group of diseases is unknown, but similar disorders have been described in animals. In the subgroup of conditions known as Hallervorden–Spatz disease, the predominant clinical features are rigidity, choreiform movements, dysarthria and intellectual deterioration. The onset of this disease is variable and late infantile, juvenile and adult onsets have been described.

On external inspection, the brain may appear normal but on cross-section there is a characteristic brown-yellow discoloration of the caudate nucleus (**7.32**), globus pallidus and substantia nigra (in the pars reticularis).

Histological examination of these sites reveals accumulation of an abnormal pigment which stains positively for iron and sometimes calcium. Numerous axonal spheroids are present at the sites, which usually give a positive PAS-staining reaction and on imunocytochemistry contain neurofilament protein. Ultrastructural examination has confirmed their axonal origin, but it is not known how this characteristic and striking lesion develops.

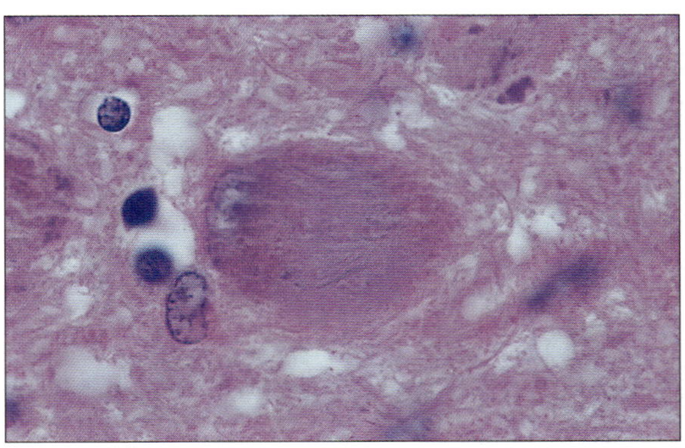

7.31 In progressive supranuclear palsy, globose neurofibrillary tangles are present within neurons in the IIIrd nerve nucleus.

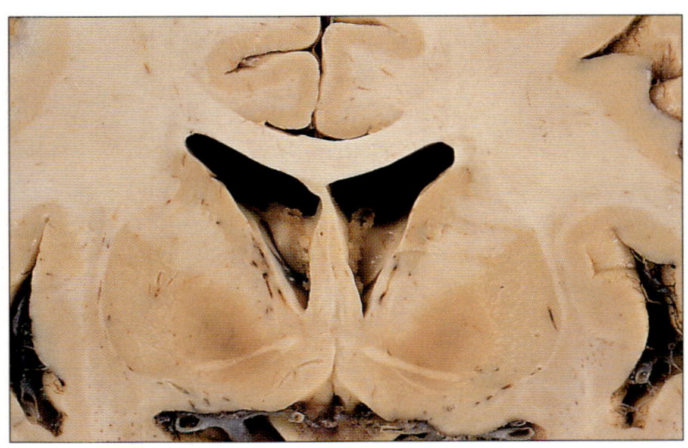

7.32 Neuroaxonal dystrophy in a male aged 24 years. The yellow-brown discoloration in the globus pallidus is characteristic of this disorder.

Corticobasal degeneration

This extremely uncommon disorder is characterised clinically by parkinsonian symptoms and signs with evidence of cortical dysfunction, including dementia. The neuropathological features are those of cell loss and astrocytosis in the cerebral cortex and basal ganglia, with variable numbers of ballooned neurons. This disorder appears to be related to Pick's disease (*see below*), but further research is needed to clarify this relationship.

Huntington's disease

Huntington's disease is considered below.

DEMENTIA

Dementia can be defined clinically as 'an acquired global impairment of intellect, reason and personality without impairment of consciousness'.

Dementia is mainly a disease of the elderly and it has been estimated that at least 15% of adults over the age of 80 years are demented. A wide range of disorders affecting the CNS may result in dementia (**7.33**), but these are usually considered in two main groups:

- organic dementia, in which there is a primary CNS disorder;
- secondary dementia occurring as part of a more generalised disease process.

The commoner diseases causing dementia are considered below.

PRIMARY DEMENTIAS

Alzheimer's disease

This common illness accounts for more than 60% of all cases of dementia in industrialised countries. Occasionally, it occurs as part of a multifactorial dementing illness in patients with severe cerebrovascular disease. In the UK, it is thought to occur in 5% of individuals over the age of 60 years, rising in incidence to 15% over the age of 80 years. Alzheimer's disease affects females almost twice as frequently as males, and usually presents over the age of 60 years with progressive dementia. The course of the illness is variable, usually lasting from 3 to 8 years, though patients with an early age of onset usually pursue a more rapid clinical course.

Although most cases occur sporadically, about 5% of cases are familial, some of which have an identifiable genetic abnormality in the Alzheimer precursor protein (APP) gene on chromosome 21. Other genetic loci are involved in some familial cases; naturally occurring polymorphisms of the gene for apolipoprotein E on chromosome 19 may also influence disease susceptibility and clinical course.

In Alzheimer's disease, macroscopic examination of the brain shows cortical atrophy, which is much more severe than in age-matched control cases, and usually most evident in the frontal and temporal lobes. The brain is reduced in weight, often down to 1kg, and there is accompanying ventricular dilatation (**7.34**). The basal ganglia may also appear atrophied, while the brainstem and cerebellum usually appear normal. The ratio for fixed tissue weights between the whole brain and hindbrain (normally 8–10:1) is therefore reduced in this disorder.

Histological examination of the brain shows extensive neuronal loss, which is most evident in the hippocampus and frontal and temporal cortex, and is accompanied by astrocytosis. These changes involve other cortical areas and subcortical grey matter structures, such as the amygdala and nucleus basalis. The characteristic histological lesions in Alzheimer's disease are the neurofibrillary tangle and neuritic plaque.

Disorders causing dementia

Disorder	Approximate frequency (%)
Primary dementias	
Alzheimer's disease	60
Pick's disease	<1
Diffuse Lewy body disease	15
Huntington's disease	1
Secondary dementias	
Vascular disorders (Chapter 4)	
Multi-infarct dementia	10
Arteriosclerotic dementia (Binswanger's disease)	5
Infective disorders (Chapter 3)	
Creutzfeldt–Jakob disease	<1
AIDS	1
Neurosyphilis	<1
Trauma (Chapter 5)	
Dementia pugilistica	<1
Chronic subdural haematoma	1
Metabolic disorders (Chapter 8)	
Myxoedema	<1
Chronic alcoholism	2
Inherited disorders	1
Miscellaneous (Chapter 1)	
'Intermittent pressure' hydrocephalus	1
Neoplastic (Chapter 10)	
Paraneoplastic syndromes	<1
Frontal lobe tumours	1

7.33 Disorders causing dementia.

Neurofibrillary tangles

These are intracytoplasmic neuronal inclusions which are most numerous in the hippocampus (**7.35, 7.36**) and temporal cortex. Tangles are elongated flame-shaped structures composed of paired helical filaments measuring 10nm in diameter with a periodicity

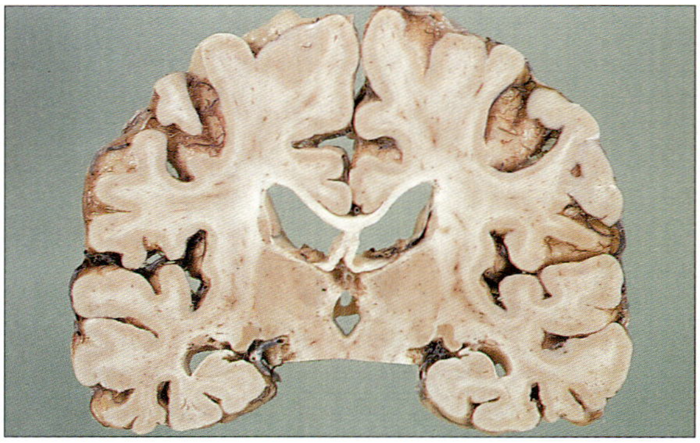

7.34 Alzheimer's disease in a male aged 66 years. The cerebrum shows global cortical atrophy, accompanied by ventricular dilatation. The hippocampi also appear reduced in size.

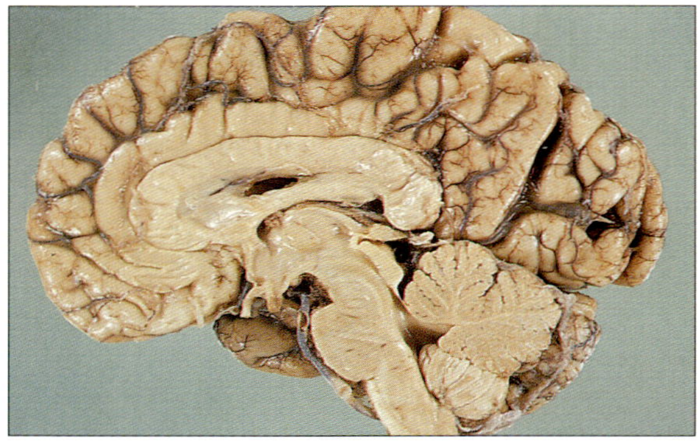

7.35 Longstanding Alzheimer's disease in a male aged 74 years showing severe atrophy of the cerebral cortex (particularly the frontal lobe). The cerebellum is of normal size.

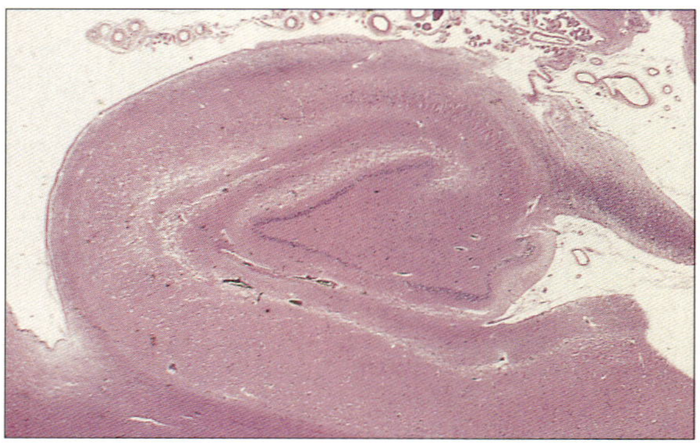

7.36 In Alzheimer's disease, the hippocampus shows a loss of nerve cells particularly in the CA1 and CA2 sectors, which appear pale at this low magnification.

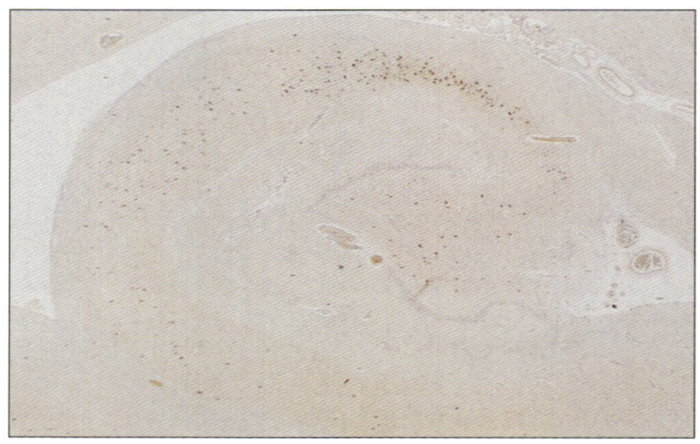

7.37 Immunocytochemistry for tau shows brown-staining neurofibrillary tangles distributed throughout the hippocampus.

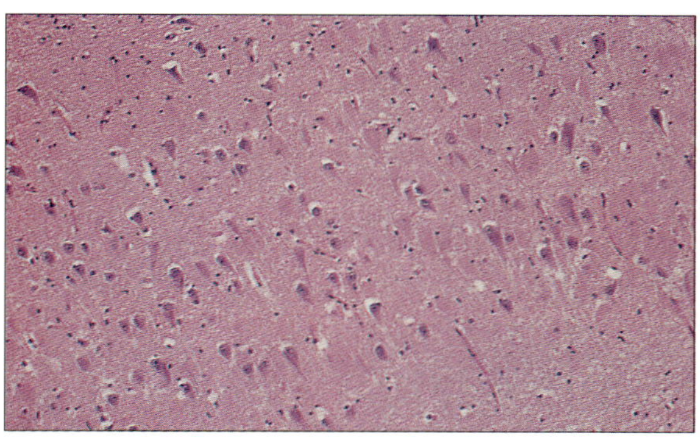

7.38 Neurofibrillary tangles are visible, after staining with haematoxylin and eosin, as elongated linear structures which appear basophilic when present within nerve cells. Tangles lying free in the neuropil have a paler eosinophilic appearance.

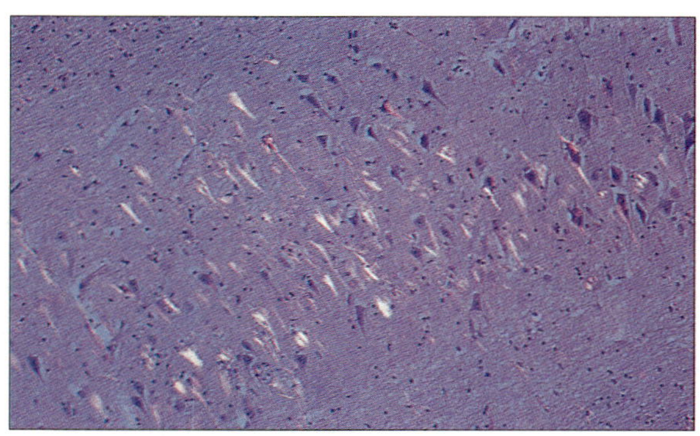

7.39 The presence of neurofibrillary tangles can be confirmed by examination of the same section as **7.38** under polarised light.

of 80nm. Their precise chemical composition is unknown; tau, a microtubule-associated protein, is present in a hyperphosphorylated form, and neurofilament protein is also present. Neurofibrillary tangles can be identified on routinely stained preparations (**7.38, 7.39**), but they are much more easily detected with the use of special staining techniques including the Congo red stain, silver impregnation techniques (**7.40**) or immunocytochemistry for tau (**7.41**) or ubiquitin. In advanced cases of Alzheimer's disease, occasional neurofibrillary tangles may be seen free within the neuropil. These are thought to represent residual inclusions from neurons that have died and undergone neuronophagia.

Neuritic plaques

These are complex extracellular structures which occur most frequently in the hippocampus and cerebral cortex (**7.42**), but are also present in deep grey matter structures, e.g. the amygdyla and nucleus basalis. Neuritic plaques may be identified on routinely stained sections but they are much more evident using special staining techniques such as the Congo red stain for amyloid, silver impregnation techniques (as mentioned above) and immunocytochemistry for Aβ protein or ubiquitin. A wide variety of plaque morphologies have been described of which three main forms can be identified:

- immature or diffuse plaque;
- mature plaque;
- burnt-out plaque.

The immature or diffuse plaque (**7.43**) consists of an apparently loose accumulation in the neuropil of the Aβ protein (a cleaved product of APP), which accumulates to form the amyloid component of senile plaques and also forms the amyloid present around

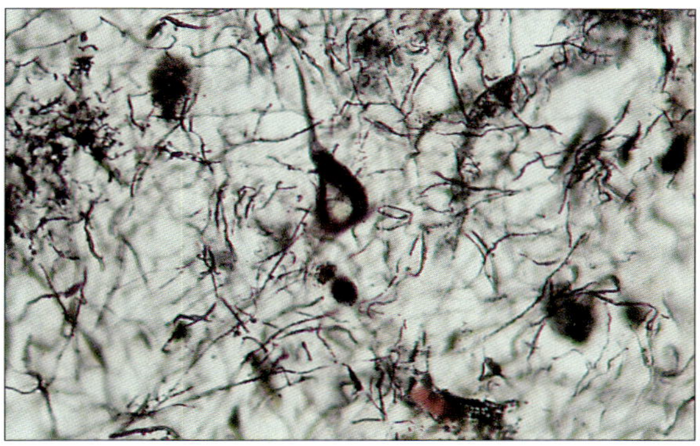

7.40 A large neurofibrillary tangle (centre) and many abnormal neuritic processes are visible in the hippocampus after silver impregnation. (Von Braunmuhl stain)

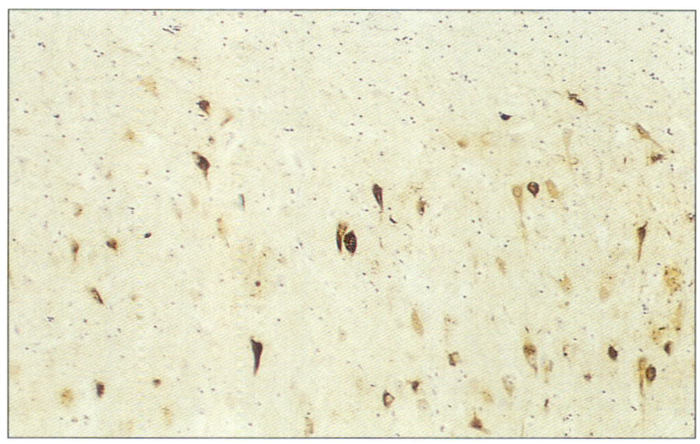

7.41 Immunocytochemistry for tau shows strong brown staining of the neurofibrillary tangles in Alzheimer's disease. There is also staining of occasional neuritic processes.

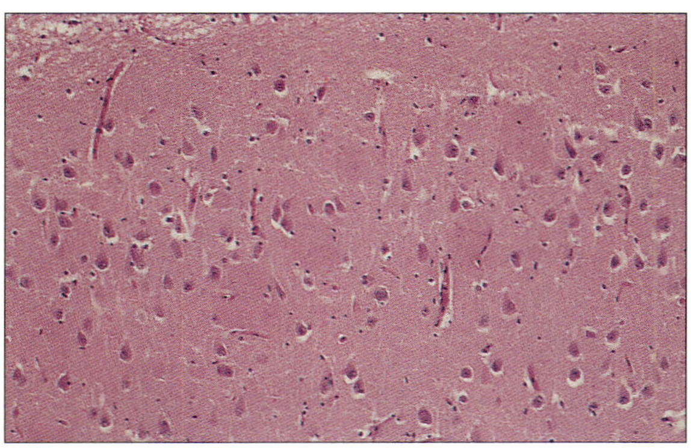

7.42 Neuritic plaques in the temporal cortex are visible, after staining with haemotoxylin and eosin, as ill-defined acellular structures (centre).

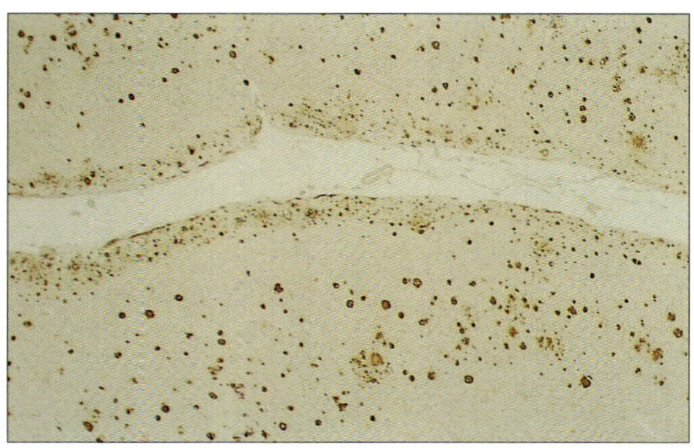

7.43 Immunocytochemistry for Alzheimer precursor protein in the temporal cortex in Alzheimer's disease shows a linear distribution of plaques. A variety of plaque morphologies are present, including ill-defined diffuse plaques and smaller mature plaques.

blood vessels in both Alzheimer's disease (**7.44**) and in normal ageing. In immature plaques, a Congo red stain for amyloid is usually negative and no neuritic components are present.

In the mature plaque, there is an amyloid core formed from the A/β protein. Around the core there is an accumulation of irregular neuritic processes apparently derived from axons (**7.45**). These distended nerve-cell processes are most evident at the edge of the plaque, but are also present within the plaque's central region. Astrocytes and microglia are present at the plaque periphery, and microglial cells may also be identified within the central region of the plaque (**7.46**). There is some evidence to suggest that these cells may be involved in the conversion of the A/β protein to the β-pleated sheet arrangement which is characteristic of amyloid.

Burnt-out plaques consist of a large accumulation of Aβ amyloid protein (**7.47**) with relatively fewer neuritic components and fewer astrocytic and microglial cells. Other abnormalities found in hippocampal nerve cells in Alzheimer's disease include:

- granulovacuolar bodies;
- Hirano bodies.

Granulovacuolar bodies are enlarged lysosome-like structures within which a central dot-like inclusion is identifiable (**7.48**). Their precise nature and mechanism of formation are unknown.

Hirano bodies are brightly stained eosinophilic inclusions with a rod-shaped structure, which are found within the cytoplasm of hippocampal neurons (**7.49**). These inclusions are composed predominately of α-actinin, but their mechanism of formation is unknown.

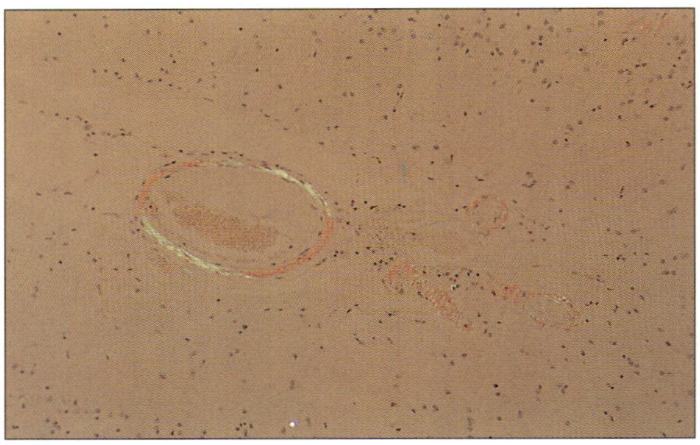

7.44 A Congo red stain shows birefringent amyloid in the walls of small subpial vessels in Alzheimer's disease. The amyloid in this congophilic angiopathy is derived from Alzheimer's precursor protein; similar changes may occur to a lesser extent in normal elderly individuals.

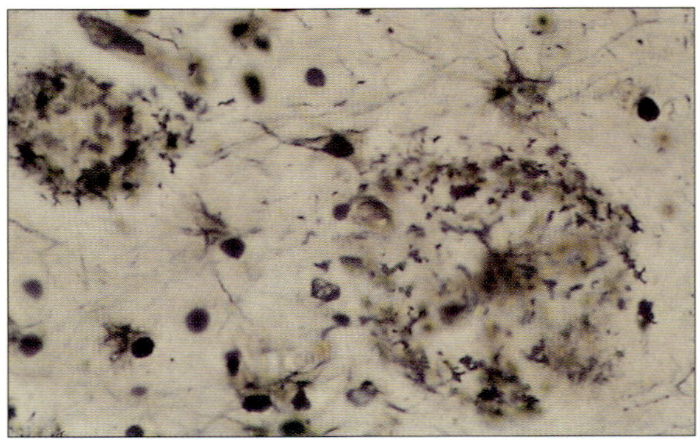

7.45 Von Braunmuhl's silver impregnation technique stains multiple neuritic processes around mature plaques in Alzheimer's disease.

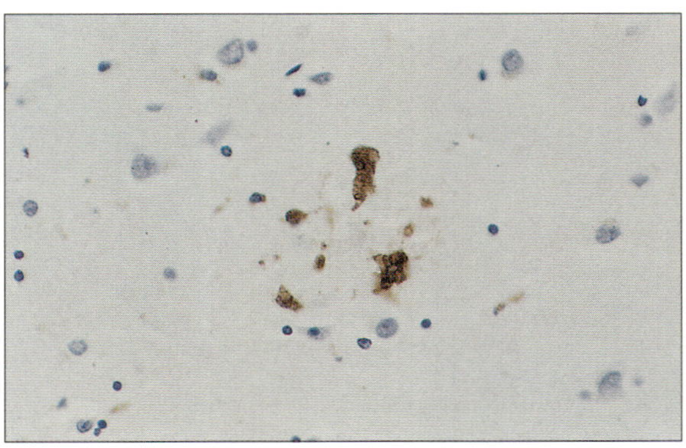

7.46 Microglial cells within a neuritic plaque are stained brown on immunocytochemistry for the CD68 epitope.

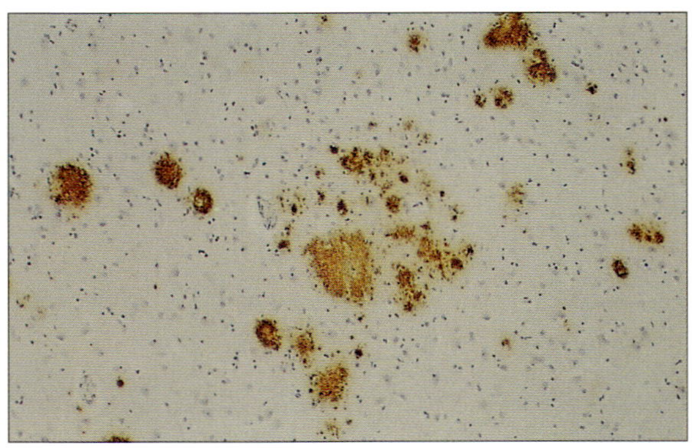

7.47 Immunocytochemistry for Alzheimer's precursor protein in the temporal cortex in Alzheimer's disease shows a large mature plaque (centre) with smaller 'burnt-out' plaques on either side.

There is enormous variability in the distribution and extent of these lesions within the CNS from patient to patient, and the severity of the histological changes must be assessed in relation to age-related changes for diagnostic purposes. Standardised criteria, such as CERAD (*see Further Reading*), have been established for the neuropathological assessment of these lesions in Alzheimer's disease.

Changes similar to those in Alzheimer's disease occur in patients with Down's syndrome (trisomy 21, *Chapter 9*) from the fourth decade onwards. These have been attributed to the extra genetic load, since APP is encoded by a gene on chromosome 21. APP can be detected by immunocytochemistry in increased quantities following diffuse axonal injury (*see Chapter 5*), but the relationship of this finding to the pathoenetic mechanisms in Alzheimer's disease is unclear.

Pick's disease

Pick's disease is an uncommon disorder that occasionally occurs as an autosomal dominant disease. It presents as a rapidly progressive dementia and affects males more frequently than females, usually in late middle-age with death occurring within 2–4 years.

Macroscopic examination of the brain in Pick's disease shows severe cerebral atrophy, the brain often weighing less than 1kg. The frontal and temporal lobes are particularly severely involved (**7.50**) and the deep grey matter structures often appear atrophied. This reduction in brain size is accompanied by compensatory ventricular dilation (**7.51**).

Histological examination in Pick's disease shows widespread neuronal loss, particularly in the frontal and temporal cortex where nerve cell loss may be so

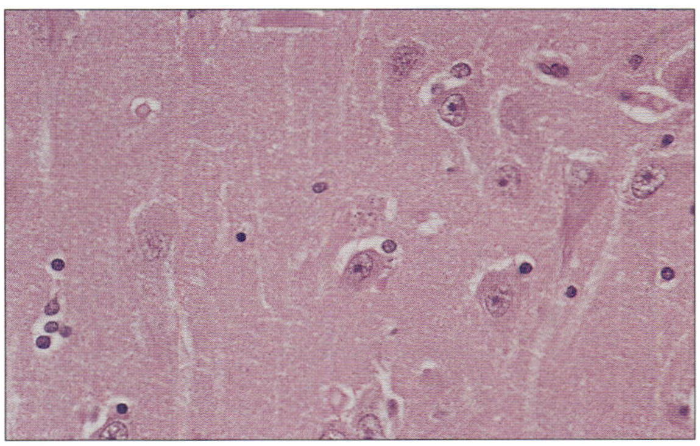

7.48 Hippocampal pyramidal neurons in Alzheimer's disease show granulovacuolar degeneration (centre), with numerous rounded inclusions containing a dot-like central core.

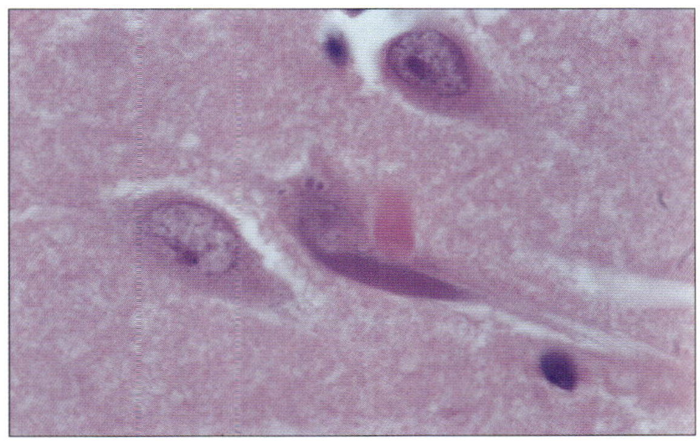

7.49 A hippocampal pyramidal neuron in Alzheimer's disease contains an eosinophilic Hirano body (centre) and a basophilic neurofibrillary tangle (bottom).

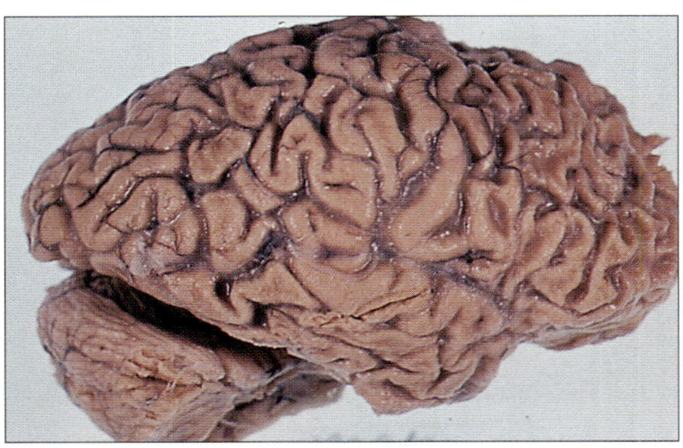

7.50 Pick's disease is characterised by circumscribed atrophy of the frontal and temporal lobes which are markedly reduced in size, in contrast to the more global atrophy present in Alzheimer's disease.

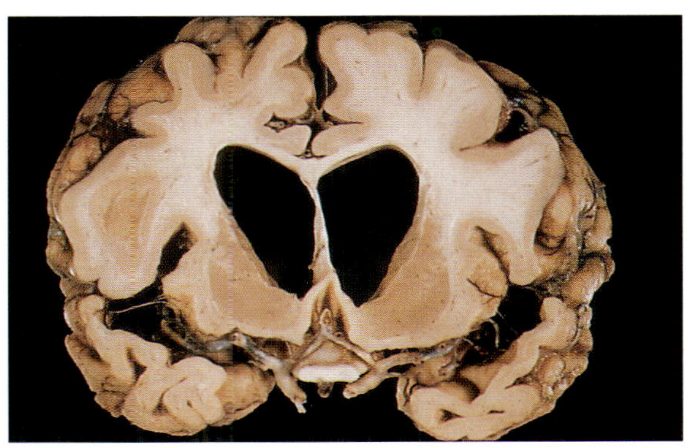

7.51 In addition to severe frontotemporal atrophy, the basal ganglia in Pick's disease are usually severely shrunken, with compensatory ventricular dilatation.

severe as to cause collapse of the cortical cytoarchitecture (**7.52**). Astrocytosis is prominent in these regions and in the underlying white matter. Surviving nerve cells may contain rounded, well-circumscribed, basophilic, cytoplasmic inclusions referred to as Pick bodies. These are argyrophilic and give a positive staining reaction on immunocytochemistry for tau (**7.53**) and ubiquitin. Other nerve cells appear enlarged with a characteristic ballooned shape, referred to as Pick cells (**7.54**). The cytoplasm of these cells is argyrophilic and may give a positive staining reaction on immunocytochemistry for neurofilament protein and αB crystallin.

Huntington's disease

This disorder is inherited as an autosomal-dominant disease affecting 4–7 per 100,000 of the population in the UK. The gene for this disorder is present on chromosome 4 and has now been cloned. The genetic abnormalities in this disorder are complex, involving numbers of insert repeat extra sequences. Genetic counselling and prospective risk assessment are now available for individuals with a family history. The disease onset usually occurs in the fifth decade of life with personality change and depression. These are accompanied by a movement disorder including chorea and myoclonus with dementia as a late feature.

The most striking abnormality on naked-eye inspection of the brain in Huntington's disease is severe atrophy of the basal ganglia, particularly the caudate nucleus, which is often concave in outline rather than convex as in normal individuals (**7.55**). Other deep grey matter structures may appear atrophied, and mild cerebral cortical atrophy is

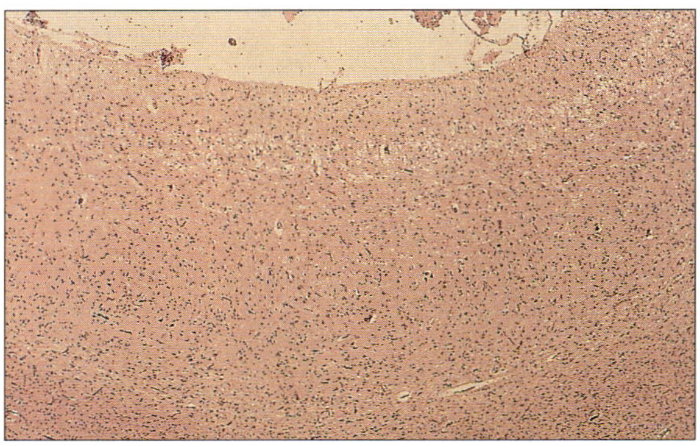

7.52 Severe neuronal loss in the temporal cortex in Pick's disease results in collapse of the cortical cytoarchitecture, with status spongiosus in layer II. The cortex appears hypercellular as a result of severe gliosis.

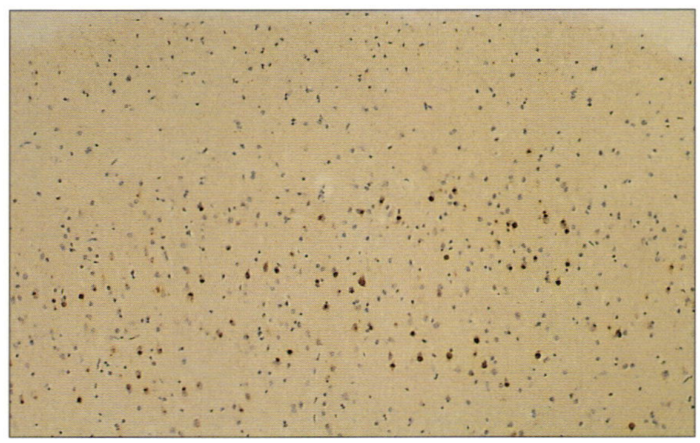

7.53 Immunocytochemistry for tau in the temporal cortex in Pick's disease shows a positive brown stain of rounded neuronal inclusions (Pick bodies).

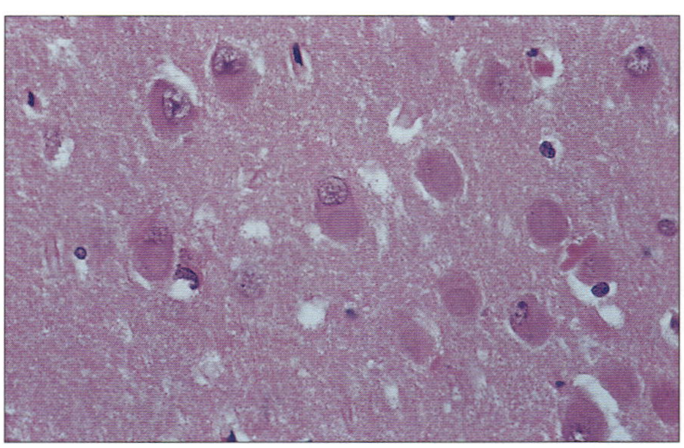

7.54 Pick bodies are visible as rounded basophilic inclusions in sections stained with haematoxylin and eosin (centre). Other neurons in Pick's disease appear swollen with no obvious cytoplasmic inclusions (right); these are referred to as Pick cells.

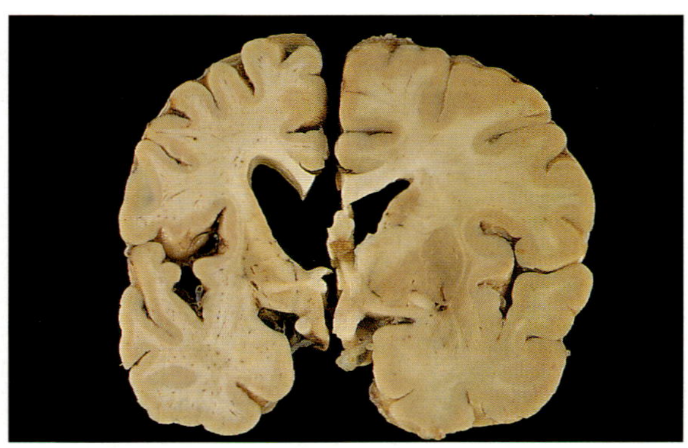

7.55 In Huntington's disease (left), the basal ganglia are markedly atrophic with a concave outline in contrast to an age-matched normal control case (right). The cerebral cortex in Huntington's disease also appears atrophic.

usually evident, though not to the same degree as in Alzheimer's disease. Other disorders may cause atrophy of the basal ganglia (**7.56**), which in itself is not specific for Huntington's disease.

On histology there is a marked loss of small to intermediate-sized neurons (mainly spiny interneurons) in the caudate nucleus accompanied by astrocytosis. Neuronal loss may be evident in other areas of the brain including the cerebral cortex, thalamus and cerebellum. No characteristic inclusions are present in the nerve cells in this disease. In the juvenile variant of Huntington's disease, cerebellar involvement may be more prominent with cerebellar atrophy being evident on naked-eye inspection and loss of Purkinje cell and granular cell neurons on histological examination. The precise mechanism of nerve cell death in this disorder is unknown, but other information on the pathogenesis of this disease is anticipated once further genetic studies are completed.

Diffuse Lewy body disease

Recent clinical and neuropathological studies have suggested that this disorder may be the second commonest form of primary dementia in the UK, after Alzheimer's disease. The clinical features of the dementia differ from those in Alzheimer's disease: visual and auditory hallucinations are common and memory loss is less severe. As its name implies, this disorder is characterised by the presence of Lewy body inclusions, not only in the pigmented nuclei in the thalamus and brainstem but in a wider distribution throughout the cerebral cortex. The cortical changes are accompanied by neuronal loss and astrocytosis, with occasional cases containing numerous Alzheimer-type senile plaques. Lewy bodies in the cerebral cortex occur in a characteristic distribution, involving particularly the frontal and temporal poles and anterior cingulate gyrus. They are sometimes difficult to identify on routinely stained sections, but can be stained by silver impregnation techniques and more effectively by ubiquitin immunocytochemisty (*see* **7.29**).

Dementia of frontal lobe type

In this uncommon syndrome, the clinical features of dementia are usually accompanied by progressive aphasia, with widespread neuronal loss and gliosis which is centred on the frontal lobe (**7.57**). A similar syndrome may also occur in patients with motor neuron disease; in these cases the filamentous inclusions which are characteristic of motor nuclei in this disorder may also occur within nerve cells of the cerebral cortex, particularly in the frontal lobes.

Parkinsonism–dementia complex of Guam

There is a high incidence of dementia in the Chamorro tribe of Guam, usually accompanied by parkinsonism and, in a few cases, clinical features of motor neuron disease (amyotrophic lateral sclerosis). This unique disorder is responsible for up to 10% of all adult deaths in this tribe. Macroscopic examination of the CNS shows cerebral atrophy and depigmentation of the substantia nigra. Histological examination shows widespread neuronal loss with numerous cortical neurofibrillary tangles but no other neuronal inclusions or senile plaques. The aetiology of this rare disorder is unknown, but a toxic substance, such as a heavy metal or the cycad seed, has been implicated in several studies.

Disorders causing atrophy of the basal ganglia
Huntington's disease
Pick's disease
Creutzfeldt–Jakob disease
Striatonigral degeneration
Multiple system atrophy
Neuroaxonal dystrophy
Chronic hepatic encephalopathy and Wilson's disease (*Chapter 8*)

7.56 Disorders causing atrophy of the basal ganglia.

Disorders associated with dementia of frontal lobe type
Pick's disease
Dementia in motor neuron disease
Diffuse Lewy body disease
Parkinsonism–dementia complex of Guam
Corticobasal degeneration

7.57 Disorders associated with dementia of frontal lobe type.

SECONDARY DEMENTIAS

Transmissible spongiform encephalopathy

This group of conditions is unique among the neurodegenerative disorders in humans because it has sporadic, infectious (iatrogenic) and genetic forms. The commonest variety is the sporadic form of Creutzfeldt–Jakob disease, which occurs in about one per million of the population per annum. This disorder is characterised by a rapidly progressive dementia accompanied by focal neurological signs, including extrapyramidal signs and myoclonus. The EEG often shows a characteristic spike-and-wave abnormality. Familial Creutzfeldt–Jakob disease is thought to account for up to 15% of all cases, and is related to another rare autosomal dominant condition, the Gerstmann–Straussler–Scheinker syndrome. These human disorders resemble similar conditions in animals (**7.58**).

All these conditions are transmissible, particularly by inoculation of CNS material from affected individuals. In humans, Creutzfeldt–Jakob disease has been inadvertently transmitted by intracerebral electrodes, corneal grafts, dura mater grafts and by subcutaneous injections of human pituitary-derived growth hormone or gonadotrophin. There is, however, no evidence at present to suggest that the related animal orders are transmissible to man.

The Fore tribe in New Guinea suffered from a disorder known as kuru, a form of human spongiform encepalopathy which was transmitted from individual to individual by ritualistic inoculation or endocannibalism.

In Creutzfeldt–Jakob disease, naked-eye inspection of the brain may show no significant abnormalities, particularly if there is a rapid clinical course. In cases with a longer history (of about two years or more), there may be marked cortical atrophy in a global distribution. Cerebellar atrophy is common, particularly in cases associated with growth hormone therapy, and in the Gerstmann–Straussler–Scheinker syndrome. On cross-section, the cerebral cortex and basal ganglia may appear atrophied (**7.59**).

Four main histological abnormalities are characteristic of this group of disorders:

- spongiform change;
- neuronal loss;
- astrocytosis;
- amyloid plaques.

Spongiform change describes the presence of small empty vacuoles within affected grey matter (**7.60**). These vacuoles measure up to 200μm in diameter and are usually present within the neuropil, but occasional neurons may contain a vacuole within the cytoplasm. In advanced cases, the vacuoles may become confluent to form larger rounded cystic structures. This abnormality is extremely variable in its severity and distribution in affected cases, but the cerebellar molecular layer is usually involved, as are the frontal cortex and basal ganglia. Prion protein (PrP) can be detected by immunocytochemistry around the spongiform vacuoles (**7.61**).

Neuronal loss accompanies spongiform change, and may sometimes be so severe as to cause collapse of the cytoarchitecture of the grey matter (status spongiosus). Cerebral cortical neuronal loss is extremely

Transmissible spongiform encephalopathies

Animal disorders	
Naturally occurring	Scrapie
Transmitted disorders	Bovine spongiform encephalopathy Feline spongiform encephalopathy Transmissible mink encephalopathy Spongiform encephalopathy in kudu and other exotic ruminants Experimental scrapie in mice and hamsters
Human disorders	
Naturally occurring	Sporadic Creutzfeldt–Jakob disease Familial Creutzfeldt–Jakob disease Gerstmann–Straussler–Scheinker syndrome Fatal familial insomnia
Transmitted disorders	Iatrogenic Creutzfeldt–Jakob disease Kuru

7.58 Transmissible spongiform encephalopathies.

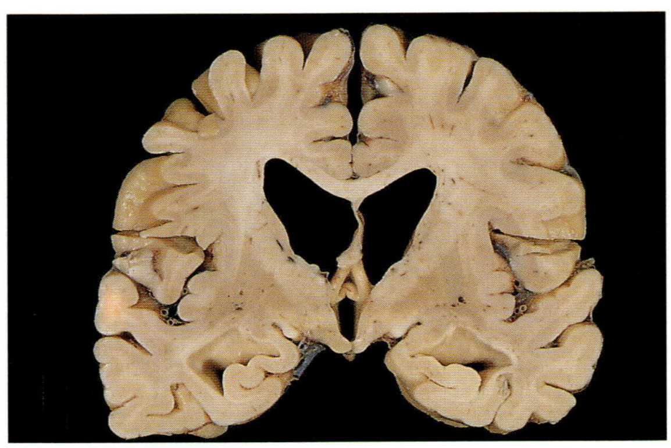

7.59 The cerebral hemispheres in Creutzfeldt–Jakob disease often exhibit cortical atrophy, with shrinkage of the basal ganglia.

variable in severity and distribution from case to case; cerebellar cortical neuronal loss is particularly severe in iatrogenic cases associated with growth hormone therapy.

Astrocytosis usually accompanies neuronal loss (**7.62**); large number of microglial cells are also evident, while amyloid plaques are present in about 15% of cases of Creutzfeldt–Jakob disease, but are much more frequent in Gerstmann–Straussler–Scheinker syndrome and in cases of Creutzfeldt–Jakob disease associated with growth hormone therapy. These amyloid plaques are most frequently found in the cerebellum, in contrast to those seen in Alzheimer's disease. Their chemical composition differs from Alzheimer-type senile plaques, being composed of PrP. This is an abnormal truncated form of a cell-surface glycoprotein encoded by a gene on chromosome 20. Many cases of familial Creutzfeldt–Jakob disease and Gerstmann–Straussler–Scheinker syndrome have identifiable mutations in this gene. The plaques will give a positive reaction with Congo red, PAS and Alcian blue techniques, and by immunocytochemistry for PrP (**7.63**).

The precise nature of the transmissible agent responsible for this group of disorders is unknown. There is substantial evidence to implicate the prion protein as an important constituent of the infectious agent, and some research groups have suggested that the protein alone is responsible for the characteristic transmissibility of the disease. The infectious agent

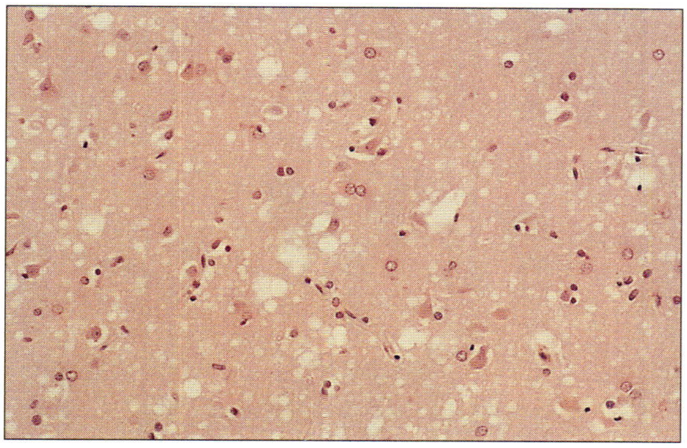

7.60 Spongiform change in the cerebral cortex in Creutzfeldt–Jakob disease is characterised by numerous small rounded vacuoles which become coalescent. Some of the vacuoles appear to be closely related to nerve cell bodies (centre). Neuronal loss and astrocytosis are accompanying features.

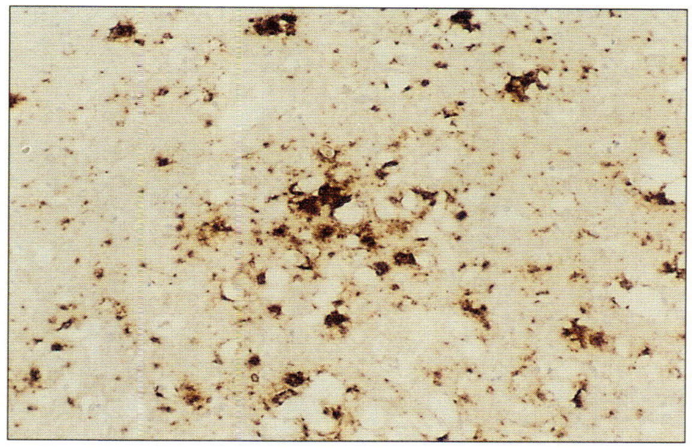

7.61 Immunocytochemistry for prion protein in the cerebral cortex in Creutzfeldt–Jakob disease shows dense brown positive staining around areas of spongiform change.

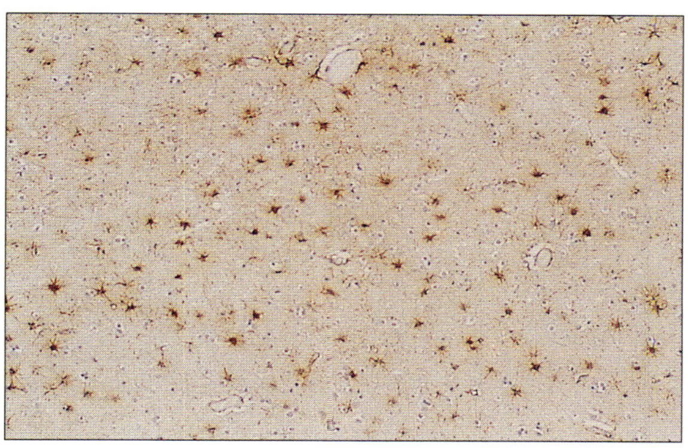

7.62 Immunocytochemistry for GFAP in a case of fatal familial insomnia, a rare human prion disease, shows widespread astrocytosis in the thalamus.

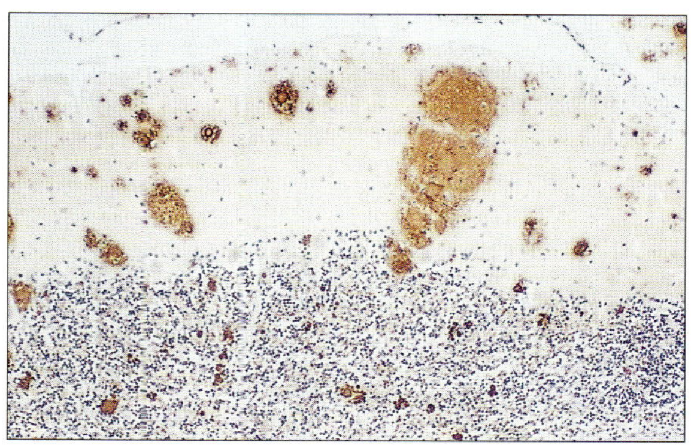

7.63 Immunocytochemistry for prion protein (PrP) in the Gerstmann–Straussler–Scheinker syndrome shows numerous brown PrP plaques within the cerebellar cortex.

resists many standard decontamination techniques, but infectivity can be substantially reduced if not abolished by exposure to 2N sodium hydroxide, 96% formic acid and autoclaving at 136°C for one hour. Protocols for autopsy procedure in suspected cases have been established (*see Further Reading*).

Vascular dementia

Cerebrovascular disease is a common cause of morbidity in the elderly. In some patients it is associated with a progressive stepwise cognitive impairment, which is usually accompanied by focal neurological disability, including stroke (*see Chapter 4*). Two main groups of vascular dementia can be recognised.

Multi-infarct dementia

Multi-infarct dementia is common, accounting for about 10–15% of all cases of dementia and may occur with Alzheimer's disease. As its name implies, this disorder is characterised by numerous infarcts in the brain, though these are markedly variable in their extent and distribution (**7.64**). In a minority of cases, there are multiple small infarcts in subcortical grey matter structures, the cerebral cortex appearing relatively spared (**7.65**). Retrospective studies have implied a relationship between the dementia and the total volume of infarction in the brain, with dementia occurring in all cases where more than 100ml of the brain has been damaged.

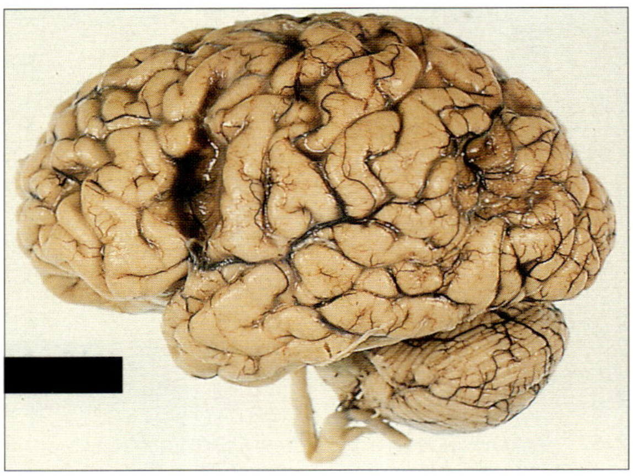

7.64 In multi-infarct dementia, numerous areas of infarction are present in a wide distribution throughout the cerebral cortex. The vertebral and basilar arteries in this case are markedly atheromatous.

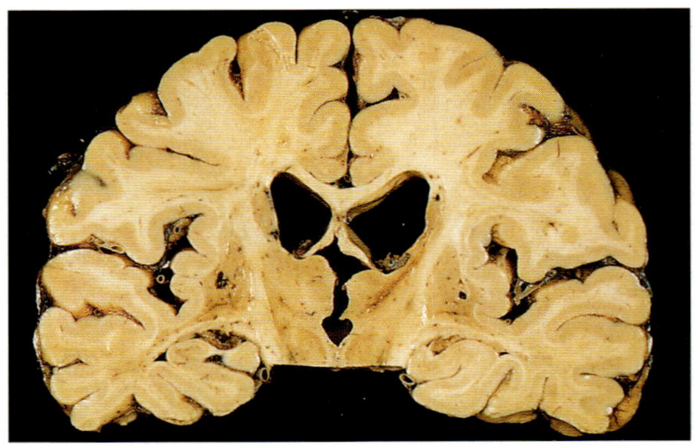

7.65 In some cases of multi-infarct dementia, there is predominant involvement of subcortical structures. This case shows evidence of infarction in the thalamus and caudate nucleus on the right and the globus pallidus and putamen on the left.

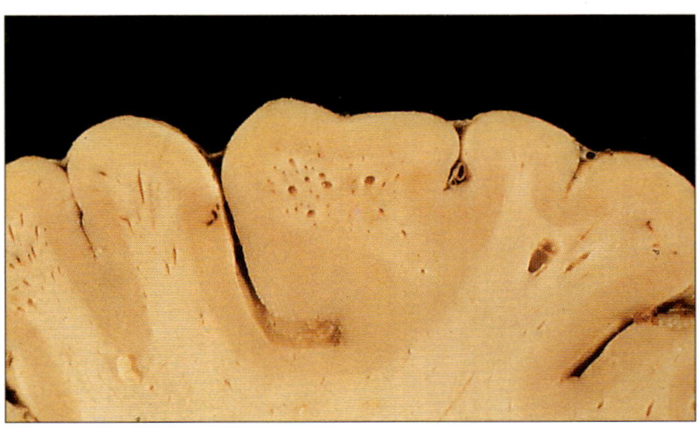

7.66 In Binswanger's disease, ischaemic damage is centred around small arteriosclerotic blood vessels in the subcortical white matter.

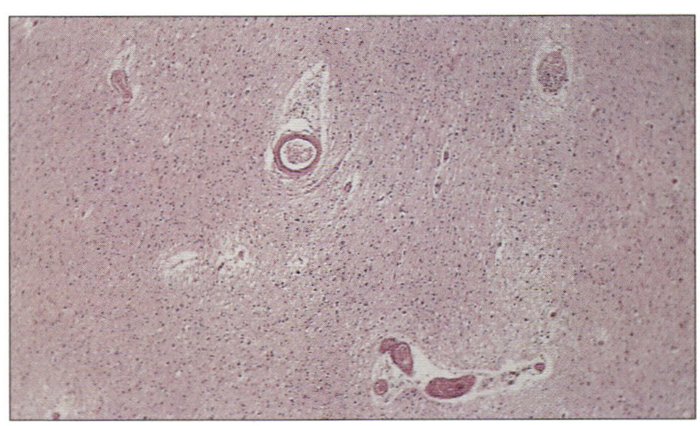

7.67 Histology of the subcortical white matter in Binswanger's disease shows marked arteriosclerosis, with widening of the perivascular space and microinfarcts.

Binswanger's disease
This uncommon form of vascular dementia occurs most fequently in the elderly and in patients with chronic hypertension and diabetes mellitus, and is associated with ischaemic damage in the subcortical white matter (**7.66**) rather than extensive cortical infarction.

Naked-eye inspection of the brain shows a reduction in the volume of the central white matter, with numerous small cavitated lesions and ventricular enlargement. This is accompanied histologically with a loss of axons and myelin with astrocytosis.

The intracerebral arterioles in these regions show marked arteriosclerosis (**7.67**). It has been suggested that progressive narrowing of the lumen of these vessels eventually diminishes cerebral blood flow to the central white matter regions, with impaired perfusion resulting in ischaemic damage.

Miscellaneous disorders

Paraneoplastic syndromes
Dementia may occur as a non-metastatic complication in patients with systemic neoplasms, particularly a small cell anaplastic ('oat-cell') carcinoma of the bronchus. In these patients, histological studies sometimes reveal evidence of a limbic encephalitis, with perivascular lymphocytic cuffing in the temporal lobe. Other patients have been shown to have a circulating antibody which binds to the nuclei of neuronal and glial cells in the CNS; this is sometimes referred to as an antiHu antibody (**7.68, 7.69**). The mechanism of host sensitisation is unknown, but this reaction may represent an antigenic cross-reaction to a tumour antigen.

AIDS
Dementia may be a prominent clinical finding in patients with AIDS, and in some cases may be a presenting feature It has been linked to HIV encephalitis, but this proposed relationship requires further research (*see Chapter 3*).

Schizophrenia
Although not usually considered as a neurodegenerative disorder, recent neuroradiological studies have demonstrated subtle structural abnormalities in the CNS, with reduced volumes of temporal lobe structures (particularly the hippocampus) and evidence of ventricular dilatation. The aetiology of these abnormalities is uncertain; both genetic and obstetric factors have been implicated.

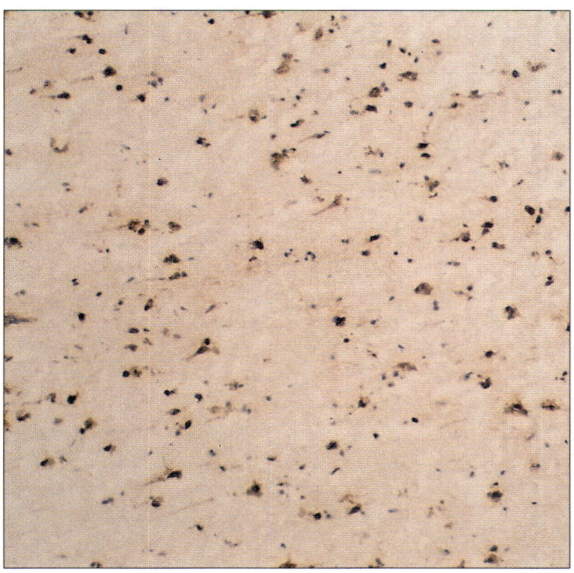

7.68 In the antiHu paraneoplastic syndrome, a circulating antibody in the serum binds to the nuclei of small cortical neurons and glial cells.

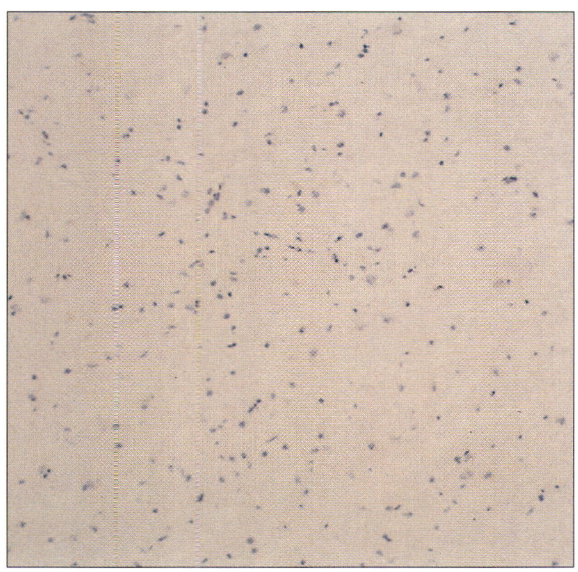

7.69 Control section of cerebral cortex for comparison with **7.68**.

FURTHER READING

Advisory Committee on Dangerous Pathogens. *Precautions for Work with Human and Animal Transmissible Spongiform Encephalopathies*. London, HMSO, 1994.

Oppenheimer DR, Esiri MM. Diseases of the Basal Ganglia, Cerebellum and Motor Neurons. In: Adams JH, Duchen LW. Greenfield's *Neuropathology*. 5th edn. London, Edward Arnold, 1992, pp 988–1045.

Mirra SS, Heyman A, McKeel D, Sumi SM, Crain BJ, Brownlee LM, Vogel FS, Hughes JP, Van Belle G, Berg L. The consortium to establish a registry for Alzheimer's disease (CERAD). Part II. Standardisation of the neuropathological assessment of Alzheimer's disease. *Neurology* **41**: 479–486, 1991.

Poirier J, Gray F, Escourolle R. *Manual of Basic Neuropathology.* Philadelphia, WB Saunders, 1990, pp 139–162.

Prusiner SB, Collinge J, Powell J, Anderton B (eds). *Prion Diseases of Humans and Animals*. Chichester, Ellis Horwood, 1992.

Rewcastle NB. Degenerative Diseases of the Nervous System. In: Davis RL, Robertson DM (eds). *Textbook of Neuropathology*. 2nd edn. Baltimore, Williams and Wilkins 1990, pp 904–961.

Roberts GW, Leigh PN, Weinberger DR. *Neuropsychiatric Disorders.* London, Mosby–Wolfe, 1993.

8. Metabolic and Nutritional Disorders

PRIMARY CNS METABOLIC DISORDERS

Many of the neurodegenerative diseases that have their onset in early life are the result of an inherited metabolic error, in which a critical enzyme system(s) is either absent or inactive due to the expression of a defective gene. This enzyme deficiency leads to early functional failure in the organ system most affected by the disorder. This is principally the nervous system in some metabolic disorders, while in others the nervous system is spared. Primary CNS metabolic diseases should be distinguished from those diseases which are secondary to functional disturbance in other organ systems, e.g. hepatic encephalopathy associated with liver disease. The secondary metabolic disorders are considered later in this chapter.

In many primary CNS metabolic disorders, the enzyme deficiency has been identified, the pathological features are well known, and in some the genetic background is now understood. In other diseases, the metabolic and genetic defects have still to be elucidated. There is considerable overlap in clinical and pathological features between individual diseases within this group. This is partly because the tissues that are most damaged are exactly similar in more than one condition. Overlap may also be caused by the presence of multiple enzyme defects, so different diseases may share one or more enzyme deficiency. The manner in which enzyme deficiency/ies leads to tissue damage is not well understood in all instances. The recent investigation of previously obscure diseases, such as the mitochondrial cytopathies, is adding to the known range of inherited CNS diseases and throwing new light on their aetiology.

CLASSIFICATION

Traditionally, these diseases have been classified on the basis of morphological abnormalities, such as the presence of neuronal storage products (storage disorders) or of white matter damage (leucodystrophies). More recently, there has been a refinement of classification, based on the subcellular localisation of the enzyme deficiency, whether it is in lysosomes, mitochondria or peroxisomes. The working classification generally adopted at present combines these two approaches, though not always satisfactorily. Some diseases which could legitimately be classified as leucodystrophies, e.g. X-linked adrenoleucodystrophy, are now known to be associated with the deficiency of a peroxisomal enzyme and might properly be reclassified in the peroxisomal group of disorders. Similarly, some mitochondrial cytopathies also show white matter vacuolation, posing as leucodystrophies. Another difficulty is that some diseases, such as adult Refsum's disease, are still poorly understood and evade proper classification despite their clear metabolic basis. Undoubtedly, there will be further modifications to the classification system in the future. In this chapter, there are synopses of clinical features, mode of inheritance and metabolic defects for each group of diseases (**8.1–8.8**). However, these synopses are indicative only and should not be regarded as either comprehensive or exclusive. The present classification includes the following groups:

- lysosomal storage disorders, the clinical features of which are summarised in **8.1–8.4**. They comprise the lipidoses, mucopolysaccharidoses, mucolipidoses, and glycogenoses;
- leucodystrophies, which can be divided into the metabolic leucodystrophies (**8.5**) and other leucodystrophies (**8.6**);
- peroxisomal disorders (**8.7**);
- mitochondrial cytopathies (**8.8**);
- other inherited disorders with a metabolic basis, including Wilson's disease, Menkes' disease, adult Refsum's disease, Lesch–Nyhan syndrome, and Lafora body disease.

CLINICAL FEATURES

Depending upon which systems are involved in the metabolic disorder, the disease may be characterised by:

- neurological symptoms alone;
- neurological symptoms in association with other systemic abnormalities;
- non-neurological symptoms in isolation.

Each disease may display a spectrum of signs and symptoms, particularly with regard to age of onset and clinical severity. Conversely, a number of different diseases may share one particular distinctive abnormality, such as the cherry-red spot of the macula which may be present in Tay–Sachs disease, Niemann–Pick disease, Farber's disease, mucolipodosis 1 and metachromatic leucodystrophy. This retinal abnormality arises non-specifically from storage of any abnormal product.

Individuals with a metabolic disease are often normal at birth and show signs and symptoms of

CNS lipidoses (lipid storage disorders)

Disease	Age of onset & inheritance pattern	Clinical features	Other organ/tissue involvement	Storage product	Enzyme deficiency
Niemann-Pick disease	Infantile, juvenile, adult Autosomal recessive	Spectrum including atypical cases; hepatosplenomegaly; dementia; cherry-red spot of macula; seizures	Liver, spleen, lymph nodes, endothelium, smooth muscle	Sphingomyelin in most	Sphingomyelinase
Gaucher's disease	Adults, juveniles, infants Autosomal recessive	Mild in adults; more severe in children; splenomegaly; fractures; failure to thrive; some intellectual decline myoclonus; no neurological deficiency in adults	Spleen, liver, lymph nodes, skeletal system	Glucocerebroside	Glucocerebrosidase
G_{M1} gangliosidosis	Infantile (type I), juvenile (type II), adult (type III) Autosomal recessive	Mental deterioration; cardiomyopathy; cherry-red spot; siezures	Spleen, liver, heart	Ganglioside G_{M1} (oligosaccharides in non-CNS organs)	β galactosidase, (low or absent in types I and II; inactive in type III
G_{M2} gangliosidosis, Tay-Sachs disease	Infantile (Tay-Sachs disease); (Sandhoff's disease) late infantile, juvenile, adult Autosomal recessive	Retardation; progressive dementia; decerebrate state spasticity; siezures; blindness; cherry-red spot	Mild hepatosplenomegaly in Sandhoff's disease	Ganglioside G_{M2} +globoside in Sandhoff's disease	Hexosaminidase A and B
Ceroid lipofuscinosis, Batten's disease	Infantile, late infantile, early juvenile, adult (Kufs) Autosomal recessive	Progressive dementia; hypotonia; myoclonus; seizures; blindness	Spleen, lymph nodes, smooth muscle, endothelium	Ceroid lipofuscin Oligosaccharides	?
Wolman's disease	Infantile Autosomal-recessive	Failure to thrive; anaemia; fever; yellow organs	Liver, spleen, adrenals	Triglycerides, cholesterylesters	Acid lipase
Farber's disease	Infantile ?	Painful joints; mental decline; respiratory problems; cherry-red spot	Spleen, lymph nodes, endothelium	Ceramide	Ceramidase
Fabry's disease	Juvenile X-linked recessive	Cutaneous telangiectasis; renal failure; impaired autonomic function; strokes; aneurysms	Skin, kidney, eye, endothelium	Trihexosyl ceramide, glycolipids	α galactosidase A

8.1–8.3 Features of lipid and glycosaminoglycan storage disorders.

CNS mucopolysaccharidoses (glycosaminoglycans storage disorders)					
Disease	**Age of onset & inheritance pattern**	**Clinical features**	**Other organ/tissue involvement**	**Storage product**	**Enzyme deficiency**
Type I MPS Hurler's disease	Infantile Autosomal recessive	Coarse facies; mental retardation; corneal clouding; mitral incompetence	Heart, liver, spleen, skeletal system	Dermatan sulphate	Iduronidase
Sheie's disease	Juvenile Autosomal recessive	Stiff joints; corneal clouding; CNS not involved	Skeletal system, heart, liver, spleen	Dermatan sulphate, heparan sulphate	Iduronidase
Type II MPS Hunter's disease	Infantile X-linked recessive	Resembles type I but milder and no corneal clouding	All involved	Dermatan sulphate	Iduronate sulphatase
Type III MPS Sanfilippo's disease	Infantile Autosomal recessive	Mental retardation; coarse facies; hirsuitism	Less than in types I and II	Heparan sulphate	Heparan sulphatase and others
Type IV MPS Morquio's disease	Infantile Autosomal recessive	Aortic disease; normal intellect; coarse facies; short stature; mild corneal clouding	As in type I; less hepatomegaly	Keratan sulphate	Sulphatase Galactosidase
Type VI MPS Maroteaux-Lamy disease	Juvenile Autosomal recessive	No mental retardation; severe bone changes; corneal clouding	As in type II; less hepatomegaly	Dermatan sulphate	Sulphatase

CNS mucolipidoses (glycosaminoglycans and lipid storage disorders)					
Disease	**Age of onset & inheritance pattern**	**Clinical features**	**Other organ/tissue involvement**	**Storage product**	**Enzyme deficiency**
Sialidosis (mucolipidosis I)	Infantile, juvenile, adult Autosomal recessive	Variable: resemble GM1 cases; myoclonus; cherry-red spot; no neurological deficiency or dysmorphism; mental retardation; visual loss	Variable, liver spleen, skeleton	Sialic-rich oligosaccharides	Neuraminadase
Mucolipidosis II I cell disease	Infantile Autosomal recessive	Similar to Hurler's skeletal deformity; intellectual retardation; inclusions in cultured fibroblasts (I cells)	Liver, spleen, skeleton and other tissues	Muco-polysaccharides glycolipid	Several acid hydrolases
Mannosidosis	Infantile, juvenile Autosomal recessive	Intellectual retardation; coarse facies; resemble MPS; prone to infection	Liver, spleen, skeleton	Mannose-rich oligosaccharides	α mannosidase A
Fucosidosis	Infantile, juvenile Autosomal recessive	Coarse facies; resemble MPS I; mental retardation; prone to infection	Liver, skeleton (focal)	Fucose-rich polysaccharides; glycosphingolipids and oligosaccharides	α I fucosidase

CNS glycogenoses (glycogen storage disorders)					
Disease	**Age of onset & inheritance pattern**	**Clinical features**	**Other organ/tissue involvement**	**Storage product**	**Enzyme deficiency**
Type I von Gierke's disease	Juvenile Autosomal recessive	Hepatomegaly; stunted growth; hypoglycaemia	Liver	Glycogen	Glucose-6-phosphatase
Type II Pompe's disease	Infantile, juvenile, adult Autosomal recessive	Hypotonia; cardiomegaly; muscle weakness	Muscle, heart, kidney	Glycogen in CNS	Acid maltase
Type III	Juvenile Autosomal recessive	Muscle weakness; hepatomegaly	Liver, muscle, heart	Glycogen	Debrancher enzyme glucosidase
Type IV	Juvenile Autosomal recessive	Hepatomegaly	Liver	Glycogen	Brancher enzyme transglucosidase
Type V McArdle's disease	Juvenile Autosomal recessive	Muscle weakness	Muscle	Glycogen	Muscle phosphorylase
Type VI	Juvenile Autosomal recessive	Hepatomegaly	Liver	Glycogen	Liver phosphorylase
Type VII	Juvenile Autosomal recessive	Muscle weakness	Muscle	Glycogen	Muscle phosphorylase
Type VIII	Juvenile X-linked recessive	Hepatomegaly	Liver	Glycogen	Liver phosphorylase

8.4 Features of glycogen storage disorders.

Metabolic leucodystrophies					
Disease	**Age of onset & inheritance pattern**	**Clinical features**	**Other organ/tissue involvement**	**Storage product**	**Enzyme deficiency**
Metachromatic leucodystrophy	Infantile, juvenile, adult Autosomal recessive	Psychomotor deterioration; behavioural and gait disturbance; psychosis; dementia; motor signs	Kidney, gall bladder	Sulphatides, cerebroside sulphate	Arylsulphatase A
Krabbe's leucodystrophy	Infantile, juvenile, adult Autosomal recessive	Psychomotor deterioration; myoclonus; blindness	None	Galactocerebroside in globoid cells	Galacto-cerebrosidase
Adreno-leucodystrophy	Juvenile, adult X-linked, usually recessive	Variable dementia; seizures; visual loss adrenal insufficiency	Adrenals	Long chain fatty acid esters	Peroxisomal lignoceroyl; co-enzyme A synthetase

8.5 Features of metabolic leukodystrophies.

neurological impairment only some months after birth. Depending on the severity and topography of CNS involvement, the affected individual may develop various symptoms, including cognitive impairment progressing to dementia, seizures, visual loss, ataxia, spasticity or peripheral neuropathy (**8.1–8.8**). Atypical cases are common and these, together with the variable age of onset and clinical severity, can make it difficult to establish an exact diagnosis unless the results of other investigations are also available.

INHERITANCE

The vast majority of these disorders are inherited in an autosomal-recessive fashion with occasional

Other leucodystrophies

Disease	Age of onset & inheritance pattern	Clinical features	Other organ/tissue involvement	Storage product	Enzyme deficiency
Canavan's disease	Infantile, juvenile Autosomal recessive	Macrocephaly; psychomotor arrest; myoclonus; seizures; blindness	None	None known	? aspartoacyclase
Alexander's disease	Infantile, juvenile, adult ? autosomal recessive ? sporadic	Psychomotor retardation; spacticity; seizures	None	None known	?
Pelizaeus–Merzbacher disease	Infantile juvenile X-linked recessive	Psychomotor arrest; nystagmus; choreoathetosis	None	None known	? defective synthesis of myelin lipids
	Adult Autosomal dominant	Psychosis; ataxia	None	None known	?
Cockayne's syndrome	Infantile Autosomal recessive	Dermatitis; dwarfism; microcephaly; retinitis pigmentosa	Skeleton, kidneys	None known	?

8.6 Features of other leukodystrophies.

Peroxisomal disorders

Disease	Age of onset & inheritance pattern	Clinical features	Other organ/tissue involvement	Storage product	Enzyme deficiency
Zellweger's syndrome	Infantile Autosomal recessive	Hypotonia; facial dysmorphism; seizures; psychomotor retardation	Liver, kidney	Abnormal bile acids, cholesterol, very long chain fatty acids	Multiple peroxisomal defects
Infantile Refsum's disease	Neonatal	Mental retardation; retinitis pigmentosa	Liver, adrenal	Phytanic acid	Multiple peroxisomal defects
Neonatal adreno-leucodystrophy	At birth Autosomal recessive	Hypotonia; seizures; failure to thrive; blindness	Adrenal, liver	?	Multiple peroxisomal defects

8.7 Features of peroxisomal disorders.

examples of X-linked recessive inheritance, and genetic counselling should be made available to families in which these diagnoses are made. Some metabolic disorders are particularly common in certain ethnic groups. For instance, Niemann–Pick 's disease, Gaucher's disease, Tay–Sachs disease and Canavan's disease are all found more commonly in Ashkenazi Jews than in other populations. The carrier rate of Tay–Sachs disease in Ashkenazi Jews is one in 30.

Among the mitochondrial diseases, sporadic cases are also recognised and some may be autosomally dominant (**8.8**). Mitochondria possess their own DNA, which is arranged on one circular chromosome and encodes cytochromes and ATPase. Many other mitochondrial activities are under the control of the nuclear genome. Multiple deletions of mitochondrial DNA may be associated with autosomal-dominant conditions. Maternal transmission is an important factor in the inheritance of mitochondrial cytopathies since mitochondria are usually passed on to progeny from the oocyte rather than the sperm.

DIAGNOSIS

In many of these diseases the metabolic pathways, enzyme deficiency and accumulating product have all been identified (**8.9**), thus increasing the accuracy of both the diagnosis in patients with clinical symptoms and antenatal diagnosis of at-risk fetuses. In storage disorders, the neurons of the peripheral and autonomic nervous systems may be involved as well as CNS neurons. Other cell types may also contain storage products, and skin, liver and rectal biopsies have all proved very useful for diagnostic purposes. Schwann cell storage may be revealed in peripheral nerve biopsies. Mitochondrial abnormalities are best seen in muscle biopsies.

Since storage products such as lipid and glycogen are vulnerable to tissue processing, they are often more reliably present in cryostat sections, especially when stained with Sudan stains (**8.10, 8.11**) or with PAS reagent. Examination at ultrastructural level for characteristic cellular inclusions also forms part of the diagnostic investigation. A diagnostic approach to individual patients with metabolic disorders is shown in **8.12**.

PATHOLOGICAL APPEARANCES OF INHERITED METABOLIC DISORDERS

The brain may appear macroscopically normal or may be severely atrophic in many of these disorders. Myelin may be absent either globally or in a patchy distribution with preferential sparing of arcuate or perivascular fibres, particularly in the leucody-

Mitochondrial cytopathies					
Disease	**Age of onset & inheritance pattern**	**Clinical features**	**Other organ/tissue involvement**	**Storage product**	**Enzyme deficiency**
Kearns–Sayre syndrome	Juvenile Sporadic	Retinitis pigmentosa; ophthalmoplegia; heart block	Muscle	None known	Mitochondrial defect
MELAS	Juvenile Autosomal dominant or recessive	**M**itochondrial **E**ncephalopathy with **L**actic **A**cidosis and **S**troke-like episodes	Muscle	None known	Mitochondrial defect
MERRF	Juvenile Autosomal dominant or recessive	**M**yoclonus **E**pilepsy with **R**agged **R**ed **F**ibres	Muscle	None known	Mitochondrial defect
Leigh's disease	Infantile Sporadic or autosomal recessive	Psychomotor regression; seizures; ataxia; blindness	None	None known	Pyruvate dehydrogenase complex and others
Alper's disease	Infantile Autosomal recessive	Seizures; blindness	Liver	?	?

8.8 Features of mitochondrial cytopathies.

strophies, but also to a lesser extent in some storage disorders. This process should be regarded as dysmyelination rather than demyelination because patients with these leucodystrophic disorders are unable to form normal myelin (*see Chapter 6*). Some diseases such as Lesch–Nyhan syndrome do not

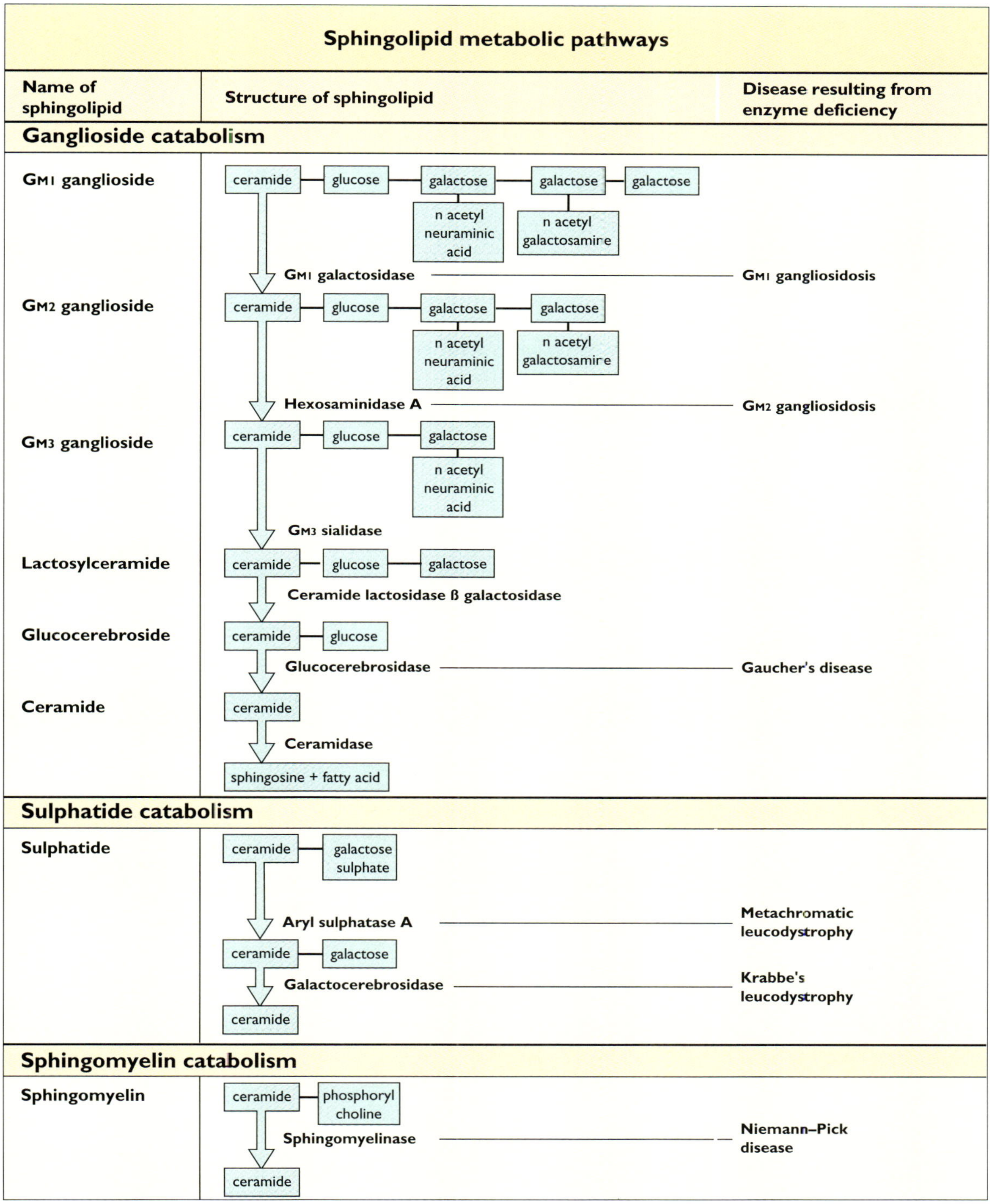

8.9 Sphingolipid metabolic pathways.

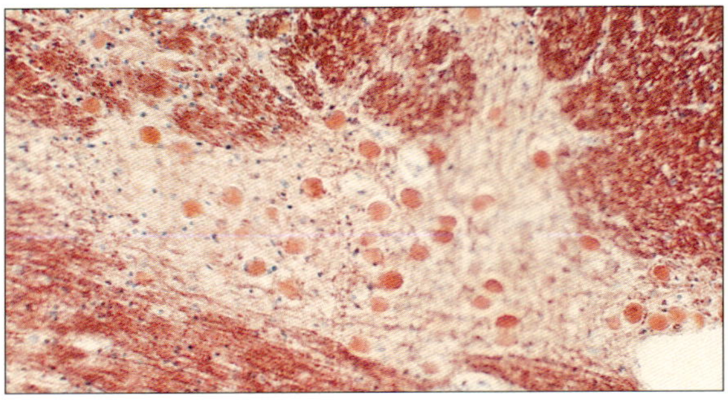

8.10 Cryostat section from the brain of a case of Niemann–Pick disease (type A) showing positive Sudan staining in distended neurons of the pons.

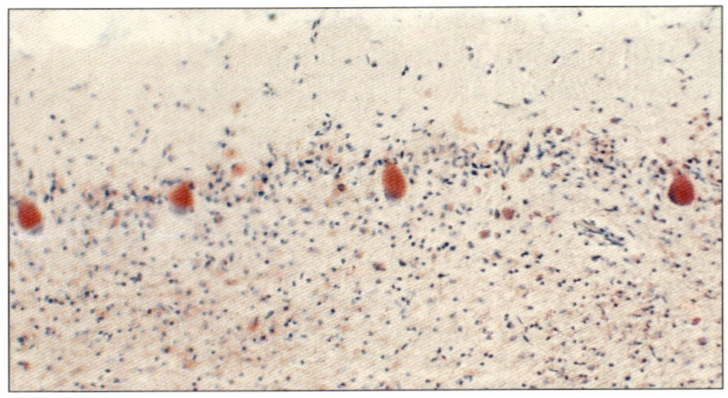

8.11 Cryostat section from the same case as in **8.10**, showing positive Sudan staining in distended neurons of the cerebellum.

Diagnostic approach to metabolic disorders		
Age, sex and ethnic background		
Clinical presentation	Physical appearance Symptoms and signs Organ systems involved Duration of illness	
Family history		
Neuroimaging		
Enzymology of blood	Cultured fibroblasts Tissues	
Lymphocyte appearances in blood film		
Histology, cryostat sections and ultrastructure	Rectal biopsy Skin biopsy Muscle biopsy Peripheral nerve biopsy (brain biopsy – last resort) Diagnostically helpful stains:	
	Oil red O and Sudan stains	Lipid
	PAS	Glycogen Carbohydrates
	Alcian blue	Mucopolysaccharides
	Luxol fast blue	Myelin
	Toluidine blue	Metachromasia
	Autofluorescence (unstained section)	Lipofuscin
Antenatal diagnosis	Chorionic villi (enzymology) Amniotic fluid cells (cultured fibroblasts) Fetal and placental tissue should be examined comprehensively for confirmation of diagnosis after termination of pregnancy (including ultrastructural examination)	
Autopsy in affected cases	Retain frozen samples of affected organs (brain, liver, spleen, etc.) Enzymology, histology of affected tissues	

8.12 Diagnostic approach to metabolic disorders.

show macroscopic or microscopic abnormalities, despite a recognised enzymatic defect.

The two major histological abnormalities in this group of disorders are storage of abnormal products

Differential diagnosis of distended neurons		
Distended neurons with storage product and ultrastructural inclusions		
Disease	**Diagnostically useful stain**	**Ultrastructure**
Niemann–Pick	PAS	Membranous cytoplasmic bodies (mcb)
Tay–Sachs (GM2) + GM1	PAS, toluidine blue	Membrance-bound concentric lamellar bodies (mcb)
Batten's	PAS, autofluorescence	Granular bodies (infantile); curvilinear (late infantile); fingerprint (juvenile)
Farber's	PAS, alcian blue	Zebra bodies
Fabry's	PAS	Membrane-bound lamellar bodies (mcb)
Hurler's (MPS I) + Hunter's (MPS I)	PAS, toluidine blue	Zebra bodies
Mucolipidoses	PAS	Membrane-bound cytoplasmic bodies (mcb)
Pompe's	PAS (diastase sensitive)	Membrane-bound glycogen
Other degenerative diseases of older age groups (see Chapter 7)		
Chromatolysis (see Chapter 2)		
Infections (see Chapter 3)		
Artefactual appearances		

8.13 Differential diagnosis of distended neurons

Differential diagnosis of vacuolation of the white matter	
Metabolic leucodystrophies	Metachromatic leucodystrophy Krabbe's leucodystrophy Adrenoleucodystrophy
Other leucodystrophies	Canavan's disease Alexander's disease Pelizaeus–Merzbacher disease Cockayne's syndrome Sudanophilic leucodystrophy
Aminoacidurias	Phenylketonuria Maple syrup urine disease
Mitochondrial cytopathies	Kearns–Sayre syndrome MELAS MERRF
Exposure to exogenous agents	Hexachlorophane Triethyltin
Cerebral oedema	
Artefactual appearances	

8.14 Differential diagnosis of vacuolation of the white matter.

in neurons and other cells, and vacuolation of white matter with myelin loss. The differential diagnoses of these two features are given in **8.13** and **8.14**. Some of the main pathological abnormalities of the more important primary metabolic disorders are listed below. Additional data are also provided in **8.1–8.8**.

CNS LIPIDOSES

Niemann–Pick disease

Various subsets of this disease are described (*see* **8.1**). In type A (early CNS involvement) and type B (mainly visceral involvement), sphingomyelinase activity is deficient whereas in types C and D sphingomyelinase activity is normal. In type A (classic) Niemann–Pick disease, the brain is atrophic and shows some demyelination. Neuronal ballooning is present in the CNS and peripheral nervous system and glial cells also show storage product (**8.15, 8.16**). The ultrastructural appearance of this condition is shown in **8.17** and **8.18.**

Gaucher's disease

In affected adults, the brain may appear normal externally and myelination is normal (*see* **8.1**). Storage

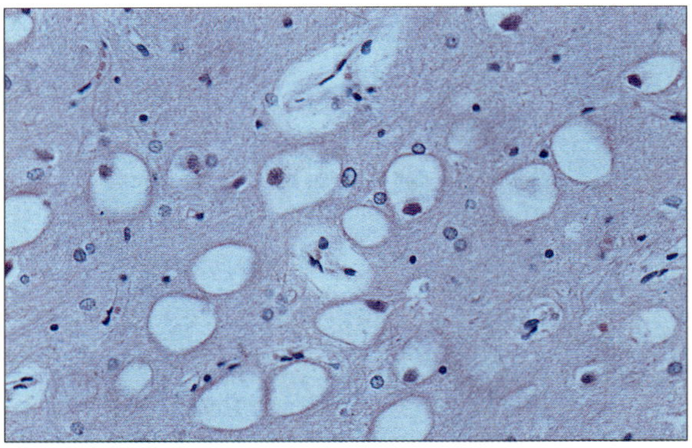

8.15 Case of Niemann–Pick disease (type A) showing distended cortical neurons in a paraffin-embedded section stained with haemotoxylin and eosin.

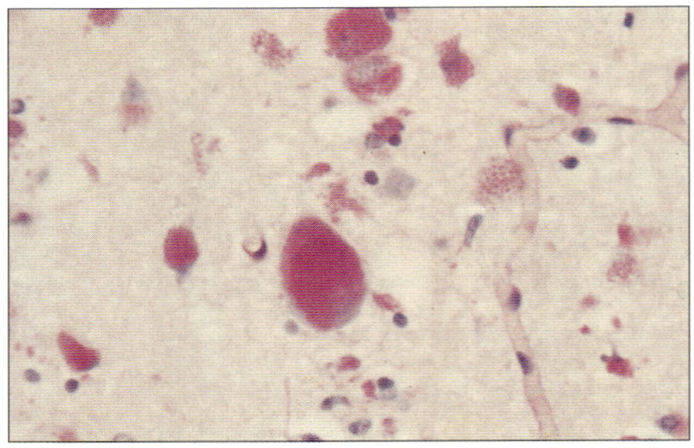

8.16 Case of Niemann–Pick disease (type A). Paraffin-embedded section showing PAS-positive distended neurons together with PAS positivity in glial cells.

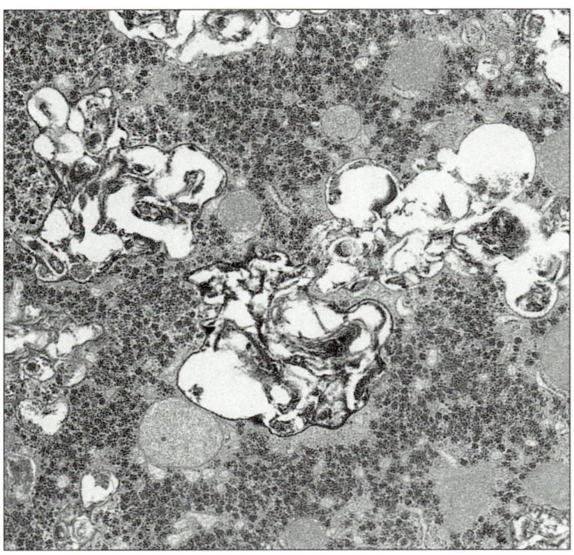

8.17 Case of Niemann–Pick disease (type B). Section of liver showing loosely arranged membranous cytoplasmic bodies together with glycogen granules (× 10,500).

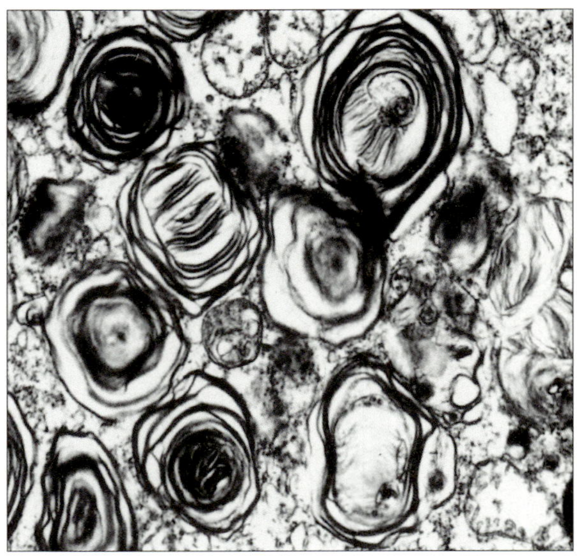

8.18 Niemann–Pick disease (type A). Ultrastructural appearances of membranous cytoplasmic bodies in a neuron in a brain biopsy (× 25,000).

cells are much more common in non-CNS organs, such as the spleen (**8.19**) and liver, but are present perivascularly within the CNS. In the more severe form in infancy, CNS neurons may also contain storage product. Membranous cytoplasmic bodies may be detected on ultrastructural examination (**8.20**).

Tay–Sachs disease (GM2 gangliosidosis)

The brain may be normal, enlarged (**8.21**), or atrophic on external examination (*see* **8.1**). Dysmyelination is present in infantile cases. Neuronal ballooning is present in the CNS and peripheral nervous system, and glial cells also show storage. Ultrastructural appearances are shown in **8.22**.

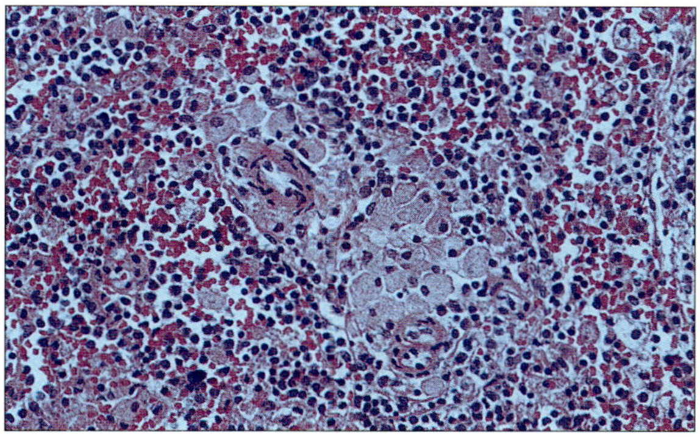

8.19 Section of spleen from a case of Gaucher's disease showing perivascular storage cells within the splenic parenchyma.

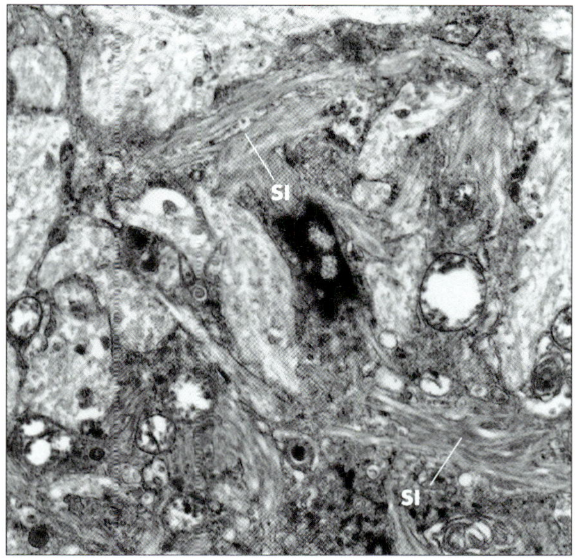

8.20 Ultrastructural appearances of striated inclusions (SI) in splenic storage cells from a case of Gaucher's disease (× 12,000).

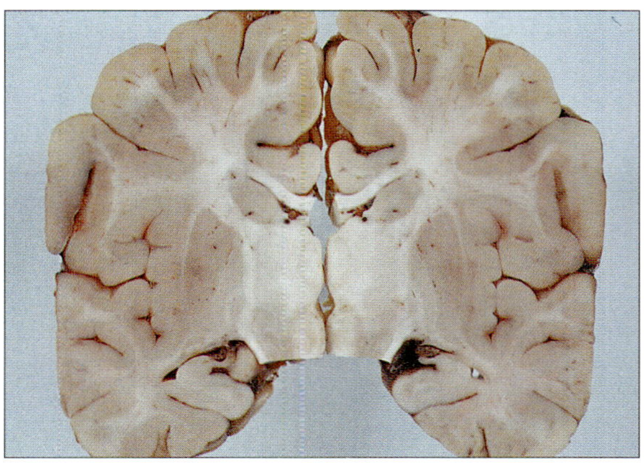

8.21 Coronal slice of brain from a patient with Tay–Sachs disease (GM2 gangliosidosis), who died in adolescence. The brain was enlarged rather than atrophic and showed pallor of the thalamus bilaterally.

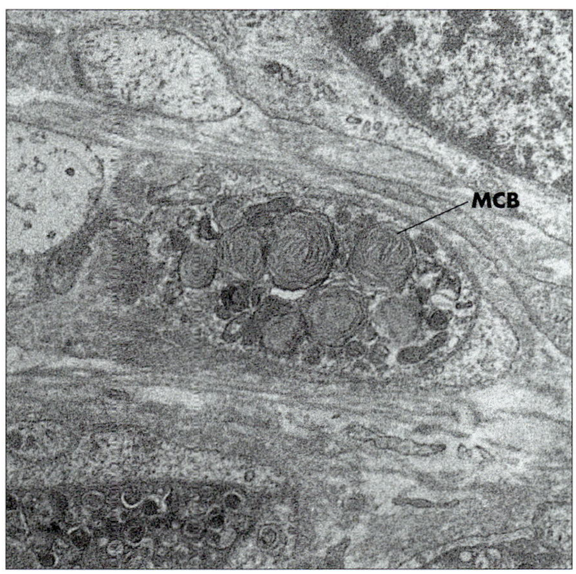

8.22 Ultrastructural appearances of membranous concentric lamellar bodies (MCB) in a case of Tay Sachs disease (× 4000).

Batten's disease (ceroid lipofuscinosis)

Cases with an early onset show microcephaly and brain atrophy (*see* **8.1**). Neurons in both the CNS and peripheral nervous system contain lipofuscin-like, autofluorescent (**8.23, 8.24**), PAS-positive material, but are not grossly distended (**8.25**). Astrocytes are also positive. The ultrastructural appearance of intracellular inclusions varies with the age of onset (**8.13, 8.26–8.28**).

Wolman's disease

The CNS is not grossly abnormal but storage cells are detected in the meninges and in the choroid plexus (*see* **8.1**). Neurons in the peripheral nervous system may contain storage product. Electron microscopy shows membranous cytoplasmic bodies.

Farber's disease

The brain is usually smaller than normal (*see* **8.1**). Storage product is present in neurons of both the CNS and peripheral nervous system (*see* **8.13**).

Fabry's disease

This multisystem disorder shows storage in many different cells including endothelial cells, and in CNS neurons (*see* **8.1**). There is a propensity for

8.23 A case of infantile Batten's disease, biopsied at the age of two and a half years. This paraffin-embedded unstained section of cortex shows autofluorescence of cortical neurons at low-power magnification.

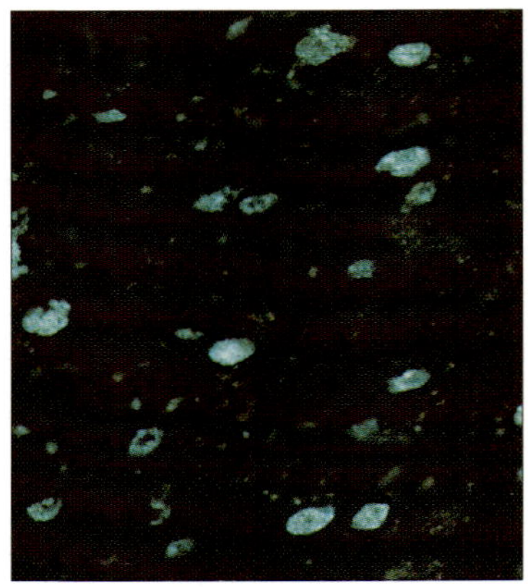

8.24 The same case of infantile Batten's disease as in **8.23** at higher magnification.

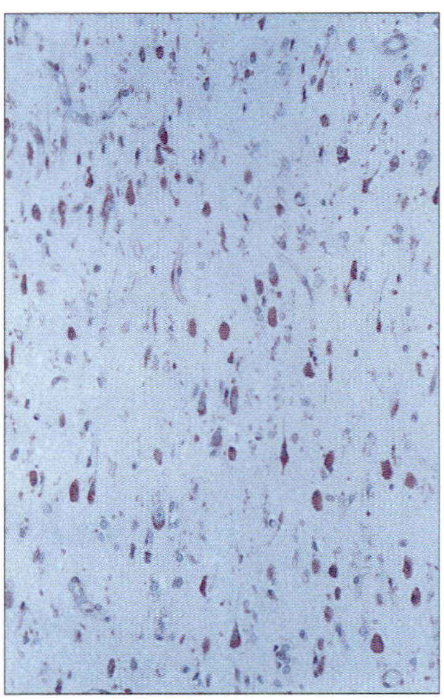

8.25 The same case as in **8.10** showing PAS-positivity but no distension of neurons in paraffin-embedded sections of the cortex.

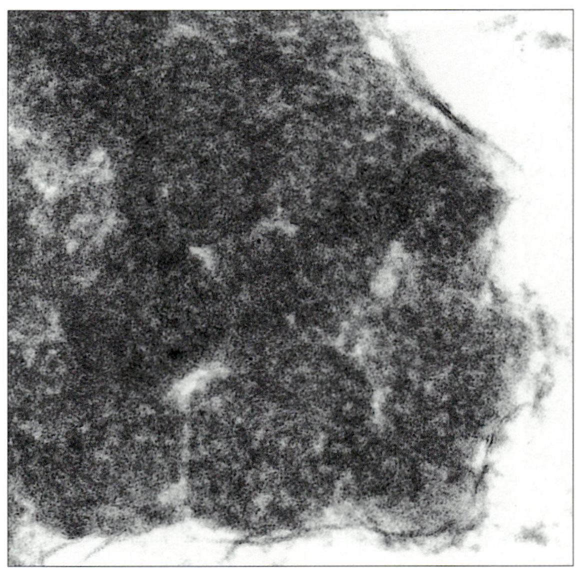

8.26 Ultrastructural appearances of the brain biopsy shown in **8.23–8.25**. The granular character of the inclusions confirms that this was an infantile case of Batten's disease (× 50,000).

aneurysm formation and thrombosis leading to infarcts (**8.29**), ischaemia and haemorrhage in the CNS.

CNS MUCOPOLYSACCHARIDOSES (MPS)

Hurler's disease (type I MPS), Hunter's disease (type II MPS), Sanfilippo's disease (type III MPS) and Morquio's disease (type IV MPS)

Brain atrophy is occasionally present in these diseases together with some dysmyelination (*see* **8.2**). Neuronal ballooning occurs in the CNS (**8.30**), but not in the peripheral nervous system. Zebra bodies (**8.31**, **8.32**) and other inclusions are seen ultrastructurally (*see* **8.13**). The CNS is not usually involved in Sheie's variant of type 1 MPS or Maroteaux Lamy disease (type VI MPS).

CNS MUCOLIPIDOSES

Mucolipidosis I (sialidosis), mucolipidosis II (I cell disease), mannosidosis and fucosidosis

The brain may be atrophic and may show dysmyelination (*see* **8.3**). Neuronal storage occurs in the CNS and peripheral nervous system and glial cells except in I cell disease, where storage is confined to non-CNS

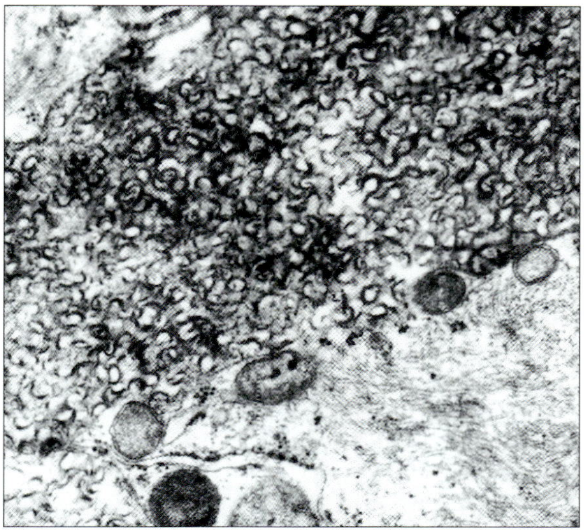

8.27 Late infantile case of Batten's disease showing typical ultrastructural appearances of curvilinear inclusions in a brain biopsy (× 30,000).

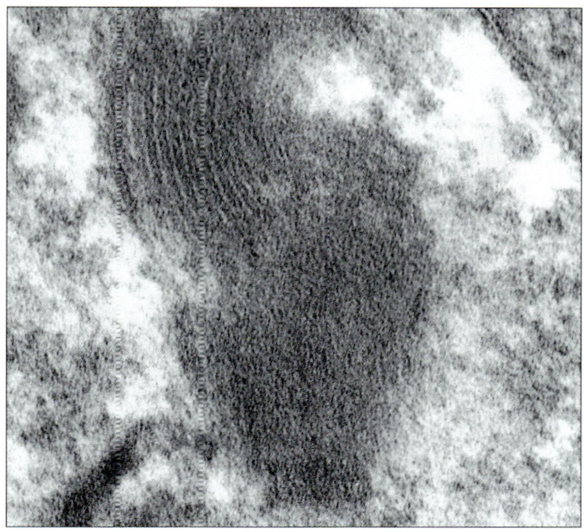

8.28 Ultrastructural appearances of inclusions in a case of juvenile Batten's disease displaying the characteristic fingerprint pattern (× 45,000).

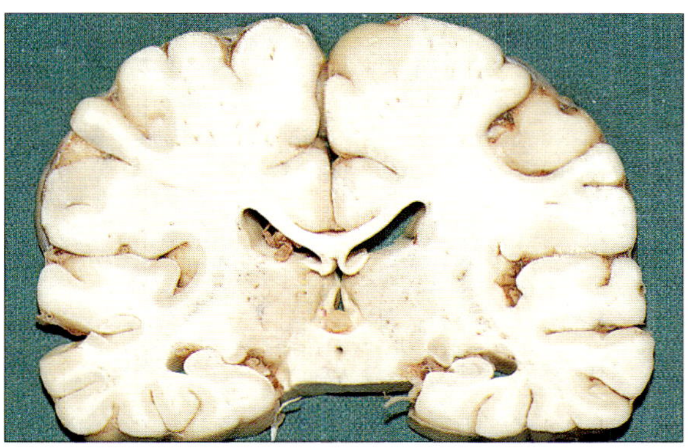

8.29 Coronal slice of brain from a patient with Fabry's disease dying in early adulthood. An old infarct is present in the left thalamus.

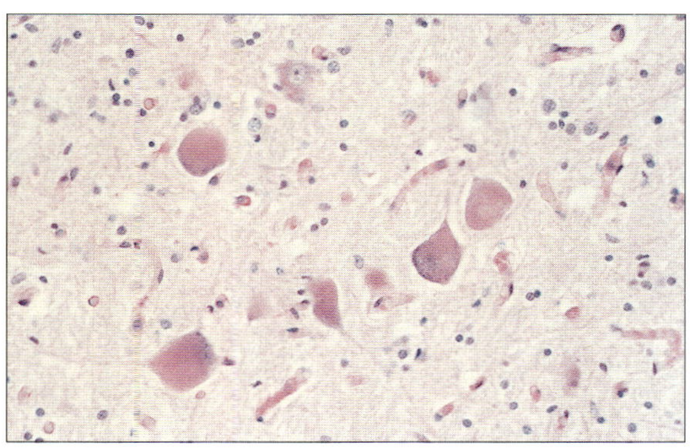

8.30 Paraffin-embedded section of the cortex in a case of Hurler's disease (type 1 mucopolysaccharidosis). The neurons are distended and are PAS-positive.

cells including cultured fibroblasts (I cells). Membrane-bound bodies are found ultrastructurally (*see* **8.13**).

CNS GLYCOGENOSES

Pompe's disease (type II glycogenosis) and type VIII glycogenosis

Brain size and myelination appear normal (*see* **8.4**). Subcortical (**8.33**) and peripheral neurons show more ballooning than do cortical neurons. Glycogen storage is also prominent in astrocytes (**8.33**).

LEUCODYSTROPHIES

Normal myelination of white matter tracts becomes visible in the CNS on the following time scale:

- At 14–24 weeks' gestation, spinal cord white matter;
- At 35–40 weeks' gestation, internal capsule, optic nerves and pons;
- At 0–3 months' postnatal, brainstem corticospinal tracts;
- At 1–2 years' postnatal, central white matter of the cerebrum.

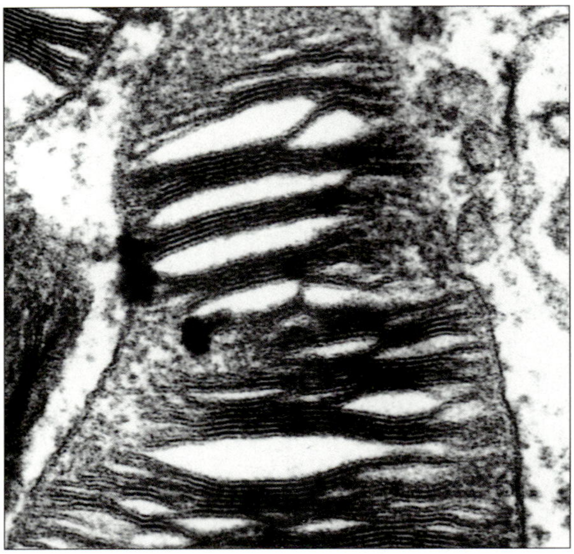

8.31 Case of Hurler's disease. Ultrastructural appearances confirming the presence of zebra bodies in skin (x 100,000).

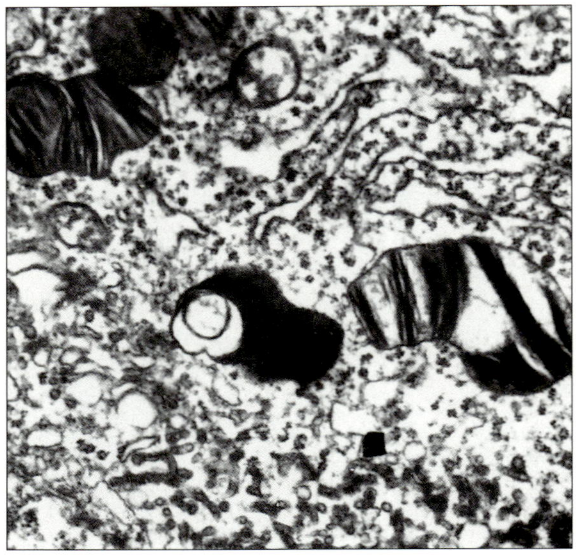

8.32 The same case as in **8.31**. Ultrastructural appearance confirming the presence of zebra bodies in brain (x 30,000).

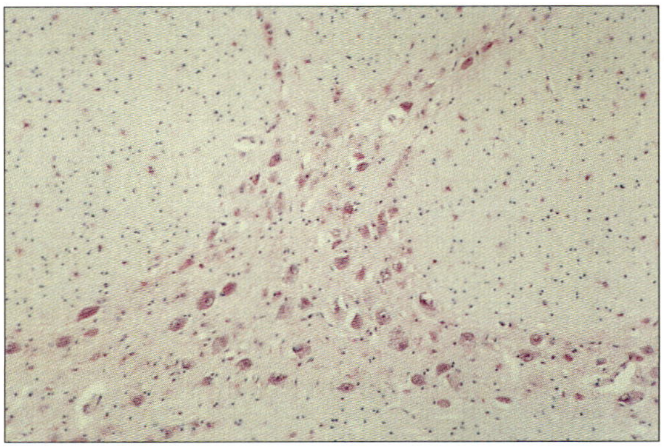

8.33 Paraffin-embedded section of pons from a case of Pompe's disease. Both neurons and glial cells are PAS-positive due to the presence of glycogen.

Dysmyelinating disorders have in common an inability to form completely normal myelin. Some inherited leucodystrophies have a known enzymatic defect, leading to accumulation of myelin-associated proteins.

The best known diseases in this category are metachromatic and Krabbe's leucodystrophies (**8.5**). In other dysmyelinating conditions, the pathogenetic mechanism is poorly understood (**8.6**) and no definite enzyme deficiencies have been demonstrated.

Vacuolation of the white matter is a prominent feature of the leucodystrophies and the differential diagnosis is shown in **8.14**. The term, sudanophilic leucodystrophy, is a potential source of confusion because it has been applied indiscriminately to more than one of the leucodystrophies and has also been used synonymously with Schilder's disease (*see Chapter 6*).

Metachromatic leucodystrophy

The brain is slightly atrophic and there is very extensive loss of central myelin (**8.34, 8.35**) with sparing of arcuate fibres (**8.36**). Metachromatic storage product is present in subcortical neurons, in white matter macrophages, and in axons and Schwann cells of the peripheral nervous system. Lamellar and membrane-bound inclusions are found in neurons and macrophages, and also in renal epithelium and in the biliary system together with metachromasia (**8.37**).

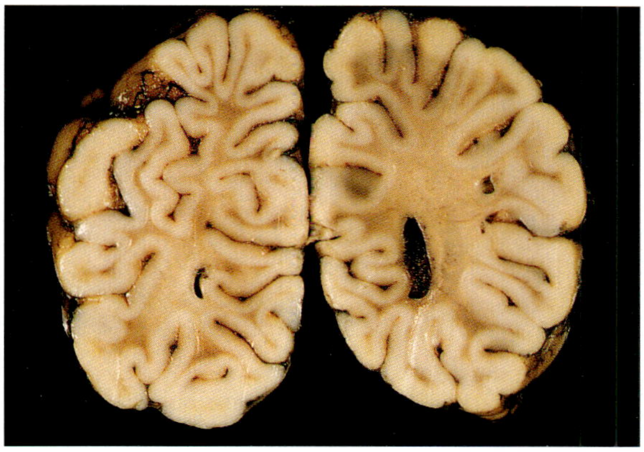

8.34 Coronal slice of brain from an infantile case of metachromatic leucodystrophy showing abnormal dysmyelinated white matter and atrophy.

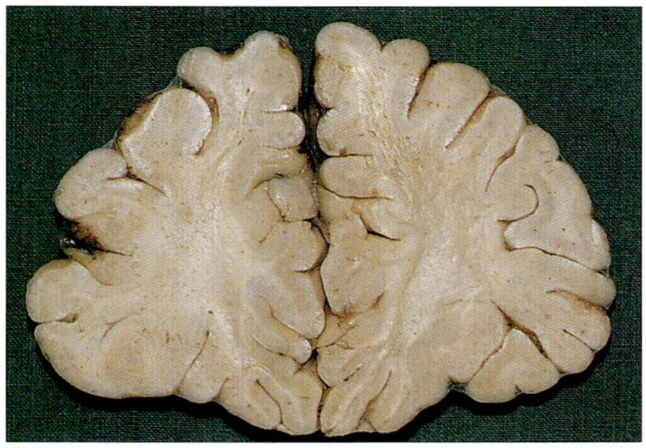

8.35 Coronal slice of brain from an adult case of metachromatic leucodystrophy. Some myelin is present but much of the central white matter is shrunken and discoloured.

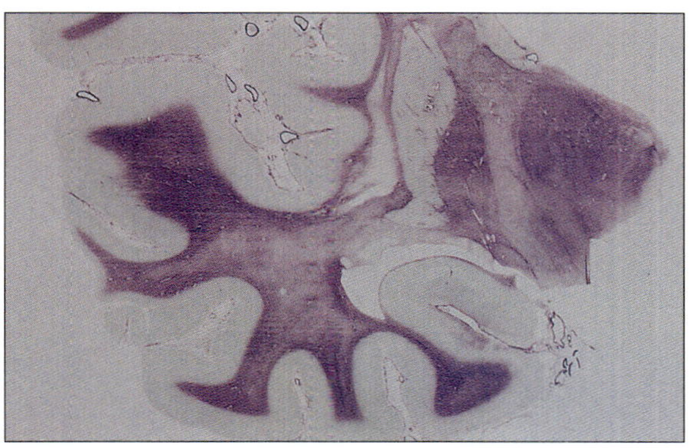

8.36 Section of temporal lobe from an adult case of metachromatic leucodystrophy, stained for myelin and showing pallor of the central white matter with sparing of the arcuate fibres. (Loyez stain)

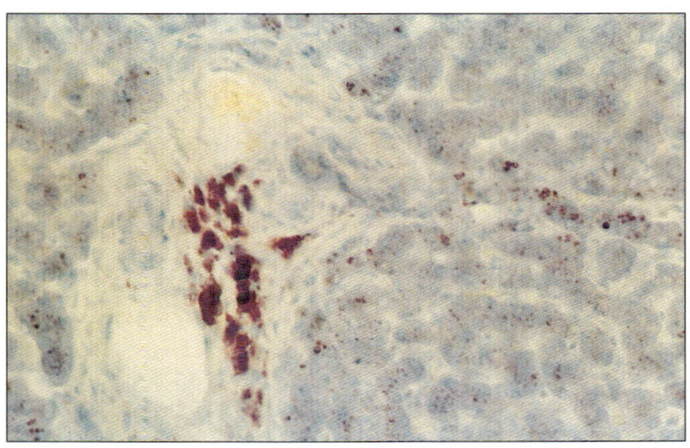

8.37 Cryostat section of liver from a case of metachromatic leucodystrophy showing metachromasia in portal-tract macrophages. (Toluidine blue stain)

Krabbe's leucodystrophy

PAS-positive globoid macrophages are scattered throughout the dysmyelinated central white matter (**8.38**). No neuronal storage is present, unlike metachromatic leucodystrophy. Tubular profiles are seen ultrastructurally in the globoid cells (**8.39**).

Adrenoleucodystrophy

Loss of myelin occurs in central white matter and in the optic nerves. Perivascular lymphocytic cuffing (**8.40**) and PAS-positive macrophages are present. No neuronal storage occurs in adrenoleucodystrophy, but characteristic curvilinear laminar bodies are seen

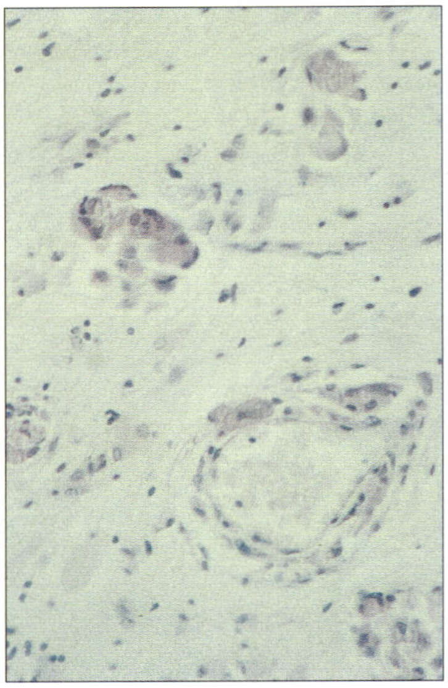

8.38 Central white matter from the brain of a patient with Krabbe's leucodystrophy. PAS-positive globoid macrophages are present in the neuropil and in the perivascular spaces.

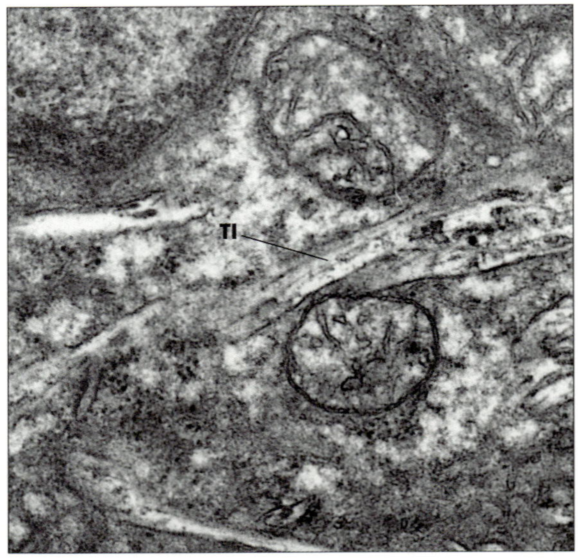

8.39 Ultrastructural appearance of tubular inclusions (TI) in a skin biopsy from a case of Krabbe's leucodystrophy (× 27,500).

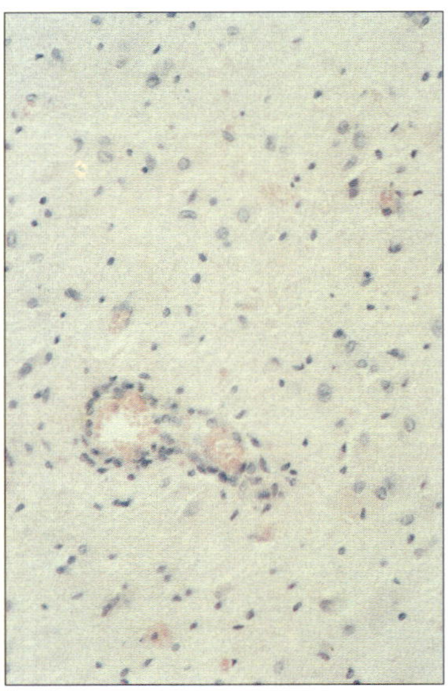

8.40 Central white matter shows perivascular lymphocytic cuffing in adrenoleucodystrophy. Gliosis is also present.

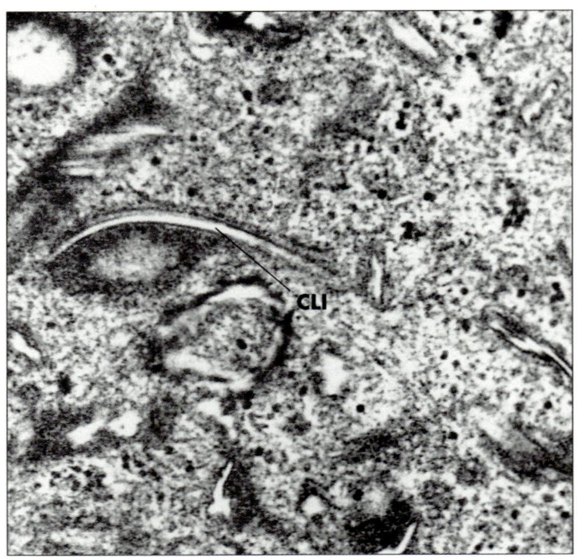

8.41 Ultrastructural appearances of curvilinear laminar inclusions (CLI) in the adrenal gland from a case of adrenoleucodystrophy (× 27,000).

ultrastructurally (**8.41**), particularly in the adrenal gland, which may be severely atrophic.

Canavan's disease
Myelin loss and central white matter vacuolation (**8.42**) are seen together with late neuronal loss and gliosis. Ultrastructural examination shows abnormally elongated mitochondria.

Alexander's disease
The unique feature in this dysmyelinating condition is the presence of subpial (**8.43**), perivascular and subependymal Rosenthal fibres which are PAS-negative. Ultrastructurally, Rosenthal bodies are composed of osmiophilic granular material, sometimes within astrocytic processes and sometimes extracellularly. The disease primarily affects astrocytes and the mechanism of myelin loss is poorly understood.

Pelizaeus–Merzbacher disease
Myelin is virtually absent in this condition (**8.44, 8.45**). The brain is atrophic and gliotic and the ventricular system is correspondingly enlarged. No specific ultrastructural features are identified in this condition.

Cockayne's syndrome
Myelin loss is patchy and prominent mineralisation may be present in the walls of blood vessels (**8.46**). No specific ultrastructural features are identified.

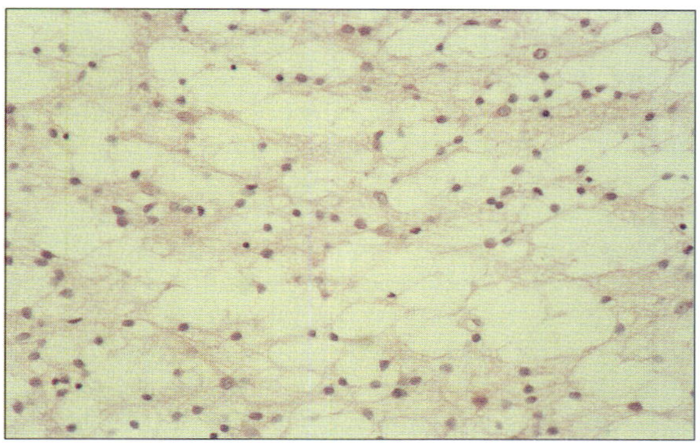

8.42 Central white matter from a case of Canavan's disease showing myelin loss and central white matter vacuolation.

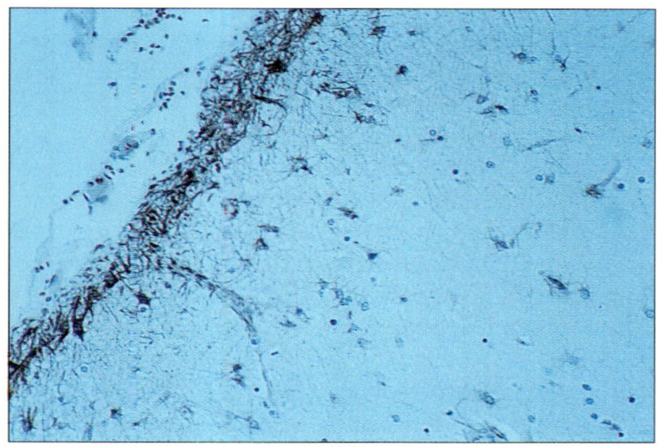

8.43 Subpial accumulation of glial fibrillary acidic protein positivity due to the presence of Rosenthal fibres in Alexander's disease.

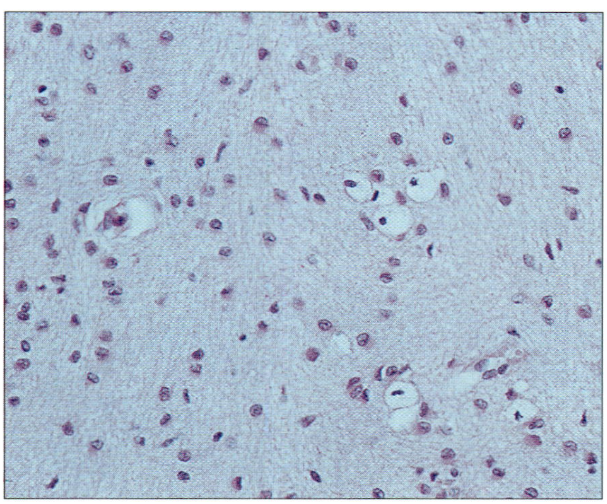

8.44 A case of Pelizaeus–Merzbacher disease stained routinely, showing virtually absent myelin in the central white matter, which is also gliotic.

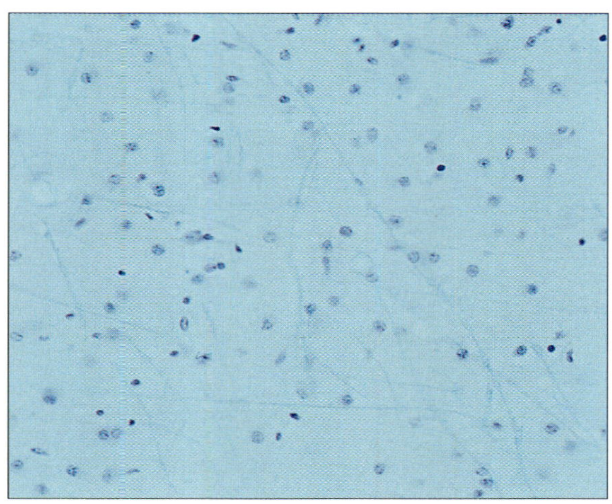

8.45 The same case as in **8.44** stained for myelin. (Luxol-fast blue)

Phenylketonuria
Microcephaly and dysmyelination occur in this aminoaciduria (**8.14**) if it is not diagnosed and treated at an early age.

The effects of the disease, including the severe mental disability, may be averted by elimination of phenylalanine from the diet.

PEROXISOMAL DISORDERS

This group of disorders is characterised by the absence, or dysfunction, of cellular organelles known as peroxisomes. These small membrane-bound bodies were first defined by their enzyme content of catalase, but it is now known that they contain a variety of enzymes concerned with the synthesis of cell-membrane proteins and bile acids, and the metabolism of long-chain fatty acids and cholesterol. The enzymes present include oxidases, dehydrogenases and aminotransferases.

The enzyme deficiencies may be single or multiple. An example of a single microsomal enzyme deficiency is X-linked adrenoleucodystrophy, but the neonatal form of adrenoleucodystrophy shows multiple peroxisomal enzyme deficiencies. The major peroxisomal disorders are shown in **8.7**, of which Zellweger's syndrome is the best-known example.

Zellweger's syndrome
This syndrome comprises hepatic cirrhosis, focal polymicrogyria (**8.47**) and grey matter heterotopias signalling neuronal migration defects. The brainstem and cerebellar nuclei may be dysplastic. Lamellar lipid inclusions are found in white matter macrophages and ultrastructural examination also confirms the absence of peroxisomes. Pseudo-Zellweger conditions have also been described in which peroxisomes are shown to be present but display functional disturbance of their constituent enzymes.

Infantile Refsum's disease
The brain is macroscopically normal, but macrophages are present in white matter and in non-CNS organs including the liver. Trilaminar inclusions are seen ultrastructurally.

Neonatal adrenoleucodystrophy
The brain shows dysmyelination and small heterotopias with macrophage infiltration. Trilaminar inclusions are seen in macrophages but are most characteristically present in the adrenal gland.

MITOCHONDRIAL CYTOPATHIES

Both functional and structural disorders of mitochondria occur and deletions and mutations of mitochondrial DNA are present in this group of diseases. Mitochondrial abnormalities are generally expressed in high-energy tissue such as CNS and muscle (*see* **8.8**). Muscle involvement is manifested as weakness, fatigue, pain and stiffness, and the characteristic histological appearance is of ragged red fibres in which accumulating abnormal mitochondria and fat are demonstrable (**8.48**). These abnormal muscle fibres show intense staining for succinate dehydrogenase and depleted cytochrome oxidase. Ultrastructurally, mitochondria may be of abnormal shape and show distorted cristae and crystalline inclusions (**8.49**).

Kearns Sayre syndrome, MELAS and MERRF
In addition to ragged red fibres, these mitochondrial cytopathies show vacuolation of the central white matter with no evidence of storage products (*see*

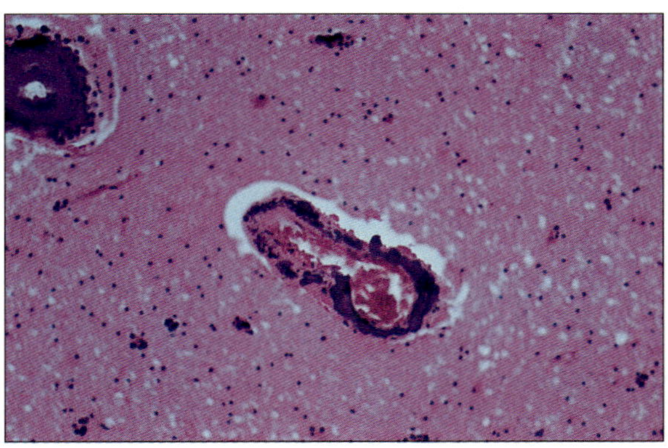

8.46 Prominent vascular mineralisation is present in Cockayne's syndrome.

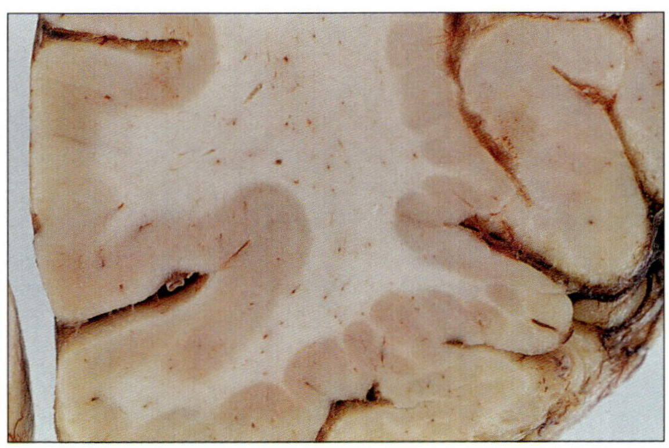

8.47 A case of Zellweger's syndrome showing polymicrogyria in the occipital lobe.

8.8). The distribution of spongy change varies between the different conditions, and grey matter may be involved (*see* **8.14**). Necrotic lesions may be present with accompanying gliosis and a variable degree of demyelination in addition to vacuolation. Mineral deposits (**8.50**) and some vascular proliferation have also been described. These cases show some similarities to Leigh's disease.

Leigh's disease

This disease is characterised by focal and symmetrical lesions in the basal ganglia (**8.51**) and brainstem. The lesions show demyelination, macrophage infiltration, gliosis and vascular proliferation (**8.52**). Mitochondrial abnormalities are observed ultrastructurally and abnormal levels of mitochondrial enzymes have been described (*see* **8.8**).

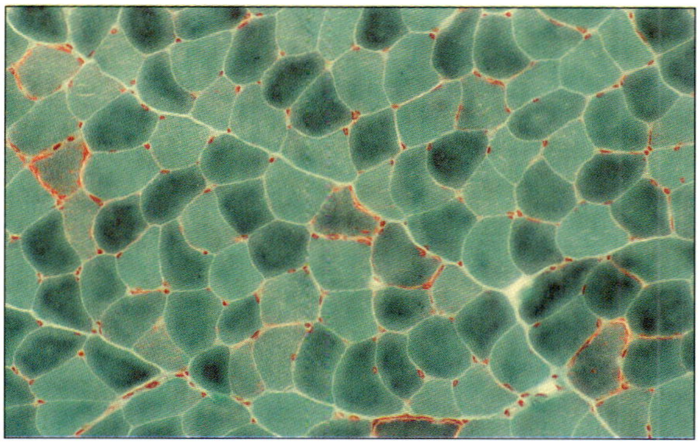

8.48 A section of muscle from a case of MELAS stained with Gomori's stain. Abnormal mitochondria and fat are demonstrated by red staining in several of the muscle fibres.

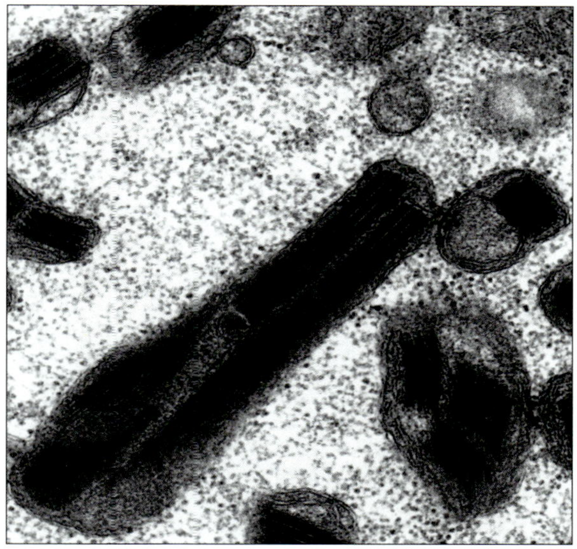

8.49 Ultrastructural appearances of abnormal mitochondria containing crystalline inclusions in a case of mitochondrial cytopathy (MELAS) (× 28,000).

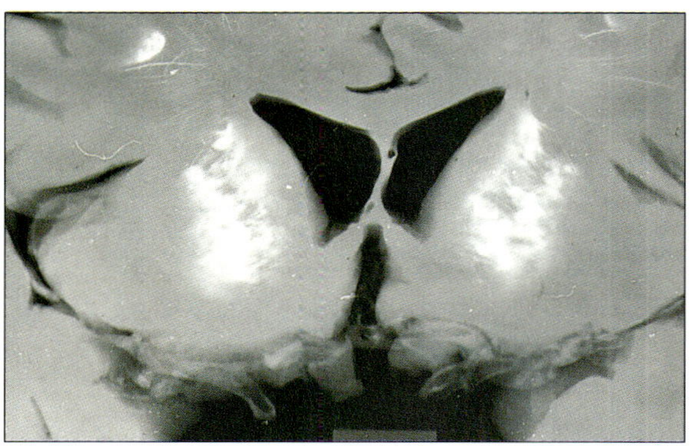

8.50 Fixed brain slice from a case of Kearns Sayre syndrome subjected to post-mortem radiological examination. Mineralisation is shown in the basal ganglia.

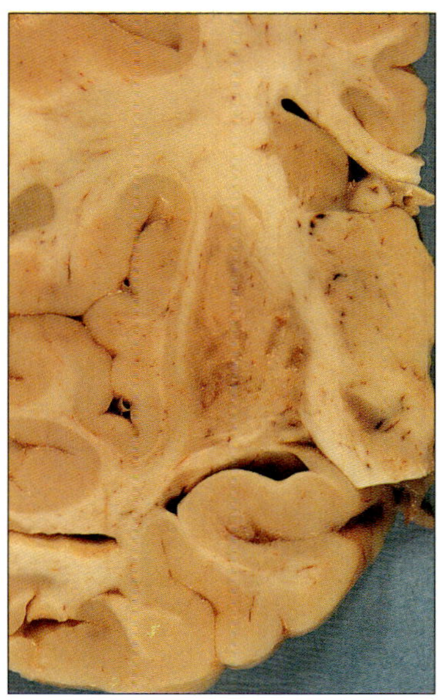

8.51 A coronal slice of brain from a case of Leigh's disease showing discoloured lesions in the basal ganglia.

Alper's disease

Early-onset microcephaly is associated with dilated ventricles and characteristically spongiform grey matter with marked loss of neurons and gliosis, giving a superficial resemblance to the pathological picture of Creutzfeldt–Jakob disease (*see Chapter 7*). Hepatic fibrosis is present in this condition and vacuolation of the brain extends to the white matter. Mitochondrial abnormalities have been described and the condition is not thought to be transmissible.

OTHER INHERITED DISORDERS WITH A METABOLIC BASIS

Wilson's disease

This autosomal-recessive condition is manifested clinically by spasticity, dysarthria and tremor arising in young adults. Copper levels are high in body tissues, but not necessarily in serum, and the accumulation of copper in the liver leads to cirrhosis (**8.53**), in the cornea to Kayser–Fleischer rings, and in the kidney to renal impairment. In the CNS, the major focus of damage is in the basal ganglia, which are shrunken and discoloured with neuronal loss, gliosis and haemosiderin-laden macrophages. Copper and haemosiderin accumulate in Alzheimer type 2 astrocytes (**8.54**).

Menkes' disease

This X-linked disease is another disorder of copper metabolism; defective transport systems in the gastrointestinal tract and elsewhere are associated with low-serum, but high-tissue, copper levels. Characteristic clinical appearances include abnormal twisted hair and growth retardation. The arteries are involved and become thickened and distorted. Abnormal Purkinje cell processes have been described (**8.55**).

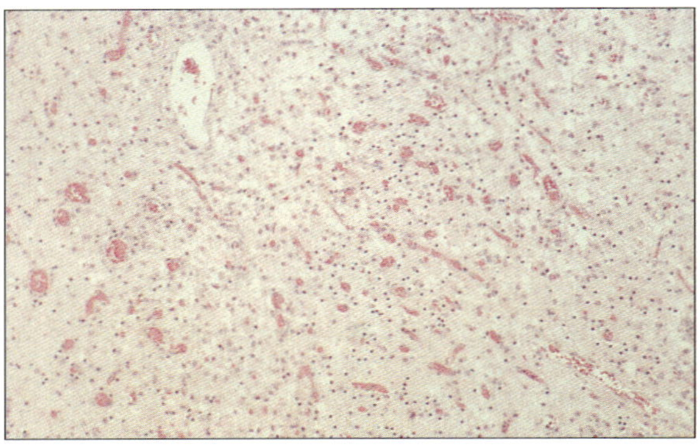

8.52 Microscopical appearances of Leigh's disease in the basal ganglia showing tissue breakdown, macrophage infiltration, vascular proliferation and gliosis.

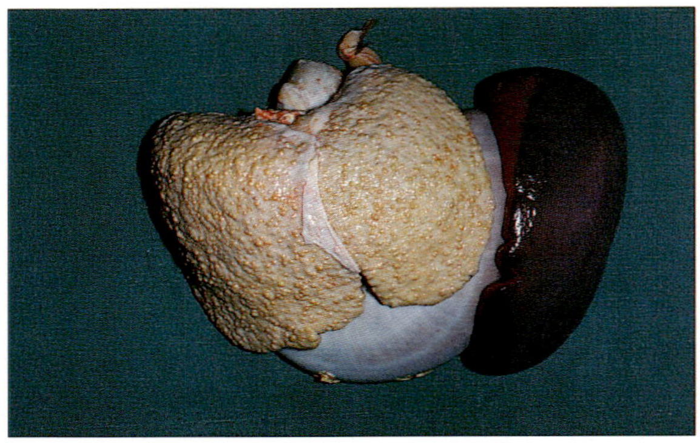

8.53 Cirrhotic liver from a case of Wilson's disease. The spleen is enlarged.

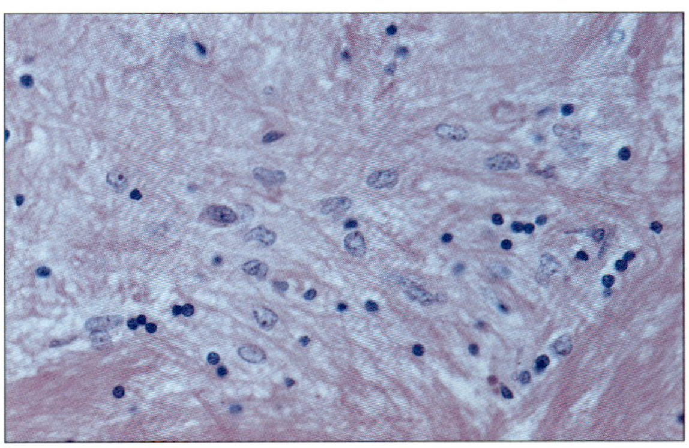

8.54 Alzheimer type 2 astrocytes in the basal ganglia of a case of hepatic encephalopathy resulting from cirrhosis of the liver.

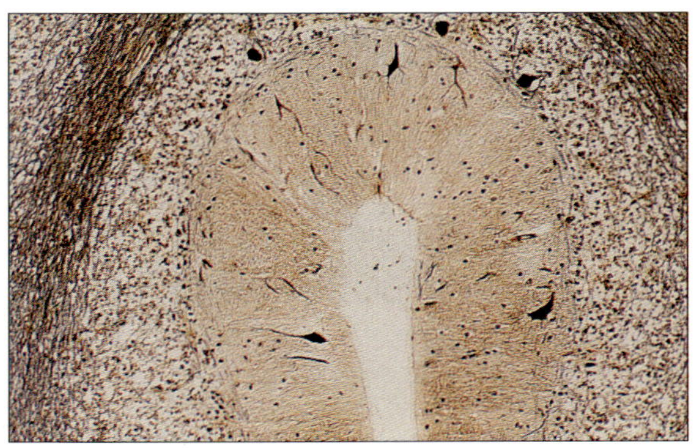

8.55 Cerebellum from a case of Menkes' disease showing silver impregnation of abnormal Purkinje cell processes in the molecular layer. (Palmgren)

The CNS shows spongiform white matter degeneration and neuronal cell death.

Adult Refsum's disease

This is an autosomal-recessive disorder characterised by retinitis pigmentosa, peripheral neuropathy, cerebellar ataxia and raised CSF protein levels. This may represent a storage disorder or possibly a microsomal or mitochondrial disorder in which phytanic acid (derived from chlorophyll) is stored as a result of reduced phytanic acid α-hydroxylase. This condition can be managed by dietary adjustment. The neuropathology is variable and non-specific. Peripheral nerves show hypertrophic changes and there may be storage within Schwann cells.

Lesch–Nyhan syndrome

This X-linked recessive disorder has its onset in the first year of life and is characterised by self-destructive behaviour. The enzymatic defect is a deficiency of hypoxanthine guanine phosphoribosyltransferase. The accumulation of uric acid produces the features of gout. Neuropathological abnormalities are not regularly found in this disorder and the defect in the CNS is likely to be biochemical, possibly involving neurotransmitters.

Lafora body disease

This familial condition, associated with myoclonic epilepsy and dementia, commences in late childhood or adolescence. The brain shows the presence of Lafora bodies in the cytoplasm of neurons, particularly in the neurons of the brainstem (**8.56**), but also in the cortex. The inclusions consist of PAS-positive polyglucosan (**8.56**). Similar inclusions may be strikingly present in non-CNS organs including the myocardium and liver.

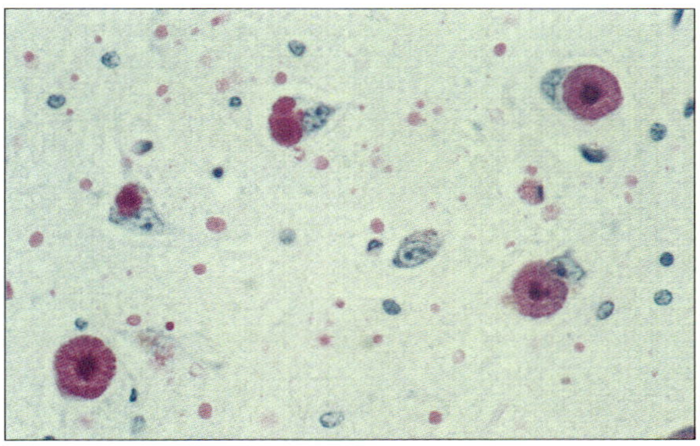

8.56 A case of Lafora body disease. PAS-positive inclusions are seen in the midbrain, both within neurons and in the neuropil.

Reye's syndrome

The basis of Reye's syndrome is poorly understood. Severe fatty change occurs in the liver (**8.57**) following a viral infection, with resulting hepatic failure, hyperammonaemia, vomiting and coma. Cerebral oedema occurs (**8.58**) and the myelin shows spongy changes. Alzheimer type 2 astrocytes (**8.54**) are observed in the brain. Mitochondrial changes have been observed in Reye's syndrome, raising the possibility that this is an intrinsic mitochondrial defect.

PRIMARY METABOLIC DISORDERS ASSOCIATED WITH VASCULAR CHANGES

These include Fabry's disease, Cockayne's syndrome, Leigh's disease and Menkes' disease. Although these diseases have different basic defects, such as storage

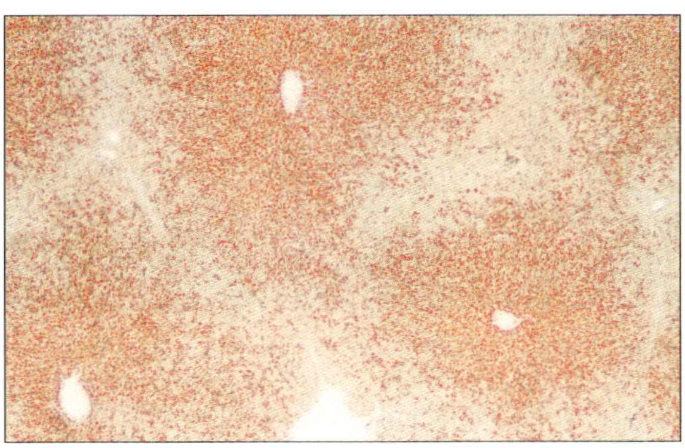

8.57 Cryostat section from the liver of a case of Reye's syndrome stained for fat which is particularly abundant around the central veins. (Oil Red O stain.)

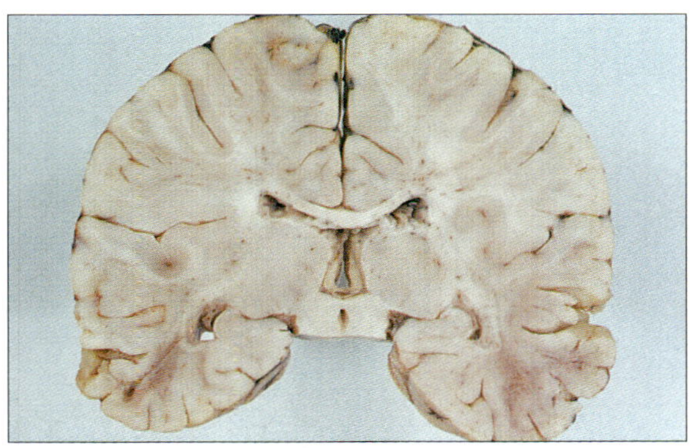

8.58 Slice of brain from a case of Reye's syndrome showing cerebral swelling and incipient hypoxic damage.

disorder, mitochondrial or peroxisomal disorders and abnormal copper metabolism, a common, significant factor in each of these disorders is blood vessel involvement. In some cases at least, this leads to haemorrhage, thrombosis and aneurysm formation.

SECONDARY CNS METABOLIC DISORDERS (DEFICIENCIES AND TOXICITIES)

Hypoglycaemia

The effects of hypoglycaemia resemble hypoxia (*see Chapter 4*) and induce cortical neuronal necrosis as well as damage to neurons in the basal ganglia (**8.59**). In contrast to hypoxia, the Purkinje cells of the cerebellum are spared. Prolonged hypoglycaemia may lead to mental disability and seizures or even death. This complication may occur in inherited disorders of carbohydrate metabolism, including Von Gierke's disease and other glycogen-storage diseases, as well as in insulin-dependent diabetes mellitus.

Hyperammonaemia

Ammonia is produced from the breakdown of amino acids and is normally excreted through the urea cycle in the liver. Hepatic disease (or more rarely inherited enzymatic deficiencies in the urea cycle) may lead to excess ammonia levels which induce the formation of Alzheimer type 2 astrocytes (*see Reye's syndrome above*). If prolonged, hyperammonaemia may also cause neuronal and myelin loss, and spongiosis of the white matter. As capillary proliferation is also a feature, the lesions resemble Leigh's disease.

Alcohol-related damage

Chronic alcohol abuse may lead to hepatic cirrhosis, which in turn leads to hepatic encephalopathy, the characteristic cellular feature of which is the presence of Alzheimer type 2 astrocytes. Alcohol may also cause, or be associated with:

- increased incidence of traumatic damage to the CNS (*see Chapter 5*);
- cerebral atrophy, particularly of the frontal lobe;
- Wernicke's encephalopathy/Korsakoff's psychosis;
- central pontine myelinolysis (*see Chapter 6*);
- cerebellar atrophy, with loss of Purkinje cells, particularly in the superior vermis (**8.60**);
- peripheral neuropathy;
- fetal alcohol syndrome (*see Chapter 9*);
- muscle disease.

Wernicke's encephalopathy

This is due to thiamine (vitamin B_1) deficiency, usually, but not exclusively, occurring in the context of alcohol abuse. Other causes include protracted vomiting, some malabsorption states, and intravenous therapy which lacks adequate vitamin B_1 cover. The lesions are centred in the mamillary bodies (**8.61**), hypothalamus, tectum of the midbrain and floor of the fourth ventricle. Acute lesions are haemorrhagic. More chronic lesions show demyelination (**8.62**), endothelial proliferation and gliosis.

Vitamin B_{12} deficiency

Absorption of vitamin B_{12} is dependent on the intrinsic factor secreted by the stomach which fails in pernicious anaemia. Malabsorption syndromes may also be associated with vitamin B_{12} deficiency. In

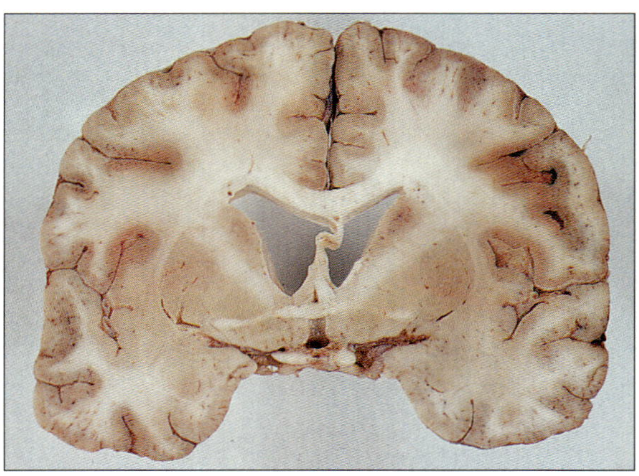

8.59 Slice of brain from a case of insulin overdose displaying the effects of fatal hypoglycaemia with evidence of necrosis in cortex and in basal ganglia.

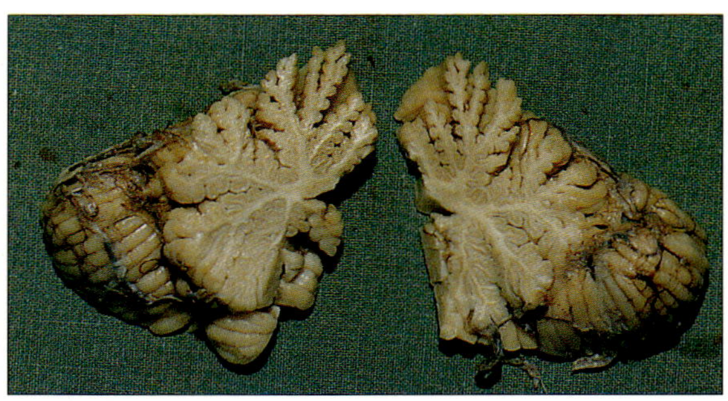

8.60 Cerebellum from a patient with a long history of alcohol abuse and cirrhosis. The cerebellum shows severe cortical atrophy which is most marked in the superior vermis.

longstanding chronic deficiency, degeneration occurs in the posterior columns and corticospinal tracts of the spinal cord (**8.63**). Vacuolation of myelin, demyelination and infiltration with lipid-laden macrophages produce the changes of subacute combined degeneration of the cord, which are closely similar to the vacuolar myelopathy seen in HIV infection (*see Chapter 3*).

Hyperbilirubinaemia

Conjugated bilirubin does not cross the intact blood–brain barrier and the brain normally remains pale in jaundiced patients. In the premature infant, or in infants with haemolytic anaemia, levels of unconjugated bilirubin rise rapidly. Since this form may enter the brain more readily, staining and damage may occur in many regions of the developing brain, particularly in the basal ganglia, giving rise to kernicterus (*see Chapter 9*).

Carbon monoxide intoxication

Exposure to carbon monoxide gas carries a very high risk of fatal cerebral hypoxia since the affinity of blood for carbon monoxide is much greater than for oxygen. Acute carbon monoxide poisoning causes a pattern of pathology which resembles that seen after cardiac arrest. Carbon monoxide exposure may lead to widespread delayed white matter damage but the effects are seen classically in the basal ganglia where focal necrosis may be seen (**8.64**).

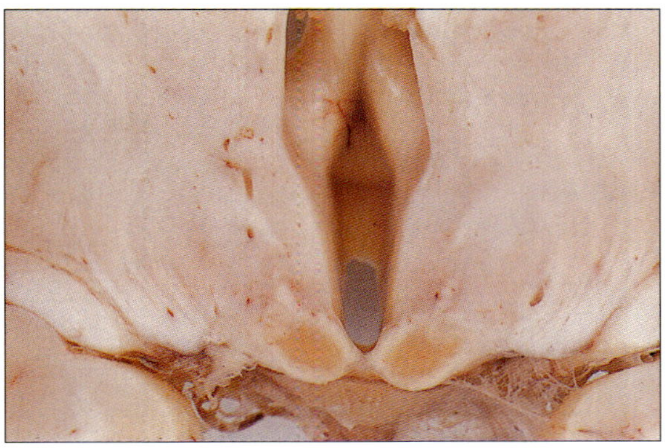

8.61 Slice of brain from a case of Wernicke's encephalopathy showing discoloration of the mamillary bodies. The discoloration and absence of haemorrhages suggests that the condition is chronic rather than acute.

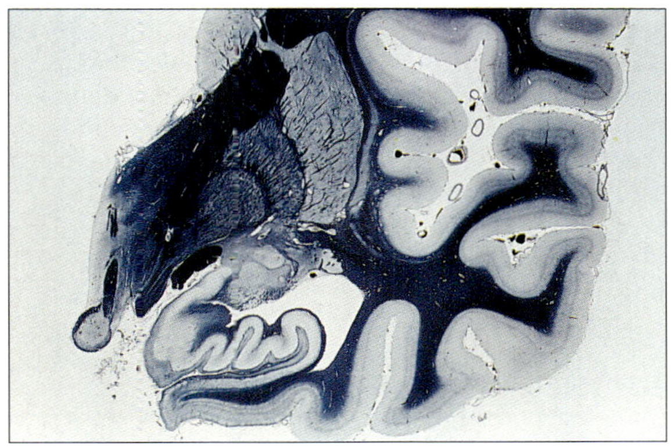

8.62 Section of temporal lobe and basal ganglia from a case of chronic Wernicke's encephalopathy, stained for myelin. The mamillary bodies are strikingly demyelinated. (Loyez stain)

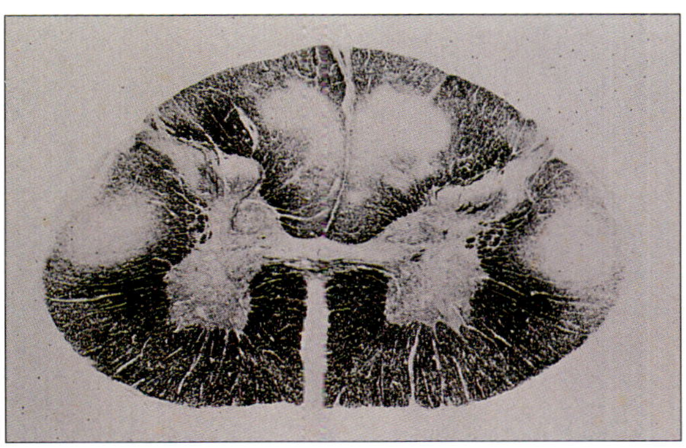

8.63 Section of spinal cord from a case of subacute combined degeneration (vitamin B_{12} deficiency) stained for myelin. Pallor of the lateral corticospinal tracts and dorsal columns is present displaying the characteristic pattern of myelin loss in this condition. (Loyez stain.)

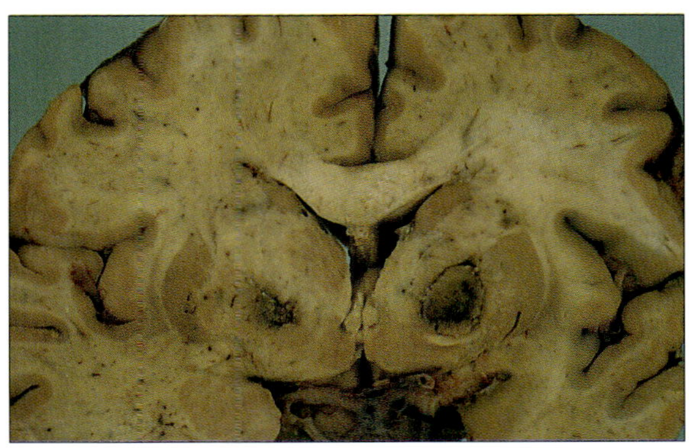

8.64 Slice of brain from a fatal carbon monoxide exposure showing brain swelling and necrosis in the basal ganglia.

Hexachlorophane intoxication

This topical cleansing agent may damage the CNS after being absorbed through the skin. Premature babies are particularly at risk. Hexachlorophane intoxication gives rise to central white matter spongy change, due to oedema of myelin sheaths (**8.14**).

Aluminium intoxication

Experimental studies have shown that aluminium intoxication may lead to neurofibrillary degeneration in animals and a link has been suggested with Alzheimer's disease. Aluminium is frequently present in the core of neuritic plaques. However, aluminium accumulation in the brains of demented patients may be a secondary rather than a primary feature, even in cases of renal dialysis dementia.

Lead intoxication

Lead poisoning may lead to encephalopathy or peripheral neuropathy. Acute intoxication leads to cerebral oedema, petechial haemorrhages and focal necrosis, probably secondary to vascular damage. The presence of PAS-positive perivascular exudate is characteristic. Chronic exposure to lead also damages cerebral vasculature.

Manganese intoxication

This occurs in manganese mine workers. Damage is centred in the basal ganglia, producing symptoms which resemble parkinsonism.

Mercury intoxication

Chronic poisoning leads to cerebral and cerebellar atrophy, neuronal loss and gliosis, and to basal ganglionic damage including the substantia nigra.

Tin intoxication

White matter vacuolation occurs after triethyltin intoxication (**8.14**). In more chronic exposure, demyelination and gliosis occur.

Calcium deposition

In pallidal siderosis, calcium and iron are deposited in the globus pallidus. In Fahr's disease, such large calcium deposits are laid down that they become visible radiographically (similar to those shown in **8.50**). Hypoparathyroidism is associated with most cases of Fahr's disease.

Effects of irradiation

These are considered in *Chapter 2*.

FURTHER READING

Becher LE, Yates AJ. Inherited Metabolic Disease. In: Davis RL, Robertson DM (eds). *Textbook of Neuropathology.* 2nd edn. Williams and Wilkins, Baltimore, 1991.

Duchen LW, Jacobs JM. Nutritional Deficiencies and Metabolic Disorders. In: Adams JH, Duchen LW (eds). *Greenfield's Neuropathology.* 5th edn. Edward Arnold, London, 1992, pp 811–880.

Friede RL. *Developmental Neuropathology.* 2nd edn. Springer-Verlag, Berlin, 1989.

Lake BD. Lysosomal and Peroxisomal Disorders. In: Adams JH, Duchen LW (eds). *Greenfield's Neuropathology.* 5th edn. Edward Arnold, London, 1992, pp 709–810.

9. Congenital and Perinatal Conditions of the CNS

GENERAL CONSIDERATIONS

The CNS develops from the enclosed hollow tube of neuroectoderm known as the neural tube (**9.1**). Mitosis at the lining layer of neuroectoderm generates cells which give rise to neurons, astrocytes and oligodendrocytes. These cells then migrate centrifugally towards the surface. Migration is guided by a structural framework of radial glial cells, which initially spans the thickness of the developing wall of the neural tube (**9.2**) and later gives rise to mature astrocytes (**9.3**). In the brain, developing neurons migrate to the surface and continue to do so throughout development, so that the youngest neurons are placed more superficially in the cortex than earlier differentiating nerve cells – the so-called inside-out arrangement.

In the spinal cord, in contrast to the brain, developing neurons do not migrate to the surface, with the result that mature grey matter is centrally placed and surrounded by white matter. Nerve cells rapidly put out processes and establish synaptic connections

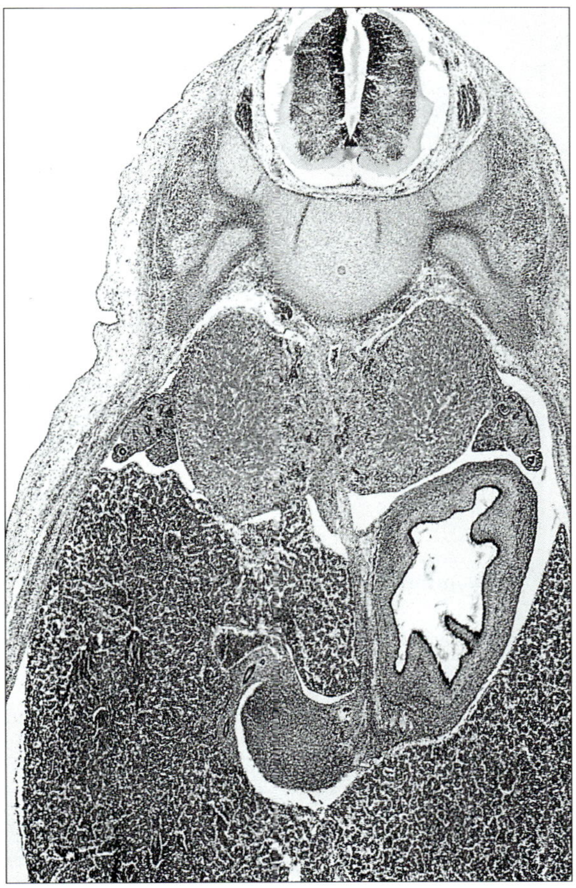

9.1 A horizontal section through an eight week embryo showing the neural tube dorsal to the developing vertebra. The ventral structures are dominated by the liver.

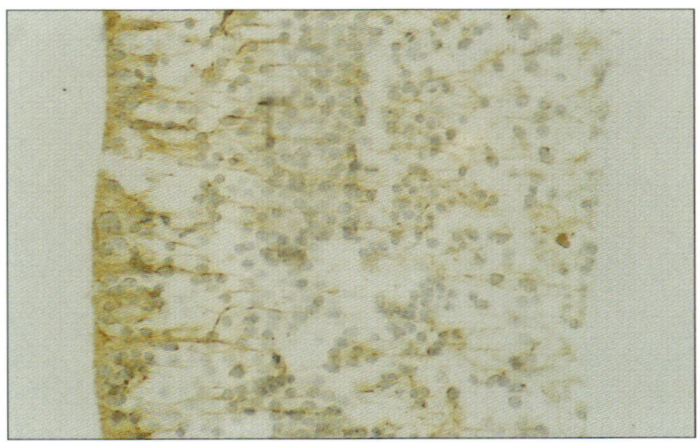

9.2 Wall of the neural tube from an eight week embryo. Radial glial fibres span the full thickness of the wall. (Stained for glial fibrillary acidic protein)

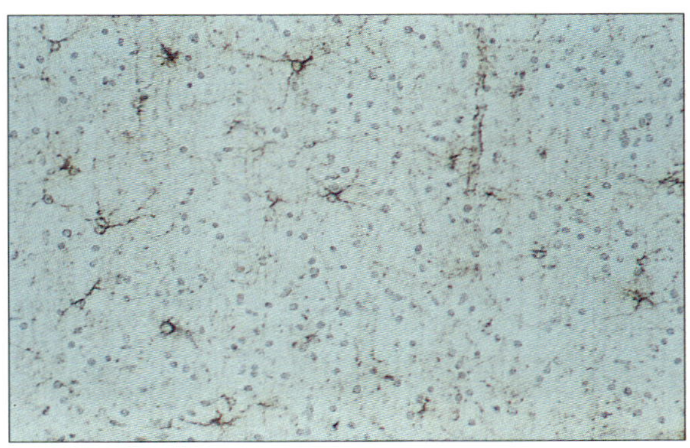

9.3 Cerebral hemisphere from a fetus of 23 weeks shows background radial glial fibres, together with mature astrocytes. (Stained for GFAP)

with other parts of the developing nervous system. Those that do not establish appropriate contacts degenerate and die by a process of apoptosis. It is estimated that up to 50% of immature neurons disappear during normal CNS development.

The mitotic generation of neurons and glial cells continues through much of fetal life in the zone of morphologically undifferentiated cells, known as the germinal matrix or subependymal zone, which lines the lateral ventricles. The germinal eminence (**9.4**) is a locally prominent part of this zone which lies adjacent to the basal ganglia. The germinal matrix is very vascular and is particularly prone to haemorrhage in the brains of those premature infants who develop respiratory distress and resultant cerebral hypoxia. Although the germinal matrix has largely disappeared in full-term infants, residual perivascular foci of migrating cells (**9.5**) are still present in the periventricular white matter and these are sometimes misinterpreted as evidence of inflammation.

Migration of cells from the subependymal zone increases the tissue mass at the cortical surface of the brain. This is associated with the establishment of gyri and sulci in the second half of gestation. Heterotopic deposits of neurons in the central white matter of the cerebrum (**9.6**) and of the cerebellum signify a failure of migration and are associated with certain CNS malformations (**9.7**). Failures of migration may also be associated with abnormal patterns of gyral formation, including abnormally large and broad gyri (pachygyria) (**9.8**), abnormally small and numerous gyri (polymicrogyria) (**9.9**), or absence of

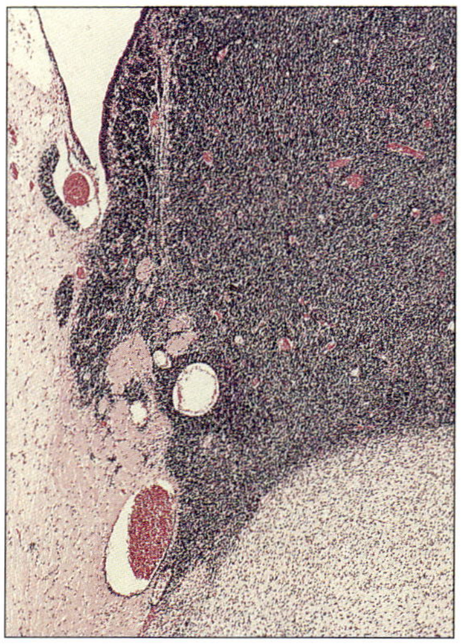

9.4 Germinal eminence in a 20-week fetus showing the relationship to the ventricular cavity. Thin-walled vessels are seen within the mass of undifferentiated cells.

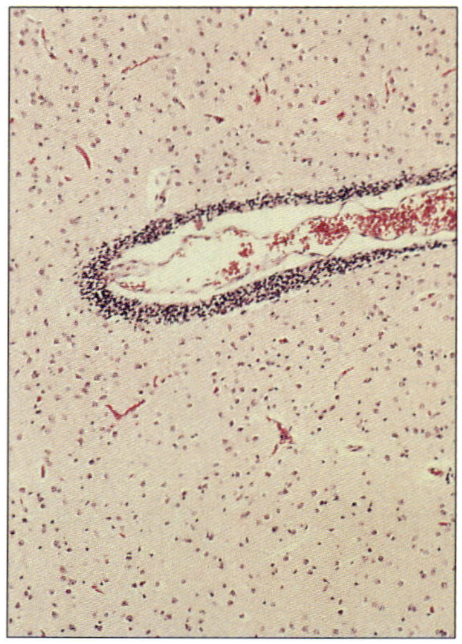

9.5 Cuff of undifferentiated cells surrounding a blood vessel in the periventricular tissues in the brain of a term neonate.

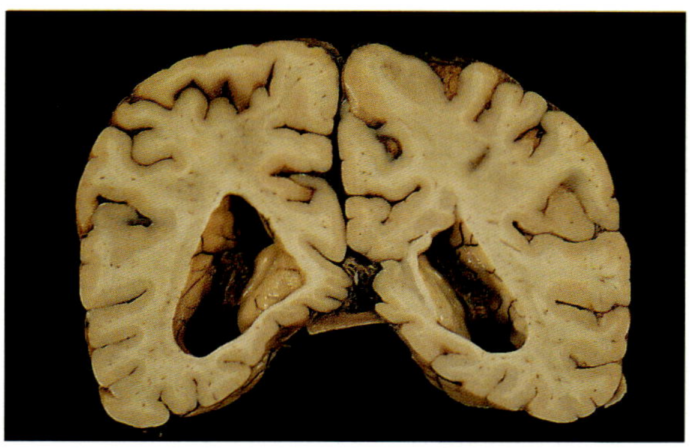

9.6 Coronal slice of brain in a child aged eight years with multiple abnormalities. Ventricular dilatation is present together with heterotopic nodules of grey matter surrounding the ventricular cavity.

Conditions associated with cerebral heterotopias	
Gyral abnormalities	Agyria Pachygyria Polymicrogyria including Zellweger's syndrome
Microcephaly	Agenesis of the corpus callosum Chromosomal abnormalities

9.7 Conditions with which cerebral heterotopias are associated.

gyri (agyria, lissencephaly). The choroid plexuses of all four ventricles show glycogen-rich epithelium in the first half of gestation (**9.10**).

The white matter of the brain is largely unmyelinated at birth, except for the internal capsule and some tracts of the brainstem *(see Chapter* 8). The white matter is very vascular during development and is more vulnerable to hypoxic insult than in the mature brain. Neurons of the basal ganglia and brainstem differentiate earlier than those of the cerebral cortex and are more likely to show hypoxic eosinophilic damage in cases of recent birth-related hypoxia, or encrustation and mineralisation in longer-term survivors *(see Chapter 2*). In the perinatal period, as in adults, the depths of sulci are more vulnerable than the crests of gyri to hypoxic damage. The brainstem nuclei, which are pigmented in the adult, are pale during the first five years *(see Chapter 2*) due to lack of neuronal melanin deposits. The cerebellum is relatively more mature than the cerebrum by the time of birth. The cortical layers of the vermis differentiate in advance of those in the hemispheres and may show selective vulnerability during mid-gestation. However, cerebellar development is far from complete at birth in that the folia are still covered by a layer of undifferentiated cells known as the external granular layer (**9.11**). From this subpial cerebellar layer, cells continue to migrate into the deeper layers of the cortex, until the external granular layer disappears at about one year of age. The leptomeninges covering both the cerebrum and cerebellum are much more cellular and vascular

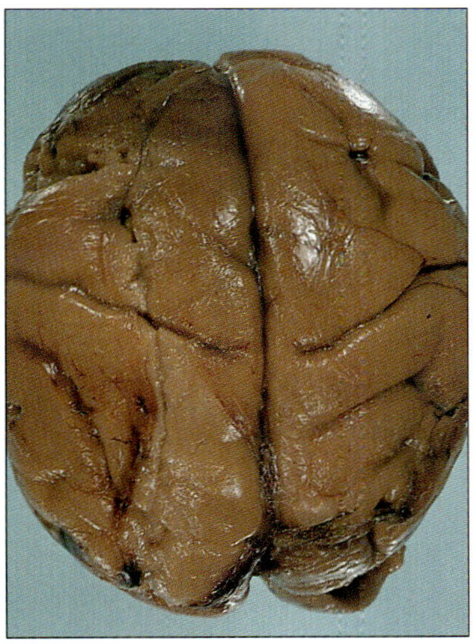

9.8 Brain from a microcephalic infant born at term. The brain shows pachygyria with abnormally broad gyral contours.

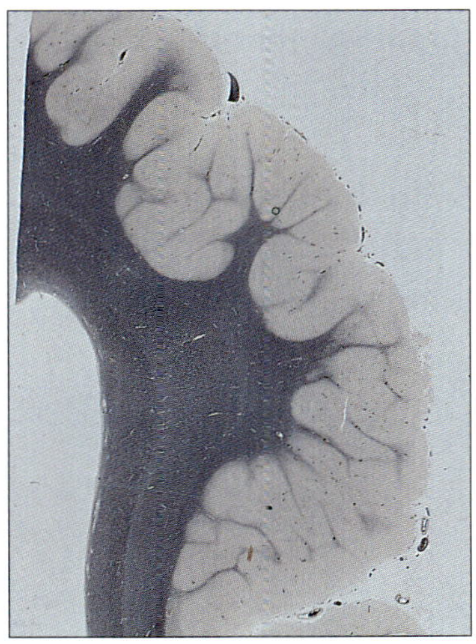

9.9 A section of cerebral cortex from a hydrocephalic brain in a case of spina bifida. The cortical ribbon shows an abnormal pattern of numerous small folds and crests – the condition of polymicrogyria.

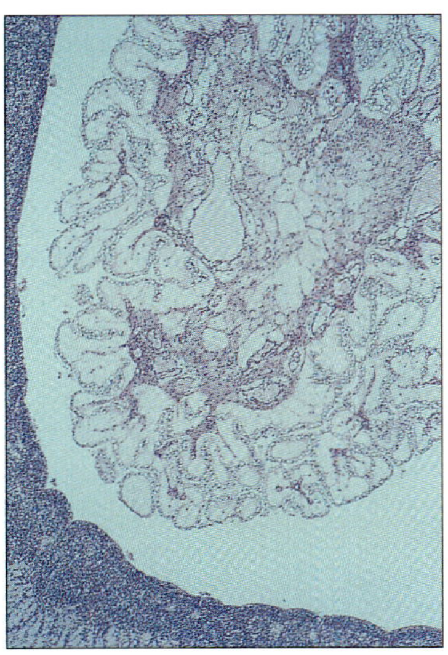

9.10 A section of the lateral ventricle choroid plexus at 22 weeks' gestation. The choroidal epithelium is pale and distended due to the presence of glycogen. The germinal matrix surrounds the ventricular cavity.

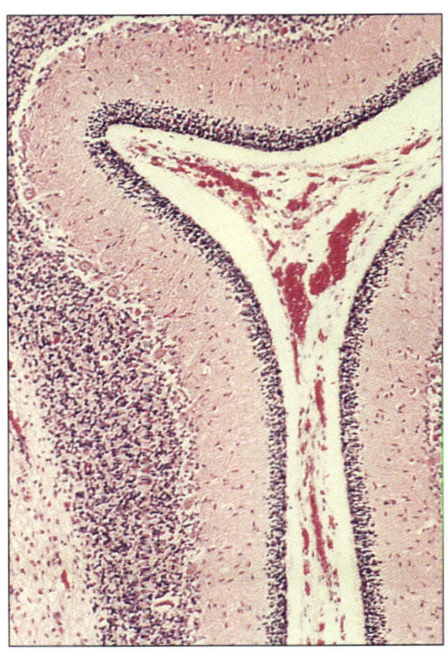

9.11 A section of cerebellum from an infant born at term. The molecular layer of the folia is covered by the external granular layer. The leptomeninges are more vascular than in the adult.

(**9.11**) during fetal life than in the adult state and contain quite a number of macrophages.

The spinal cord is relatively well-differentiated by the time of birth and many of the tracts are myelinated. The central canal is widely patent and shows a caudal dilatation, sometimes named the terminal ventricle, at the level of the conus. The central canal is usually obliterated by ependymoglial cells during the second or third decade. At birth, the most caudal segment of the spinal cord lies below the adult level of L2 and this has implications for the safety of lumbar puncture in the neonate.

ABNORMALITIES OF THE DEVELOPING NERVOUS SYSTEM

Insults which interfere with the normal development of the nervous system are shown in **9.12** and are separated according to the timing of maximal damage.

Possible insults to CNS development	
Intrauterine	Genetic Chromosomal Malformations Infections Immunological Vascular Teratogenic drugs Irradiation Metabolic Tumours Neurodegenerative
Perinatal	Vascular Infections Trauma Tumours Metabolic

9.12 Possible insults to CNS development.

The phases of CNS development include neuroectodermal mitosis, migration, differentiation and establishment of contacts. Insults produce a pattern of damage which reflects more the timing of damage than the nature of the insult. This is particularly true of hypoxic damage in the developing nervous system (*see below*). Some insults may be operative from the moment of conception, such as chromosomal and some genetic abnormalities, while others have an effect from early prenatal life, such as neural tube defects. Others are much more likely to occur around the time of birth, such as vascular accidents.

Some genetic abnormalities may be expressed only in middle-to-late adult life after many years of apparently normal CNS function, such as Huntington's disease and familial prion diseases (*see Chapter 7*). The incidence of conditions which have a clear genetic basis decreases with advancing age. Chromosomal abnormalities occur in approximately 5% of all conceptions, with trisomy 21 having an incidence of greater than 1% of births to mothers aged 40 years and more. Neural tube defects occurred in about 0.5% of births before the advent of antenatal diagnosis. Prion diseases occur with a frequency of 0.5 per milion of the population.

GENETIC ABNORMALITIES

An abnormal genetic make-up may reveal its influence on the development of the nervous system only late in life. Development may proceed at first in an apparently normal fashion, as in most of the genetically determined storage and other metabolic disorders considered in *Chapter 8*. Alternatively, other genetic conditions may be obvious by the time of birth, such as microcephaly in the offspring of consanguinous marriages (**9.13**). It is important to note that microcephaly may be the end-result of

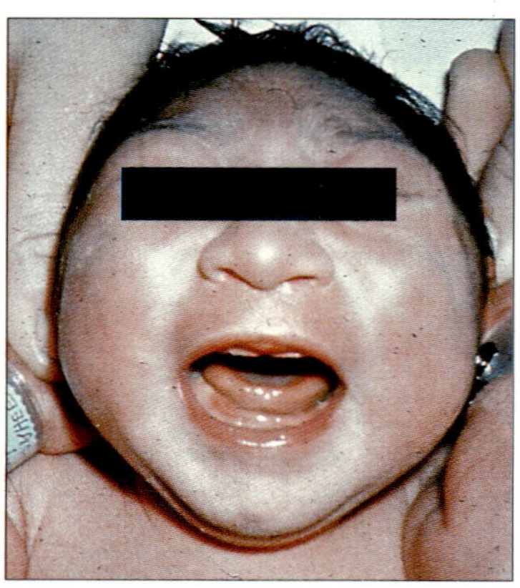

9.13 Microcephalic infant born from a consanguinous marriage.

Causes of microcephaly
Genetic/familial causes
Hypoxic/ischaemic causes
Fetal alcohol syndrome
Intrauterine infections
Irradiation

9.14 Causes of microcephaly.

several different possible causes (**9.14**) which should be considered in the differential diagnosis. Some other examples of genetic abnormalities affecting the CNS include the following.

X-linked mental retardation

This disorder, which occurs in one per 1000 liveborn males, is the most common cause of reduced intelligence after Down's syndrome and is characterised by an excess trinucleotide repeat sequence on the X chromosome. The neuropathology of this condition is not well understood, although anomalous synapses and structural abnormalities of the brainstem have been described in some individuals.

Von Recklinghausen's disease

This inherited condition occurs in two forms, both associated with pigmented skin lesions described as café-au-lait spots and a tendency to form tumours associated with peripheral nerves. These may be benign, but they also show a tendency for malignant transformation *(see Chapter 10)*. In the central form of the disease, bilateral schwannomas occur on the acoustic nerves. The peripheral form shows multiple schwannomas associated with nerve roots or cutaneous nerves.

Huntington's disease

This is determined by an abnormal genetic locus on chromosome 4 which is inherited in an autosomal-dominant pattern. Affected individuals show progressive cell loss in the basal ganglia, particularly in the caudate nucleus, and this leads in middle life to dementia and abnormal involuntary movements *(see Chapter 7)*.

Tuberous sclerosis

Affected individuals show abnormal focally expanded gyri known as tubers (**9.15**) and have a propensity to develop CNS tumours of different varieties, including gliomas and subependymal astrocytomas *(see Chapter 10)*. These may be associated with tumours in other organs, particularly in the kidney and myocardium.

Meckel–Gruber syndrome

This syndrome is manifest at birth and is characterised by the presence of an encephalocele, polydactyly and polycystic kidneys. Survival is short in this autosomal recessive inherited condition.

CHROMOSOMAL ABNORMALITIES

Many spontaneous abortions are associated with abnormal numbers of chromosomes in the conceptus (**9.16**). Autosomal trisomies and triploidy are common, and are often associated with failure of development in multiple systems, including the CNS, leading to early miscarriage. However, certain abnormalities, involving particularly the sex chromosomes, such as Turner's syndrome (monosomy X), are compatible with long life and do not appear to affect CNS development. This is in contrast to the following three varieties of trisomy, which have a profoundly damaging effect on the CNS.

Trisomy 21 (Down's syndrome)

Individuals with Down's syndrome are mentally disabled. The structural basis for the mental deficit is not well understood. The brain may be macroscopically normal or may show an unusually small

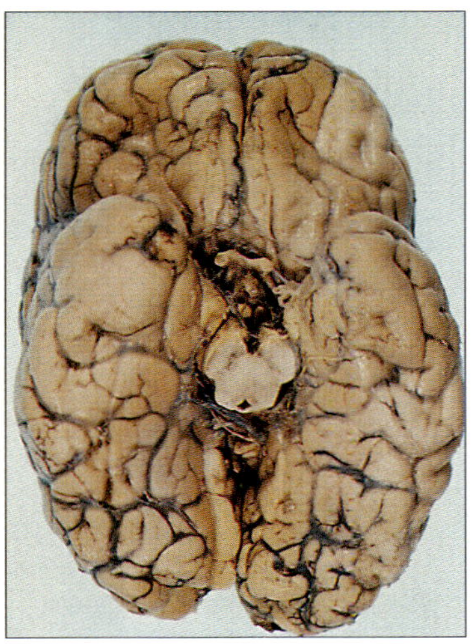

9.15 A ventral view of the brain in a case of tuberous sclerosis showing tubers of both temporal lobes, right more than left, and of the left frontal lobe.

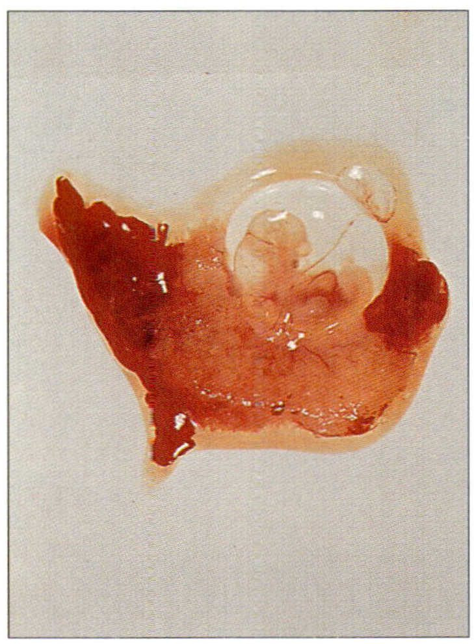

9.16 Spontaneous abortion at seven weeks showing intact amniotic sac and surrounding placenta and yolk sac. The embryo is abnormal and has only one centrally placed eye below a bulging forebrain. Chromosomal analysis showed triploidy. Cyclops deformity was confirmed in the embryo after opening the sac.

superior temporal gyrus in some cases (**9.17**). Some neurons may have poorly developed dendritic trees and a paucity of connections. The facial appearance is characteristic and individuals with trisomy 21 have early-onset Alzheimer's disease *(see Chapter 7)*.

Trisomy 18 (Edwards' syndrome)

Fetuses with trisomy 18 do not survive for long after birth. Microcephaly may be present and there is an association with spina bifida malformations.

Trisomy 13 (Patau's syndrome)

Fetuses with this trisomy show a variable degree of facial and CNS malformation. The spectrum of abnormality ranges from cyclops deformity (**9.16**) at one extreme to near normal facial appearances at the other, although the classical phenotype consists of cleft lip and palate together with hypotelorism and severe underlying CNS malformation. The cerebral hemispheres fail to develop separately from the forebrain with the result that there is a single ventricle and variably fused central grey matter, globes and optic nerves – a condition known as holoprosencephaly (**9.18**). The least severe malformation in this spectrum is arrhinencephaly, where the first cranial nerves may be absent as an apparently isolated phenomenon. Infants with trisomy 13 rarely survive for long after birth.

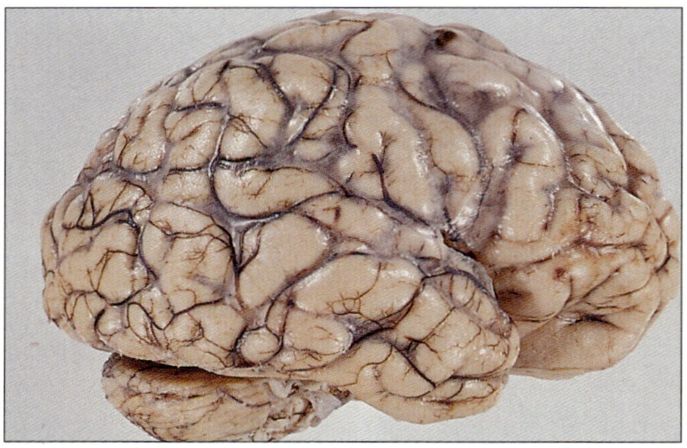

9.17 Lateral view of the brain from an adult with Down's syndrome. The superior temporal gyrus is narrower than usual – an abnormality present in approximately one half of cases of Down's syndrome.

MALFORMATIONS

Neural tube defects

Neural tube defects are among the most common congenital malformations. Before the advent of antenatal screening, the incidence of these defects varied between 0.1% and 0.5% of live births, being more common in some parts of the world, including the UK, than others. The major varieties of neural tube defects include:

- spina bifida (**9.19**);
- anencephaly;
- anencephaly combined with complete spina bifida.

It is generally assumed that these defects arise from a failure of closure of the neural tube and that they occur in the first four weeks of embryonic development. This is supported by descriptions of neural

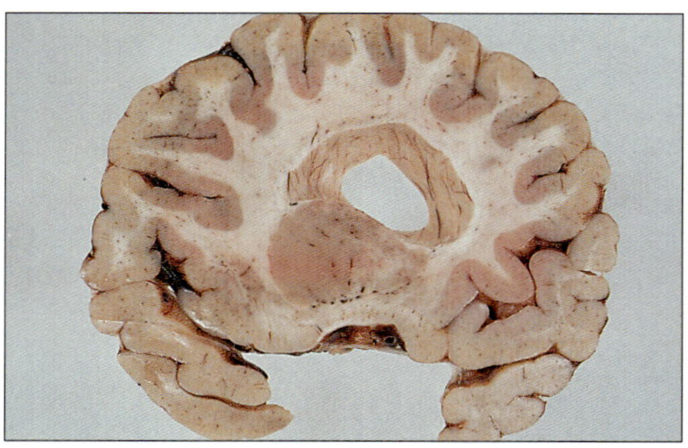

9.18 Holoprosencephalic brain showing a single ventricle and a fused mass of deep grey matter. There is no division of the cerebral hemispheres.

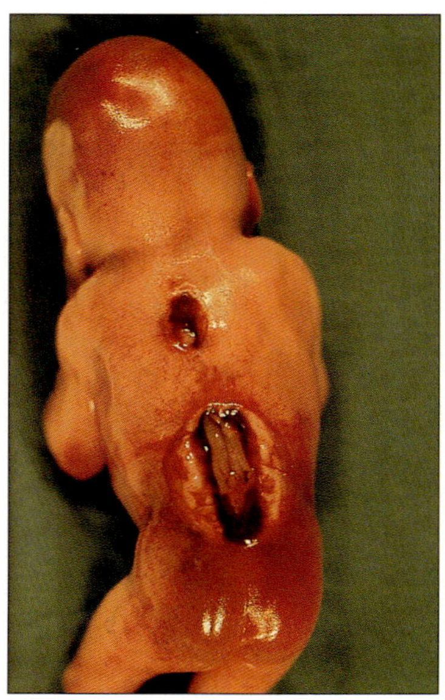

9.19 Fetus of 20 weeks' gestation with spina bifida detected antenatally, followed by termination of pregnancy. There are two spina bifida lesions. The thoracolumbar lesion is a typical open myelocele with an abnormal spinal cord displayed at the base of the open lesion. The presence of a second lesion in the thoracic region is unusual.

tube defects in human embryos aborted before eight weeks of gestation. Most of these abnormalities may now be detected before birth through leakage of fetal proteins, particularly alphafetoprotein, into the amniotic fluid and thence into maternal blood. Ultrasound screening is also used extensively in antenatal detection. The birth incidence of these defects has fallen considerably through termination of affected pregnancies. Although the cause of neural tube defects is not well understood, it is clear that genetic factors play a part in the aetiology. Female fetuses are more frequently affected than males and the defects tend to occur in families with a rising risk of recurrence (5–10%) after one or more affected pregnancies.

While anencephaly is incompatible with postnatal survival, spina bifida does not usually lead to death in the neonatal period. In spina bifida occulta, the bifid vertebral lesion is skin-covered, and that skin may be hairy, or may display a naevus or a sinus tract. In the more serious defect of open spina bifida, the spinal cord itself is abnormal and is either exposed on the body surface (myelocele) (**9.20**), or covered wholly or in part by meninges (meningocele or myelomeningocele). These apparently localised spina bifida lesions are often complicated by other conditions such as hydrocephalus and Arnold–Chiari (Chiari type II) malformation.

Hydrocephalus

Enlargement of the ventricles occurs by mid-gestation in approximately half of the fetuses with spina bifida. This is not at first associated with enlargement of the head, which generally occurs only by the time of birth (**9.21**). However, spina bifida is only one cause of hydrocephalus arising during prenatal life (**9.22**). Any abnormality which interferes with the circulation of CSF may lead to hydrocephalus. They include aqueduct stenosis which may be due to:

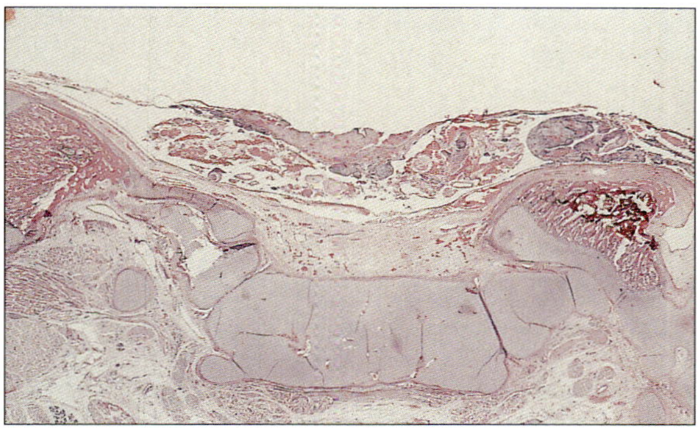

9.20 A section of a spina bifida myelocele showing abnormal spinal cord exposed on the dorsal surface of a vertebral body. The spinal cord tissues are in continuity through thin membrane with skin at the edge of the lesion.

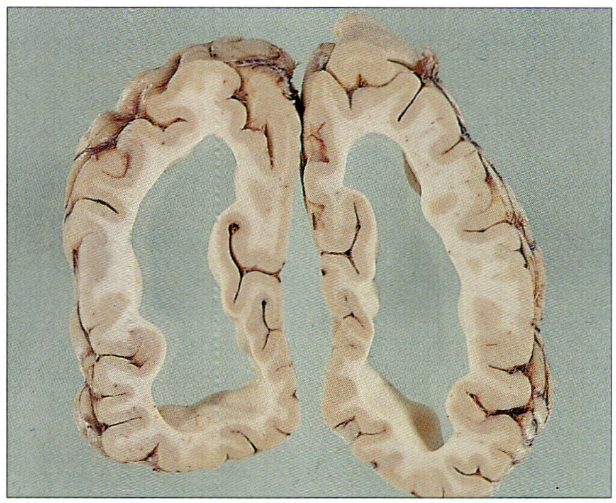

9.21 Coronal section through the occipital lobes of a hydrocephalic brain in an infant born at term with spina bifida who survived for 18 months.

Causes of hydrocephalus

- Spina bifida
- Arnold–Chiari malformation
- Aqueduct stenosis
  - Sex-linked
  - Acquired
- Dandy–Walker malformation
- Intrauterine infections
- Intrauterine CNS haemorrhage

9.22 Causes of hydrocephalus.

- an inherited defect affecting males only;
- secondary to intrauterine infection or haemorrhage (**9.23**);
- present with no obvious causation.

In the Dandy–Walker malformation, the roof of the fourth ventricle is imperforate. This leads to cystic dilatation and obstruction of the CSF pathway (**9.24**).

Arnold–Chiari malformation

There are several different types of malformation in which posterior cranial fossa structures are displaced downwards through the foramen magnum. The one most commonly associated with spina bifida is the Chiari type II malformation, in which a shallow posterior cranial fossa is associated with the displacement of vermis and brainstem downwards into the cervical spinal canal (**9.25**), with characteristic kinking of the brainstem (**9.26**), and upper cervical nerves passing upwards to reach their exit foramina (**9.25**). The type I malformation consists of chronic but asymptomatic elongation of cerebellar tonsils, without displacement of brainstem or vermis (**9.27**). In the type III malformation, a bony defect is present in the posterior wall of the foramen magnum allowing cerebellar herniation.

Other conditions associated with neural tube defects

Several different abnormalities of the brain and spinal cord may occur in isolation, but are most commonly

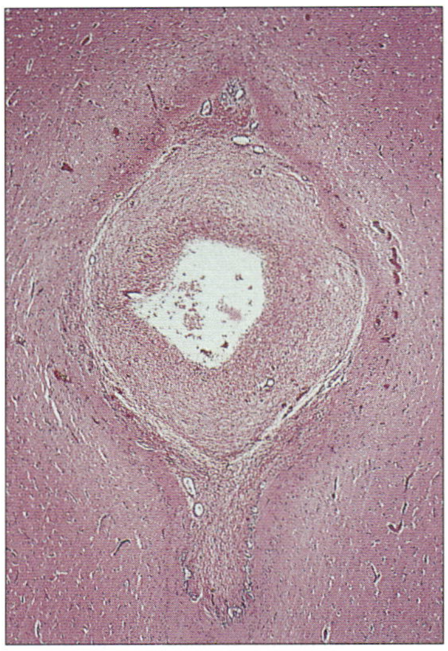

9.23 A section of the midbrain from a case of aqueduct stenosis. The original outline of the aqueduct is visible and the lumen is considerably narrowed by the presence of gliosis. A small residual channel is present centrally.

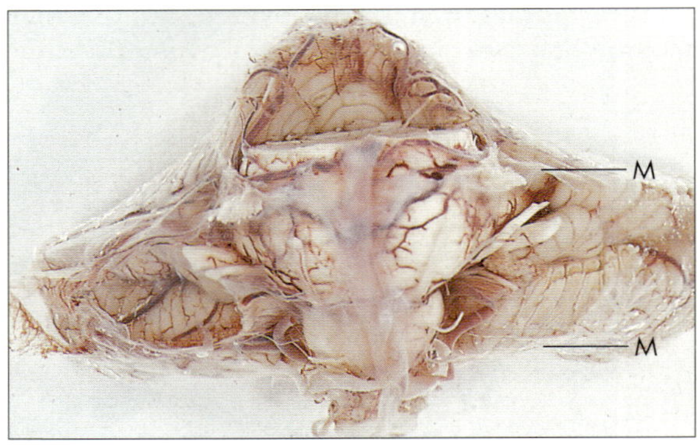

9.24 Brainstem and cerebellum from a case of Dandy–Walker syndrome. The remains of the cystic dilatation of arachnoid mater are present as a torn edge of membrane (M).

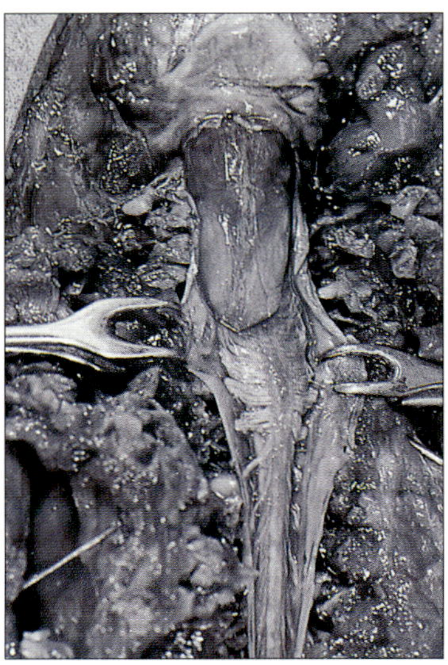

9.25 Dorsal view of the cervical spinal canal in a case of Arnold–Chiari (type II) malformation. The vermis is elongated. The upper cervical roots pass upwards towards their exit foramina.

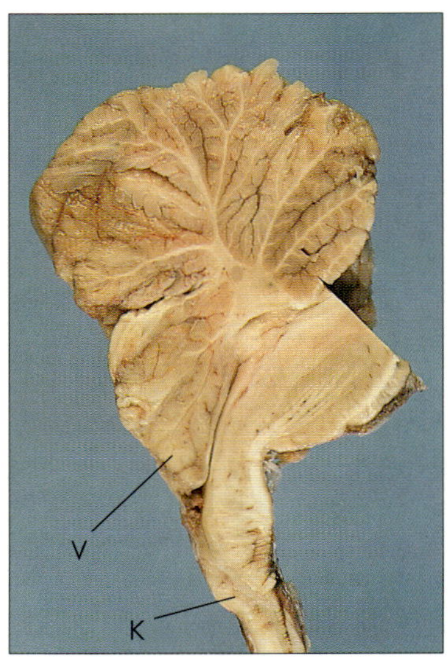

9.26 Sagittal section through the brainstem and cerebellum in a case of Arnold–Chiari malformation. The vermis (V) is elongated below the level of the foramen magnum dorsal to the abnormally kinked brainstem (K).

seen in the context of neural tube defects. These include the following.

- Agenesis of the corpus callosum (**9.28**).
- Partial splitting of the spinal cord (diplomyelia), possibly associated with a bony or cartilaginous spur (diastematomyelia). The central canal may be duplicated (**9.29**).
- Intraspinal cysts and lipomas. The cysts may be lined with epithelium of respiratory or gastrointestinal type.
- Hydromyelia. In this condition, the central canal is distended beyond what is normal for fetal life.

Syringomyelia

An abnormally dilated central canal continues laterally as a split in the parenchyma of the spinal cord (**9.30**). A similar abnormality may extend into the brainstem (syringobulbia). These may be congenital malformations, but some cases in later life have an associated history of trauma *(see Chapter 5)*.

Amniotic band syndrome

The fetus may be abnormally adherent to parts of the cord or placenta, and a widely based attachment to the head can mimic anencephaly.

CONGENITAL INFECTIONS

Immune mechanisms in the fetus are immature and the fetus may be vulnerable to certain maternal infections which cross the placenta.

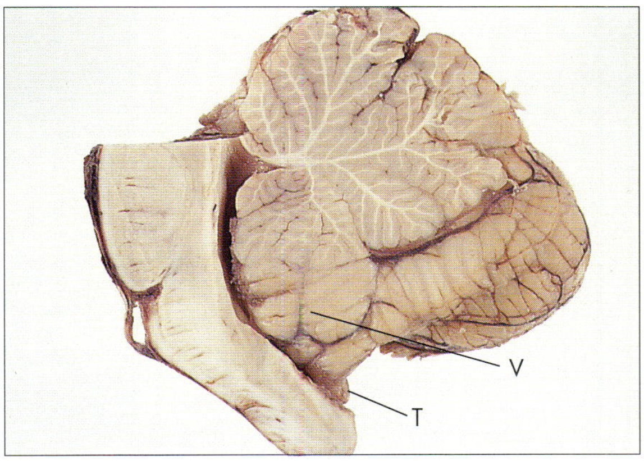

9.27 Sagittal section through brainstem and cerebellum in a case of Chiari type I malformation. The brainstem is not kinked and it is the cerebellar tonsils (T) which are elongated caudally rather than the vermis (V).

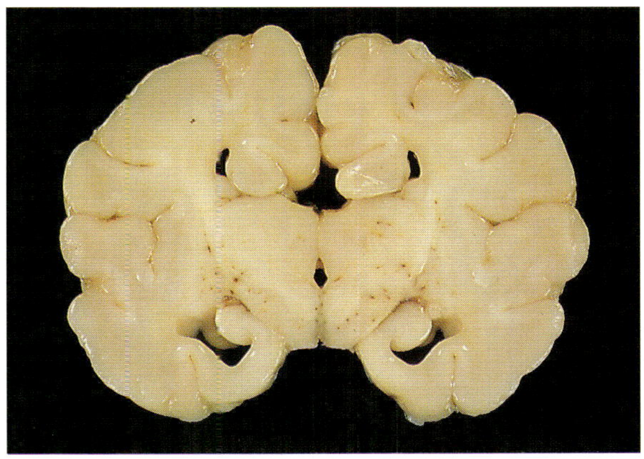

9.28 Coronal section through the brain of a slightly premature microcephalic infant in whom the corpus callosum is absent. The lateral ventricles show the characteristic 'batwing' shape.

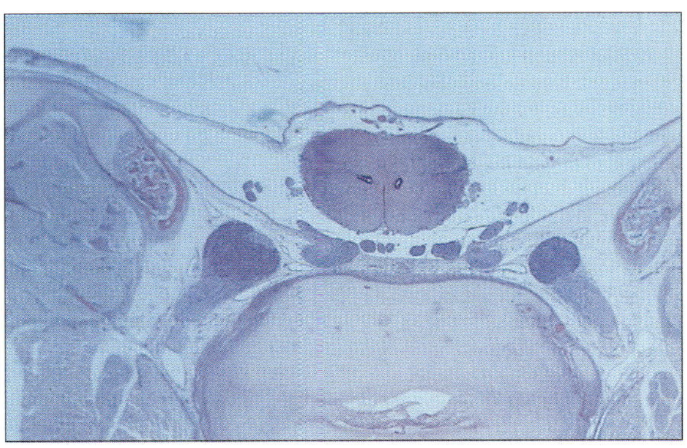

9.29 Spinal cord from a 20 weeks' gestation spina bifida fetus. The cord is covered by a thin membrane above the level of the myelocoele and the central canal is duplicated.

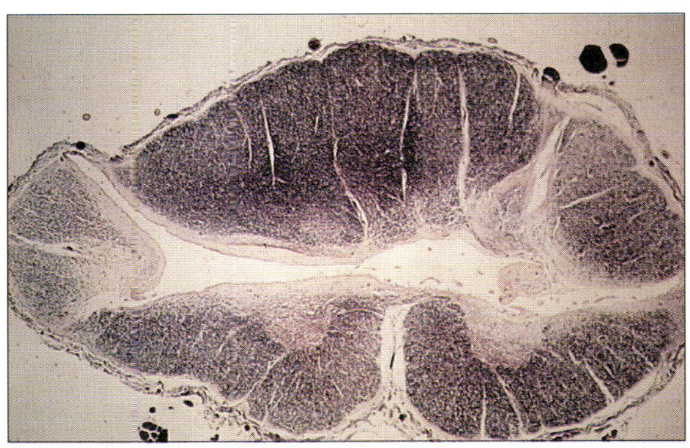

9.30 Transverse section through the cord of a case of syringomyelia. The cord is stained for myelin. The central canal is distended laterally in continuity with a cyst reaching the pial surface. (Loyez stain)

The major infections found in fetal life are listed in **9.31**. Syphilis is no longer a numerically significant fetal hazard. With other infections, maternal infections may be silent or clinically overt, but even in recognised maternal illness, fewer than half the exposed fetuses display evidence of damage. Cytomegalovirus (**9.32**) and *Toxoplasma* are particularly damaging organisms and can cause fetal encephalitis, with necrosis and calcification, particularly in the basal ganglia (**9.33**). Fetal infection with *Listeria monocytogenes* causes small necrotising granulomas in many different tissues (**9.34**), including the CNS.

HIV infection is transmitted vertically in less than 20% of affected pregnancies in industrialised countries. The rate is higher in Africa. The timing of mother-to-infant transmission is still unclear and may well occur around the time of birth, or even during breast feeding, as well as earlier in pregnancy. Fetal HIV infection does not inflict visible damage in the CNS, but HIV encephalitis is a well-recognised complication of paediatric AIDS (**9.35**). The major effects of HIV in the CNS are described in *Chapter 3*. Paediatric cases differ from adult cases in that CNS opportunistic infections and lymphomas are less common complications, but vasculitis, white matter pallor (**9.36**) and mineralisation of blood vessels are more common (**9.37**).

Perinatal infections of the CNS may be manifested in immunosuppressed or in normal neonates. They include meningitis and encephalitis caused by organisms such as *Escherichia coli*, *Haemophilus influenzae*, *Candida* and other fungal and viral infections (**9.38**).

Intrauterine CNS infections	
Rubella	Affects eye, ear, heart and CNS
Cytomegalovirus	Haemolytic anaemia CNS infections and calcification
Toxoplasmosis	Haemolytic anaemia CNS infections and calcification
Human immunodeficiency virus	
Listeria monocytogenes	
Syphilis	

9.31 Intrauterine infections of the CNS.

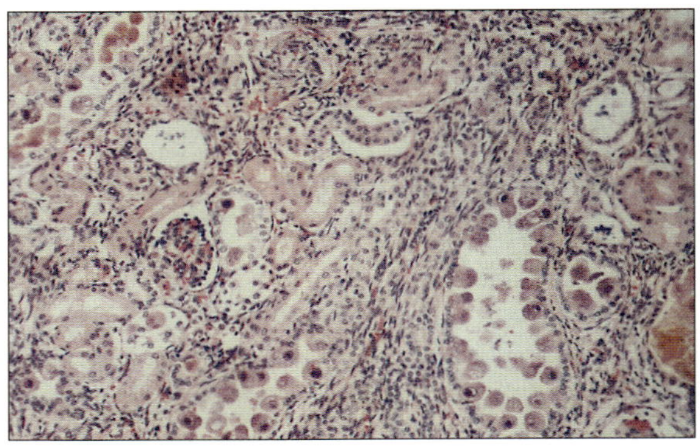

9.32 A section of kidney from a full-term infant found to be suffering from intrauterine cytomegalovirus infection. Many cells distended with viral inclusions are present within the renal tubules.

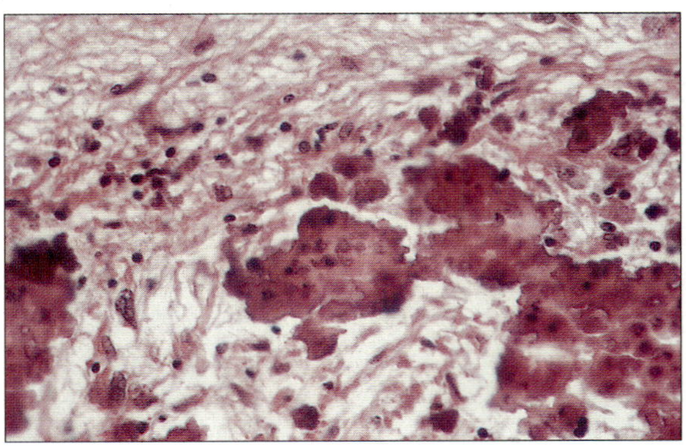

9.33 A section of basal ganglia from the brain of an infant with congenital toxoplasmosis. Calcification is widespread and organisms are hard to identify.

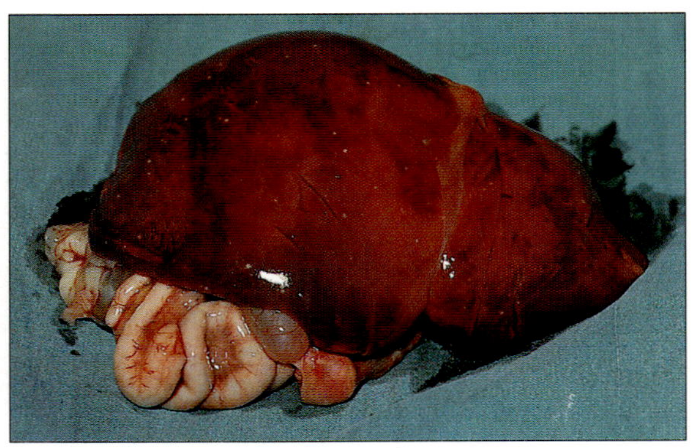

9.34 Liver from an infant with congenital listeriosis. Numerous very small white granulomata are present on the surface of the liver indicative of systemic listeriosis.

IMMUNOLOGICAL INSULTS

Only rarely does the fetus become a target of maternal immunological attack. This may occur in cases of fetal–maternal rhesus incompatibility and occasional cases of ABO incompatibility. In severe cases, the fetus may display haemolytic anaemia and jaundice with the threat of neonatal kernicterus (*see below*).

VASCULAR INSULTS

The developing CNS is vulnerable to hypoxic and ischaemic damage at all stages, both in intrauterine life and about the time of birth. The incidence of perinatal asphyxia with consequent brain damage and neurological signs and symptoms is not declining, despite improved obstetric care, and probably affects 0.2–0.4% of live births. It is undoubtedly true that hypoxic episodes related to birth events can give rise to pathological changes in the CNS, and the pattern of these depends on the developmental maturity at the time of birth.

Premature infants

In premature infants, who may be liable to respiratory distress syndrome, the resulting hypoxia leads to endothelial necrosis and subependymal haemorrhage (**9.39, 9.40**) from thin-walled vessels in the germinal matrix. These haemorrhages are graded in severity and may show evidence of rebleeding and reactive changes (**9.41, 9.42**). In more severe cases, the subependymal haemorrhage ruptures into the ventricular system (**9.39**). Intraventricular haemorrhages are associated with a high risk of long-term brain damage, particularly hydrocephalus. These conditions are

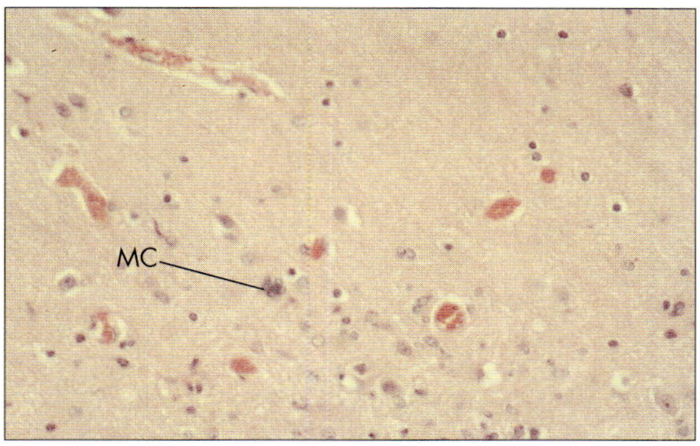

9.35 Multinucleated cells (MC) in the brain of a 9-month-old infant dying of AIDS. Multinucleate cells with very inconspicuous cytoplasm are described particularly in paediatric HIV encephalitis and have been called cluster cells.

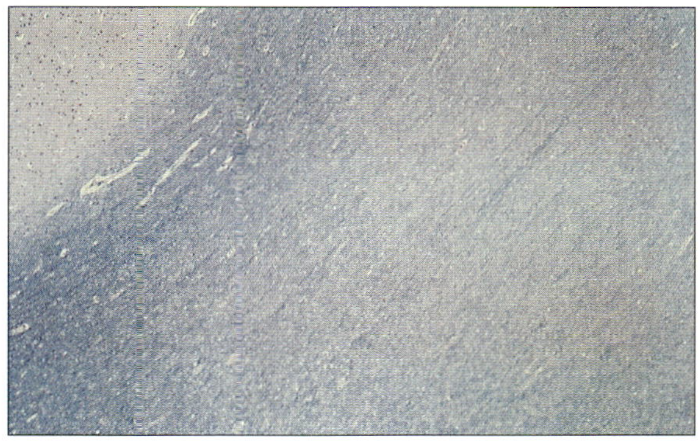

9.36 White matter shows myelin pallor in the case shown in **9.35**. (Luxol fast blue)

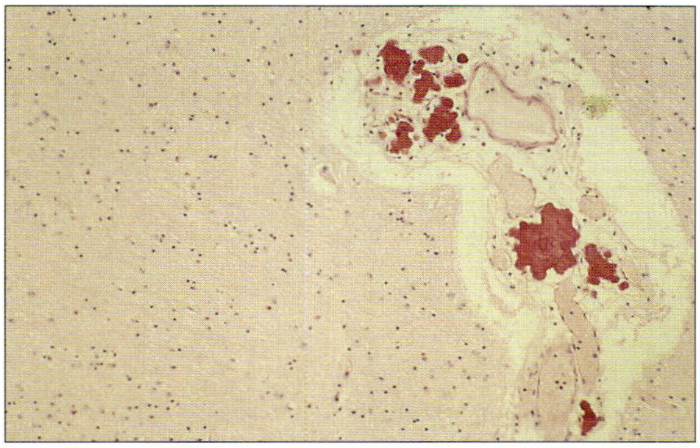

9.37 Perivascular calcification is a non-specific but frequent finding in cases of HIV encephalitis in paediatric AIDS.

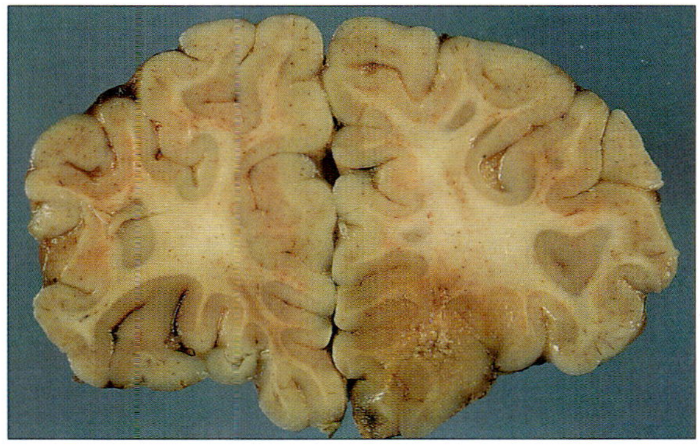

9.38 Coronal sections of the frontal lobes from an infant with perinatally acquired *Candida* infection. The lesion in the inferior surface of the right frontal lobe is an infarct associated with fungal infection.

readily diagnosed on CT scanning. In premature infants, the periventricular white matter is also a target of hypoxic damage (**9.43**), and this is characterised either by widespread necrosis or by focal white matter lesions showing axonal loss, accumulation of microglia and macrophages, and mineralisation of residual processes – the characteristic lesions of periventricular leucomalacia (**9.44**). Hypoxic damage may lead to localised cysts within the white matter (porencephaly) (**9.45**), or may result in extensive symmetrical loss of white matter and sometimes grey matter, as seen in cystic encephalomalacia (**9.46**).

Full-term infants

In the infant born at term, the pattern of hypoxic damage is different and is characterised by diffuse neuronal damage (**9.47, 9.48**), particularly in neurons of the brainstem and basal ganglia which are relatively mature. This is in contrast to the pattern of hypoxic damage in the adult, in whom the basal ganglia are not particularly vulnerable. Excitatory neurotransmitter overactivity provoked by hypoxia may be a significant contributing factor. It has been claimed that pontosubicular lesions, combining neuronal changes in the subiculum and in the pons,

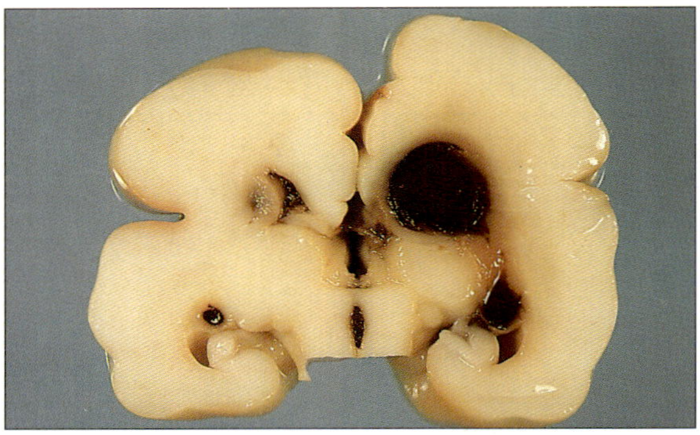

9.39 Brain from an infant born at 28 weeks' gestation who survived for five days. Subependymal haemorrhage is identified in both hemispheres and is particularly well seen in the left cerebral hemisphere. On the right side, intraventricular haemorrhage has also occurred due to rupture of the subependymal haemorrhage.

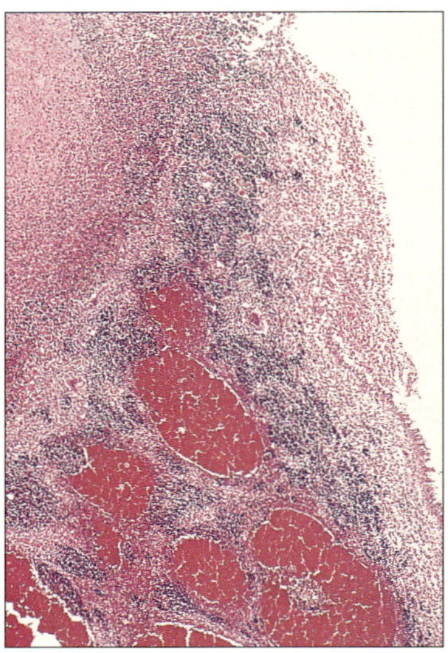

9.40 A section from the germinal eminence of a premature infant showing subependymal haemorrhage.

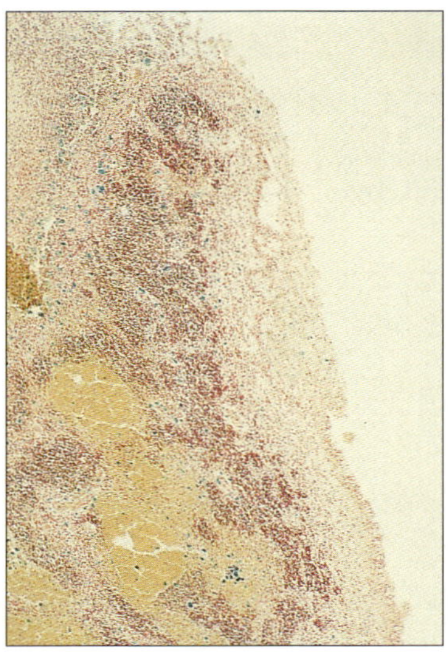

9.41 A section through the subependymal haemorrhage shown in **9.40**, stained for haemosiderin and demonstrating evidence of previous haemorrhage.

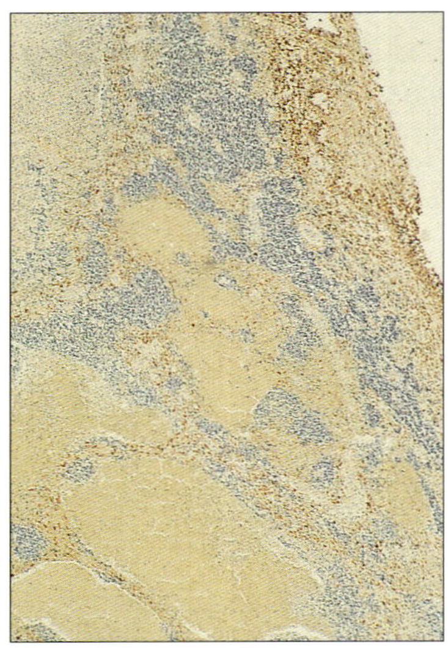

9.42 A section through the subependymal haemorrhage shown in **9.40**, stained for GFAP, demonstrating the astrocytic response to the presence of subependymal haemorrhage.

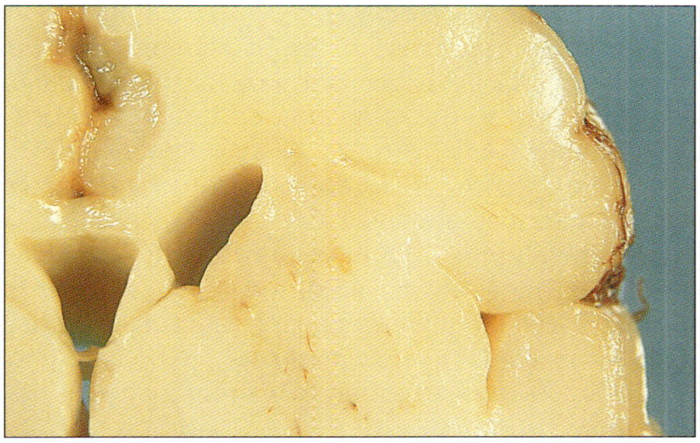

9.43 Brain from an infant born at 33 weeks' gestation who survived for two weeks, showing slightly pigmented lesions in the periventricular white matter which proved histologically (**9.44**) to be periventricular leucomalacia.

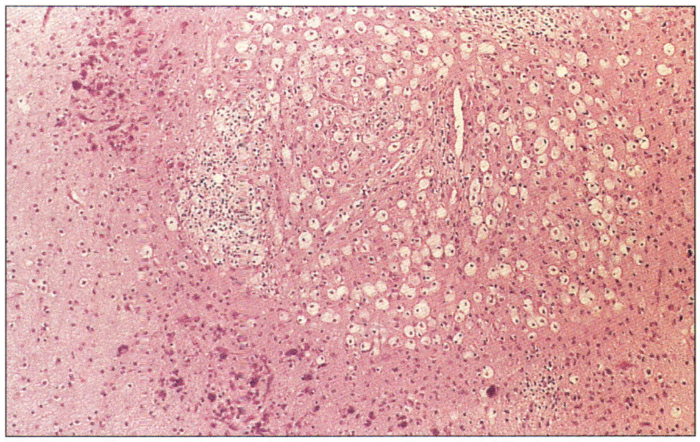

9.44 Microscopic appearances of periventricular leucomalacia. A central mass of foamy macrophages is surrounded by a zone of mineralised axons and microglia.

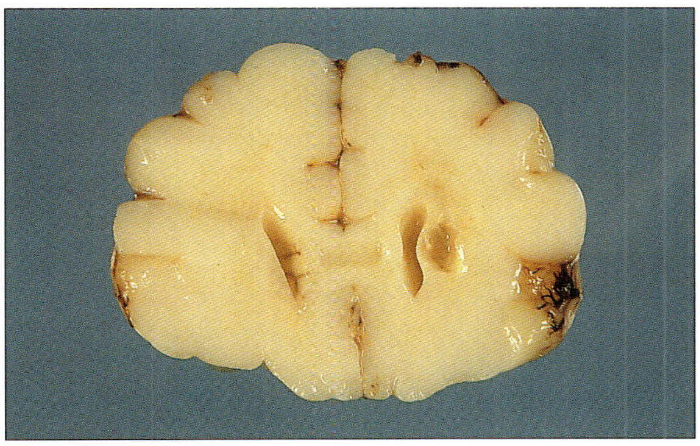

9.45 Brain from a premature infant born at 29 weeks' gestation who survived for three weeks. A small porencephalic cyst is present lateral to the right lateral ventricle.

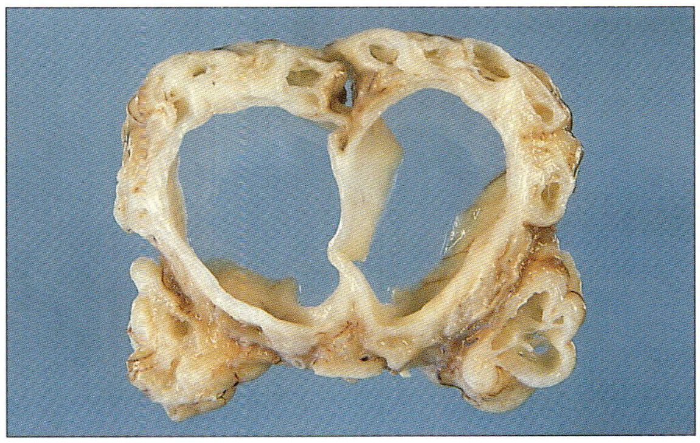

9.46 Cystic encephalomalacia in an infant suffering perinatal hypoxia. The infant survived eight months after birth.

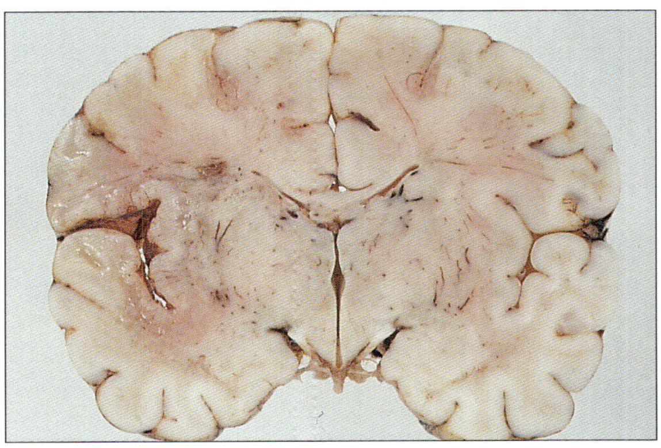

9.47 Perinatal hypoxia in an infant born at term who survived for three days. The brain is swollen and shows global hypoxic changes with frank infarction in both insular regions.

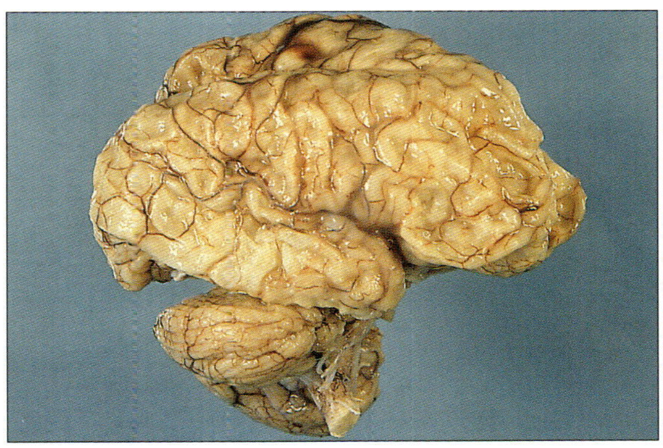

9.48 Infant born at term who suffered perinatal hypoxia and survived for nine weeks. The brain is shrunken and section showed gross dilatation of ventricles and loss of brain tissue.

are characteristic of perinatal asphyxia in the term infant. Dead neurons in the basal ganglia show a peculiar propensity for encrustation and mineralisation *(see Chapter 2)*. In surviving infants, a brisk astrocytic response is also seen and there may be abnormal myelination of non-neuronal processes, particularly in the basal ganglia – so-called status marmoratus (**9.49**). Some of these lesions are peculiar to the developing brain and have no counterpart in adult neuropathology, but occasionally an adult pattern of infarction in arterial distributions is also seen . These have been attributed to emboli from placental infarcts (**9.50**).

Hypoxia in the perinatal period may result in ulegyria in which the crests of gyri are preferentially preserved, while the depths of sulci show profound neuronal loss (**9.51**), indicating the heightened vulnerability of some cortical neurons to oxygen deprivation. After six months of age, paediatric brains show, for the most part, adult responses to ischaemic and vascular insults.

While perinatally associated vascular insults cause recognisable patterns of brain damage in the developing CNS, it has become clear that these do not generally lead to the clinical condition of cerebral palsy. Most cases of cerebral palsy originate in fetal life, and only a few cases are associated with intrapartum and postnatal events.

The developing CNS is vulnerable during intrauterine existence to any condition which deprives it of oxygenated blood. Placental infarcts and abruptio, twin/twin transfusion, maternal hypoxia, and congenital heart disease may all cause damage to the fetal nervous system.

Investigation of stillborn infants shows that nearly half have evidence of hypoxic brain damage, usually in the white matter, which is visible at the time of birth. Thrombosis of the CNS dural sinuses leads to venous thrombosis (**9.52, 9.53**) as in the adult. Infection and dehydration are predisposing factors.

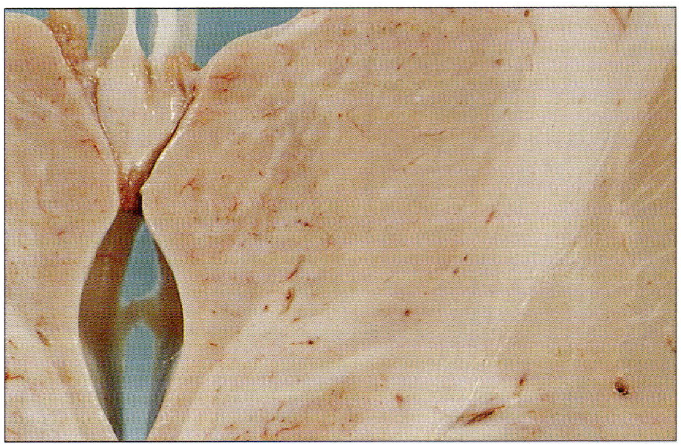

9.49 Thalamus showing status marmoratus in a three-year-old child who displayed neurological deficit following birth hypoxia.

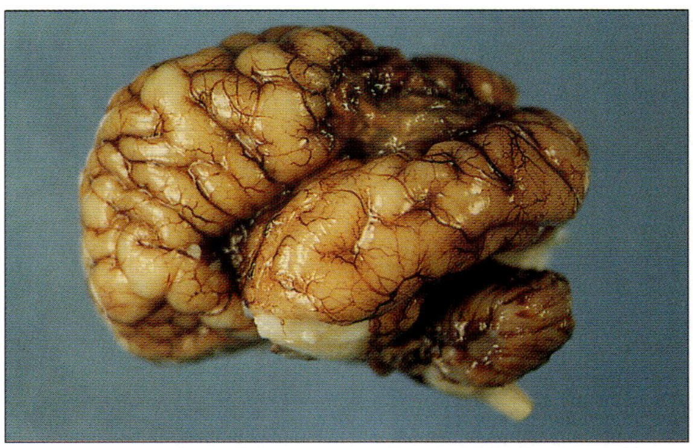

9.50 Focal deficit in the middle cerebral artery distribution of an infant born at term with placental infarcts.

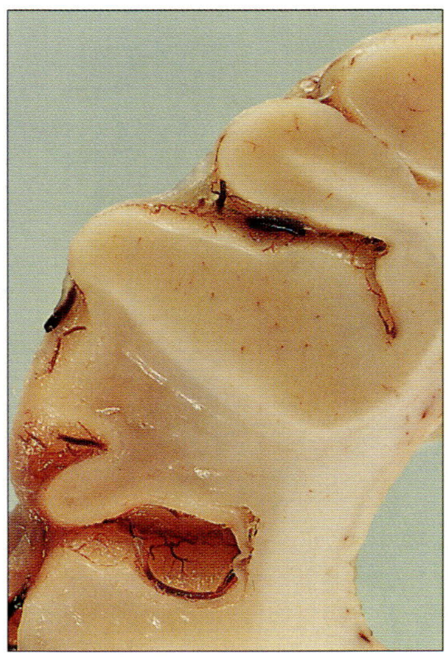

9.51 Coronal slice of brain showing the lesions of ulegyria in an infant suffering birth asphyxia. The depths of the sulci show cystic cavitation of the grey matter.

TERATOGENS AND IRRADIATION

Not all drugs cross the placenta, but some of those that do are capable of causing fetal malformations. The best known of these is thalidomide which may cause shortening and deformity of the limbs in addition to other deformities. This effect may be mediated through abnormal neural crest development. Sodium valproate, which is used in the treatment of epilepsy, is associated with an increased risk of neural tube defects. Alcohol, especially episodic drinking, can give rise to the fetal alcohol syndrome, in which microcephaly and mental disability may be present. Irradiation can lead to microcephaly due to the sensitivity of neuroblasts during migration. Because of these risks to fetal development, exposure to all unnecessary drugs and to radiation should be avoided, especially during the first half of pregnancy.

METABOLIC INSULTS

Metabolic disorders are described in detail in *Chapter 8*. However, there are some extrinsic metabolic insults, which particularly affect early CNS development.

Hyperbilirubinaemia

In the premature infant, or in infants with haemolytic anaemia, levels of unconjugated bilurubin rise rapidly. Since this form may cross the blood–brain barrier, staining and damage may result in many regions of the developing brain, particularly in the basal ganglia, giving rise to kernicterus.

Maternal iodine deficiency

This is endemic in certain inland areas such as central China. It can lead to hypothyroidism-induced maldevelopment of the CNS, manifested clinically as cretinism.

Maternal malnutrition

Although the fetal nervous system is largely protected when the mother is malnourished, a significant degree of malnutrition may delay or impair myelin formation. This may also occur in postnatal development when the infant itself is at direct risk of protein and micronutrient deprivation.

TRAUMA

Traumatic damage to the developing nervous system is very rarely seen before birth. Birth trauma to the CNS is usually an unfortunate consequence of assisted delivery, particularly high-forceps delivery, and is only seen occasionally nowadays *(see Chapter 5)*. While skull fracture is rather unusual in the neonate, the presence of sutures and the consequent potential for deformation of the immature skull, may lead to intracranial haemorrhage and damage to neural tissue. Excessive twisting of the head and neck during delivery may result in tears in the falx or the tentorium, and lead to subdural haemorrhage *(see Chapter 5)*.

Accidental and non-accidental injuries are also seen in neonates, infants and young children. Non-accidental injury may be suspected in children with suspicious patterns of bruising, particularly in those

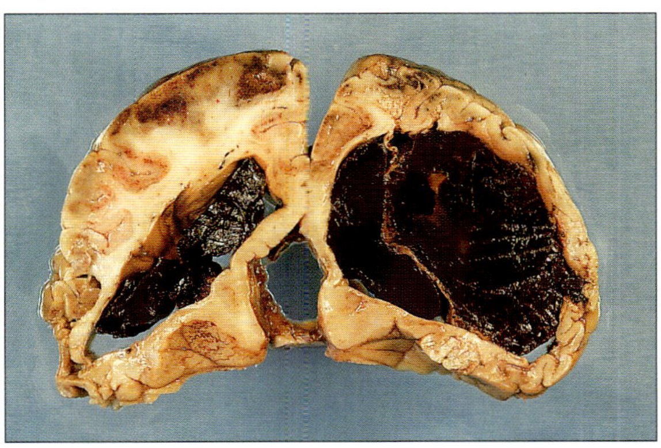

9.52 Venous infarction of the brain associated with massive haemorrhage in a five-month-old infant with extensive dural sinus thrombosis, resulting from aneurysmal dilatation of the vein of Galen.

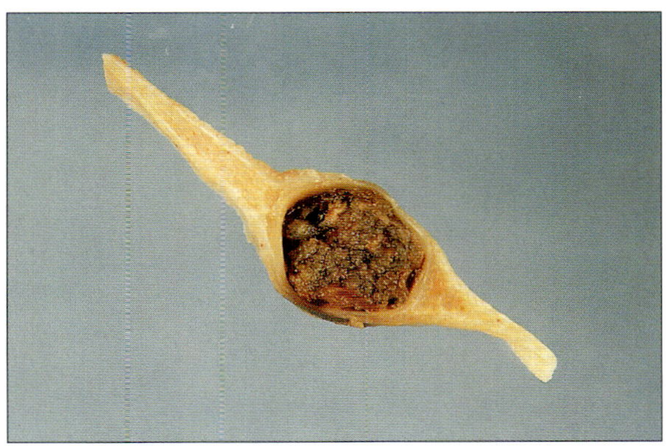

9.53 A section of superior sagittal sinus containing organised thrombus associated with venous infarction of the brain (**9.52**).

with evidence of previous or healing injuries, visible externally or detected on radiological examination. A particular form of non-accidental injury results from shaking, which may lead to intracranial haemorrhage, particularly subdural haemorrhage and/or axonal damage. The presence of retinal haemorrhages is a pointer to this kind of trauma. Chronic subdural haemorrhages may become encapsulated and contain only clear fluid, the so-called subdural hygroma *(see Chapter 5)*.

TUMOURS

Tumours of the immature nervous system are among the commonest form of malignancy of childhood *(see Chapter 10)*. Rarely, they may arise before birth and give rise to hydrocephalus. The commonest malignant intracranial neoplasm of childhood is medulloblastoma and an association with the external granular layer of the cerebellum has been suspected (**9.54**). Malignant tumours of childhood are frequently composed of primitive neuroectodermal cells and may possibly arise in pluripotential stem cells, which are more numerous in the developing CNS than in adults. Occasionally, benign tumours arise within the nervous system during development (**9.55**). These overlap with heterotopias and congenital malformations.

INFANTILE DEGENERATIONS

Rarely, particular subsets of neurons degenerate at an early stage of development, in contrast to the more general deterioration seen in the inborn errors of metabolism. One example of infantile system degeneration is Werdnig–Hoffmann disease, in which motor nerve cells, and some thalamic neurons degenerate soon after birth, leading to degeneration of anterior spinal roots (**9.56**) and denervation of skeletal muscle, and death from respiratory tract infection within the first year or two of life. The appearances in the nervous system are similar to those of other types of spinal muscular atrophy *(see Chapter 7)*.

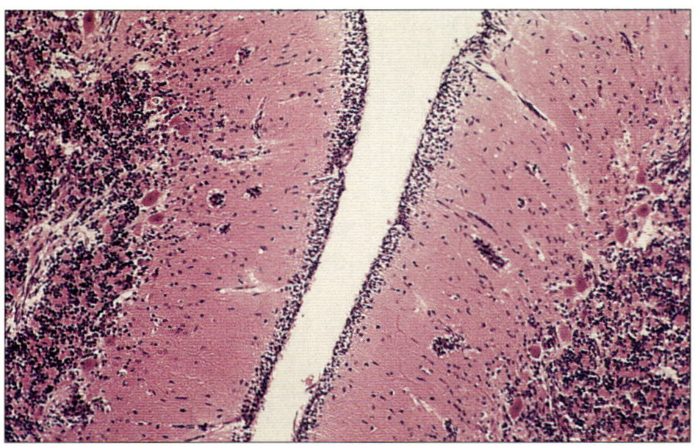

9.54 Cerebellar cortex from a three-month-old infant showing dysplastic foci of undifferentiated cells in the molecular layer. The external granular layer is slightly irregular in thickness.

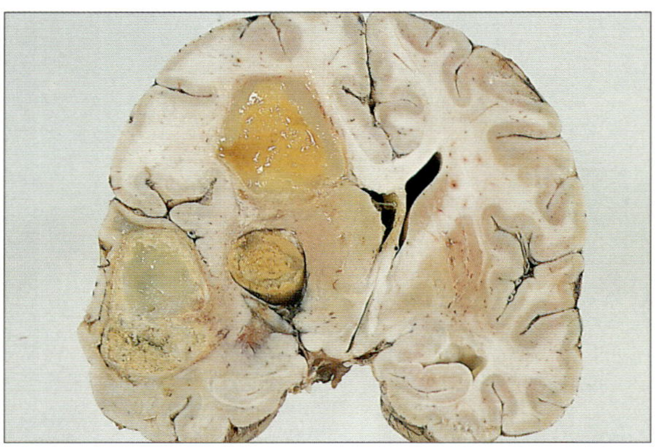

9.55 Coronal slice of a brain showing an extensive congenital dermoid within the left cerebral hemisphere causing midline shift.

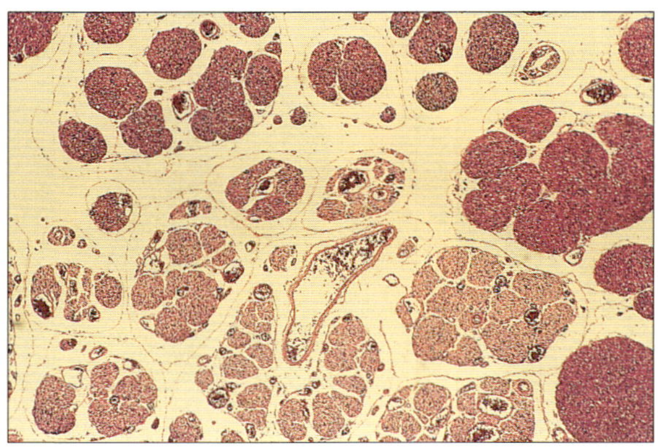

9.56 Transverse section through the cauda equina nerve roots showing pallor and atrophy of the anterior roots in a case of Werdnig–Hoffmann disease.

SUDDEN INFANT DEATH SYNDROME

This major cause of mortality in the first year of life affects one in 2000 of liveborn infants, particularly males. Although the incidence has fallen in the last few years, the cause remains mysterious and CNS malfunction is suspected. Gliosis of the central white matter and brainstem has been described, but is neither confined to, nor consistently present in, cases of sudden infant death syndrome.

FURTHER READING

Duckett S. *Pediatric Neuropathology*. Baltimore, Williams & Wilkins, 1995.

Friede RL. *Developmental Neuropathology*. Berlin, Springer-Verlag. 1989.

Harding BN. Malformation of the Nervous System. In: Adams JH, Duchen LW. Greenfield's *Neuropathology:* Chapter 10. 5th edn. London, Edward Arnold, 1992, pp 521–638.

Rorke LB. Anatomical features of developing brain implicated in pathogenesis of hypoxic–ischaemic injury. *Brain Pathol*, 1992; **2**: 211–221.

10. CNS Tumours

The diagnosis of CNS tumours accounts for a large part of the clinical workload in most neuropathology laboratories. Precise figures for the incidence of primary CNS tumours are difficult to obtain through either local or national registries. Recently published figures for Scotland indicate a frequency of around nine per 100,000 of the general population (**10.1**); this is comparable to similar epidemiological surveys in other industrialised countries. Within this figure, there is a wide variation in the incidence of CNS neoplasms in relation to age, with two peaks of high incidence in the first decade of life and in the sixth and seventh decades (**10.2**). There is evidence to suggest that the incidence of intrinsic CNS tumours is increasing, and that these tumours occur most commonly in individuals in higher (least deprived) social class groups. In children, CNS tumours are the commonest variety of solid tumours and represent

Tumour type	No. of cases/100,000 population/year
All primary intracerebral tumours	9.0
Glioma + medulloblastoma	7.6
Secondary intracerebral tumours	13.6
Benign intracranial extracerebral tumours	5.5
Meningioma	2.5
Pituitary adenoma	2.4
Acoustic schwannoma	0.6
Others	0.3

10.1 Incidence of intracranial tumours in Lothian region, Scotland, UK. Gliomas and medulloblastomas account for the vast majority of primary intracerebral tumours, while meningiomas and pituitary adenomas constitute the two main groups of benign intracranial extracerebral tumours. Further information on the subtypes of secondary intracerebral tumours is given in **10.87**.

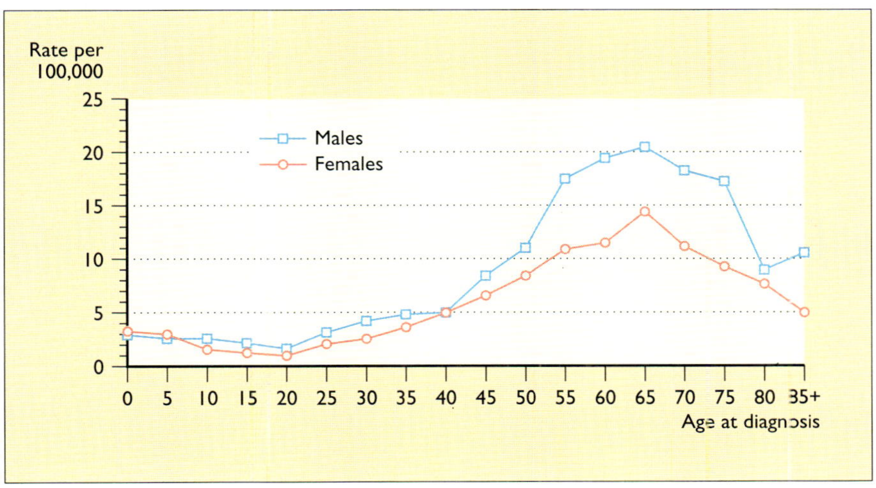

10.2 Incidence graph of CNS tumours in relation to age. (*Adapted from: Cancer Registration Statistics, Scotland, 1981–1990.*)

the second commonest group of all tumours after leukaemias. In adults, the relative incidence of CNS tumours is more difficult to estimate, but they probably rank as the eigthth most common group of solid tumours (**10.3**). There is a marked difference in the incidence of various histological subtypes of CNS neoplasms in children and adults (**10.4**), which has important implications for therapy and prognosis.

Commonist registered cases of site-specific tumours in Scotland in 1983–1987 in different age groups (excluding leukaemias and lymphomas)

Age < 65 years	Age < 55 years	Age < 45 years	Age < 15 years
Lung	Breast	Breast	**Brain**
Breast	Lung	Cervix	Bone/soft tissue
Bowel	Bowel	Testis	Kidney
Bladder	Cervix	**Brain**	Testis
Stomach	**Brain**	Bowel	
Cervix	Melanoma	Melanoma	
Ovary	Testis	Lung	
Brain	Bladder	Bone/soft tissue	

10.3 Registered cases of site-specific tumours in Scotland from 1983–1987 in different age groups (excluding leukaemias and lymphomas), arranged in ascending frequency.

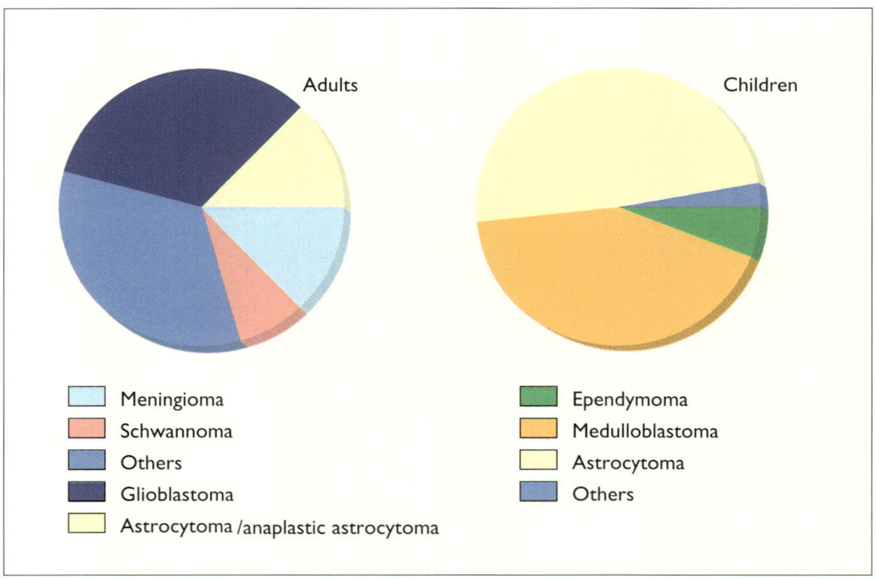

10.4 Comparison of the relative incidence of histological subtypes of CNS neoplasms in adults and children.

CLINICAL FEATURES

The clinical features of a CNS neoplasm relate primarily to its site and rate of growth rather than its histological type. Characteristic signs and symptoms include the following.

- Non-specific effects of raised intracranial pressure with headache (characteristically most severe in the morning), nausea and vomiting (particularly with posterior fossa tumours), and visual disturbances as a consequence of papilloedema.
- Epilepsy is a common presenting feature, particularly for infiltrative intrinsic tumours.
- False localising signs, including IIIrd and VIth cranial nerve palsies, due to intracranial herniation and raised intracranial pressure respectively.
- Localising signs and focal disabilities which are usually of slow onset and progressive.

Many CNS neoplasms are associated with oedema in the surrounding brain which potentiates the mass effect of the tumour. Occasionally, haemorrhage into a CNS tumour, particularly a glioblastoma, results in an acute presentation resembling a stroke (**10.5**). Obstruction of the cerebrospinal fluid (CSF) pathway by an expanding neoplasm will result in hydrocephalus. This is particularly common with tumours of the posterior fossa in children, which will readily compress the cerebral aqueduct or fourth ventricle (**10.6**).

DIAGNOSIS AND CLASSIFICATION

Most patients with suspected CNS neoplasms undergo neuroradiological examination, usually either CT scanning or MRI. These techniques are now able to provide accurate anatomical localisation of intracranial tumours which can be used to plan surgical investigation, e.g. stereotactic biopsy. Most patients with CNS neoplasms undergo biopsy for accurate histological classification.

A variety of classification schemes has been employed for CNS neoplasms, the most recent of which is the revised WHO classification (*see Further Reading*), which is based on the presumed histogenesis and differentiation (**10.7**). The widespread use of specialised investigative techniques, including electron microscopy and immunocytochemistry, has allowed a far greater diagnostic accuracy over the past decade than was previously possible. Antibodies commonly used as an aid to diagnosis of CNS neoplasms are listed in **10.8**.

CNS tumours are classified on a histopathological basis alone, but it is clinically relevant and convenient to consider two main categories:

- intrinsic tumours (arising within the CNS);
- extrinsic tumours (arising from cranial and spinal nerves and the coverings of the nervous system).

Tumours arising from adjacent structures (including the pituitary gland) and metastatic tumours will be considered separately.

INTRINSIC TUMOURS

Intrinsic tumours account for virtually all CNS neoplasms occurring in children and for around 60% of all primary CNS neoplasms in adults. Of these, by far the commonest are astrocytic tumours, which include

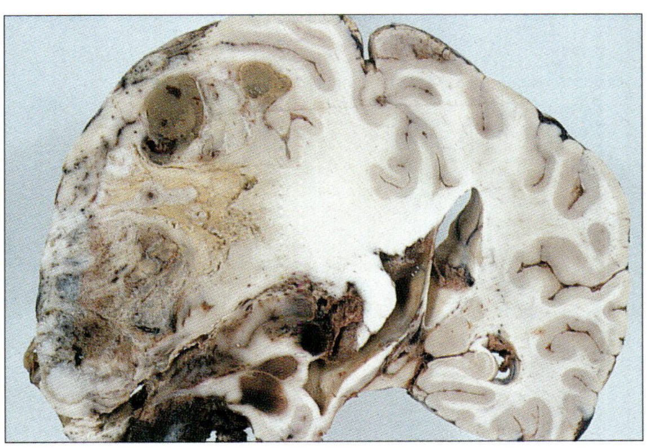

10.5 Male aged 64 years with a massive left cerebral glioblastoma. There is extensive haemorrhage and an acute presentation resembling a stroke.

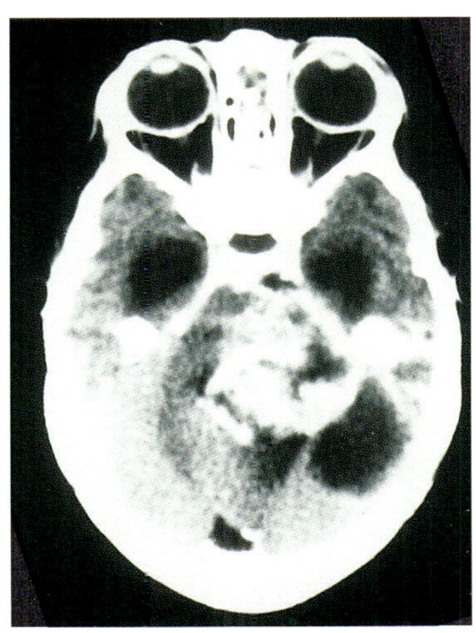

10.6 CT scan of a posterior fossa tumour (choroid plexus carcinoma) in a four-year-old male, who presented with the features of hydrocephalus accompanied by cerebellar ataxia and vomiting (*see also* **10.32**).

a variety of neoplasms with markedly different behaviours and prognoses.

Many classification schemes for these tumours provide a numerical grade, usually ranging from 1–4, with Grade 4 tumours being the most aggressive (**10.7**). Tumour grading is often considered to be a subjective exercise, but it has been shown that some recently developed grading systems, e.g. the St Anne system, are reproducible and can provide information of prognostic significance (**10.9**) for astrocytic tumours. Grading of small tumour biopsy specimens remains a major challenge in diagnostic practice.

ASTROCYTOMA

Astrocytomas are composed of well-differentiated astrocytic cells which usually express GFAP on immunocytochemistry. Various subtypes of astrocytoma are recognised on clinical and morphological grounds.

Pilocytic astrocytoma

This is the commonest astrocytic tumour to occur in children and young adults. Most arise in the cerebellar hemisphere (**10.10**), but some also occur

Simplified WHO classification of CNS tumours

Description	WHO grade
Astrocytic tumours	
Astrocytoma	
Fibrillary	II
Protoplasmic	
Gemistocytic	
Anaplastic astrocytoma	III
Glioblastoma and variants	IV
Pilocytic astrocytoma	I
Pleomorphic xanthoastrocytoma	II
Subependymal giant cell astrocytoma	I
Oligodendroglial tumours	
Oligodendroglioma	II
Anaplastic oligodendroglioma	III
Ependymal tumours	
Ependymoma and variants	II
Anaplastic ependymoma	III
Myxopapillary ependymoma	I
Subependymoma	I
Mixed gliomas	
Mixed oligoastrocytoma	II
Anaplastic oligoastrocytoma	III
Choroid plexus tumours	
Choroid plexus papilloma	I
Choroid plexus carcinoma	III
Neuronal and mixed neuronal–glial tumours	
Gangliocytoma	I
Ganglioglioma	I–II
Embryonal tumours	
Medulloblastoma and variants	IV
Primitive neuroectodermal tumours	IV
Tumours of cranial and spinal nerves	
Schwannoma	I
Neurofibroma	I
Malignant peripheral nerve sheath tumour	III–IV

Description	WHO grade
Tumours of the meninges	
Meningioma and variants	I
Atypical meningioma	II
Papillary meningioma	I–III
Anaplastic meningioma	III
Capillary haemangioblastoma	–
Lymphomas and haematopoetic neoplasms	
Primary malignant lymphoma	–
Germ cell tumours	
Germinoma	–
Embryonal carcinoma	–
Yolk sac tumour	–
Teratoma and variants	–
Tumours of the sellar region	
Pituitary adenoma	–
Pituitary carcinoma	–
Craniopharyngioma	I
Cysts and tumour-like lesions	
Rathke's cleft cyst	–
Epidermal cyst	–
Dermoid cyst	–
Local extensions from regional tumours	
Paraganglioma	–
Chordoma	–
Metatastic tumours	
Carcinoma	–

10.7 Simplified WHO classification of CNS tumours.

Antibodies used in diagnostic neuro-oncology	
Antibody	Tumour specificity
Glial fibrillary acidic protein (GFAP)	Astrocytomas, ependymomas, glioblastomas
Leu 7	Oligodendrogliomas, nerve sheath tumours
S100	Nerve sheath tumours, chordoma
Transthyretin	Choroid plexus tumours
Carbonic anhydrase type II	Oligodendrogliomas, choroid plexus tumours
PGP 9.5	Ganglion cell tumours, primitive neuroectodermal tumours
Synaptophysin	Desmoplastic medulloblastomas, pineocytomas, ganglion cell tumours
Vimentin	Meningiomas, mesenchymal tumours, chordoma
Epithelial membrane antigen	Meningiomas, metastatic carcinoma
CAM 5.2 (cytokeratins)	Meningiomas, metastatic carcinoma, chordoma
Desmoplakins	Meningiomas, metastatic carcinoma
Leucocyte common antigen T and B cell markers	CNS lymphoma
Placental alkaline phosphatase Human chorionic gonadotrophin Alphafetoprotein	Germ cell tumours
Growth hormone Prolactin Adrenocorticotrophic hormone Thyroid-stimulating hormone Luteinising hormone Follicle-stimulating hormone Glycoprotein hormone α-subunit	Pituitary tumours

10.8 Antibodies used in diagnostic neuro-oncology.

Features used in the St Anne grading system for astrocytic tumours
Nuclear pleomorphism
Mitoses
Necrosis
Vascular endothelial proliferation

10.9 The St Anne grading system for astrocytic tumours. (*Adapted from: Daumas-Duport C, Scheithauer B, O'Fallon J, Kelly P. Grading of astrocytomas. A simple and reproducible method.* Cancer *1988;***62***:2152–2165.*)

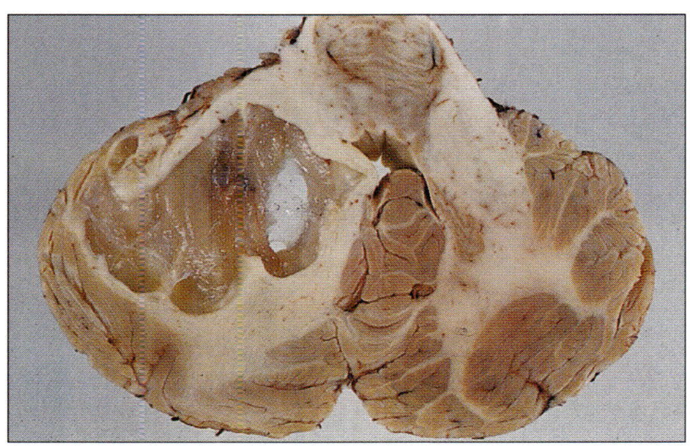

10.10 Male aged 13 years with a cystic astrocytoma in the left cerebellar hemisphere. The cyst has an irregular nodular lining and the adjacent white matter is compressed, but not extensively infiltrated.

around the region of the third ventricle, hypothalamus and in the optic nerve. Tumours of this type in the region of the optic nerve and hypothalamus are particularly associated with neurofibromatosis type 1. These tumours are often well-circumscribed, and in the cerebellum are particularly amenable to complete surgical resection. In the cerebellum, pilocytic astrocytomas often include cystic spaces which are admixed with solid areas of tumour. Histologically, the tumour cells are arranged in a composite compact and spongy pattern. The cells are usually bipolar and form parallel bundles (**10.11**). Rosenthal fibres and granular bodies are usually present within the tumour matrix. Endothelial proliferation is not uncommon in these tumours, but has no sinister prognostic significance. Mitotic figures and focal necrosis are absent, but a moderate degree of nuclear pleomorphism is commonly noted.

Diffuse infiltrating astrocytomas

These can be further subclassified into fibrillary, protoplasmic or gemistocytic types, according to the morphology of the predominant tumour cell population. These tumours typically occur in childhood and early adult life and may occur in any site within the CNS including the spinal cord (**10.12**). In adults, most astrocytomas involve the cerebral hemispheres (**10.13**), but in children the brainstem is commonly involved (**10.14**). The commonest histological subtype is the fibrillary astrocytoma composed of elongated process-bearing cells in a loose fibrillary matrix (**10.15**). In the protoplasmic astrocytoma, the tumour cells have a small cell body with relatively few processes (**10.16**) and often give a weak or even negative reaction on immunocytochemistry for GFAP. In contrast, the tumours cells within a gemistocytic astrocytoma are larger with more abundant eosinophilic cytoplasm and a variable number of cell processes. A strongly positive reaction on immunocytochemistry for GFAP is characteristic (**10.17**).

Anaplastic astrocytoma

This group of tumours may arise *de novo* or as a consequence of focal dedifferentiation within a well-differentiated astrocytoma. In the anaplastic astrocytoma, the neoplastic cells exhibit a wide range of nuclear atypia and cellular pleomorphism with mitotic activity and increased cellularity (**10.18**). Vascular endothelial proliferation may be conspicuous but necrosis is absent.

The anatomical localisation of anaplastic astrocytomas corresponds to those for diffuse infiltrating well-differentiated astrocytomas; these tumours tend to occur in adults within the cerebral hemispheres (**10.19**). The extent of neoplastic infiltration within the brain is often more extensive on histological examination than suggested by neuroradiological studies.

Glioblastoma

This is the commonest variety of astrocytic tumour in adults (accounting for over 50% of primary CNS

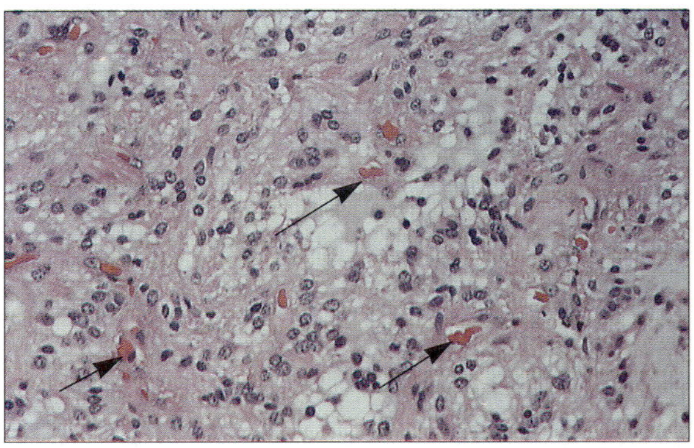

10.11 Histology from the tumour in **10.10** shows the features of a pilocytic astrocytoma, with small cystic spaces and elongated tumour cells arranged in a composite 'spongy' and dense arrangement. Occasional Rosenthal fibres (arrows) are present.

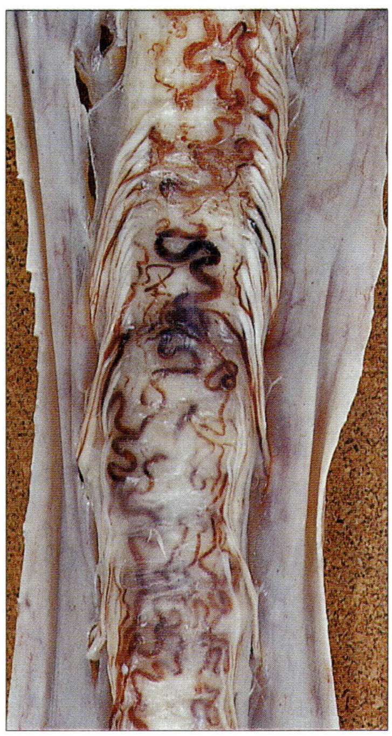

10.12 Male aged 24 years with a diffuse astrocytoma of the spinal cord. The spinal cord is irregularly swollen in the upper thoracic and lower cervical segments, with distortion of the overlying vessels.

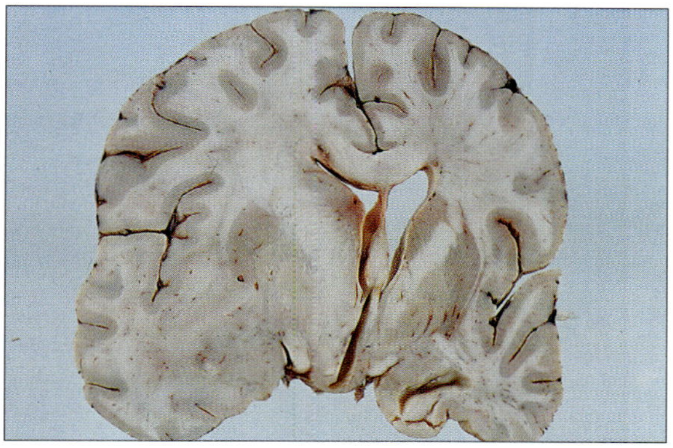

10.13 Male aged 25 years with a diffuse astrocytoma involving the left cerebral hemisphere. This tumour has considerably expanded the region of the temporal lobe, basal ganglia and central white matter, with infiltration into the corpus callosum which is markedly thickened.

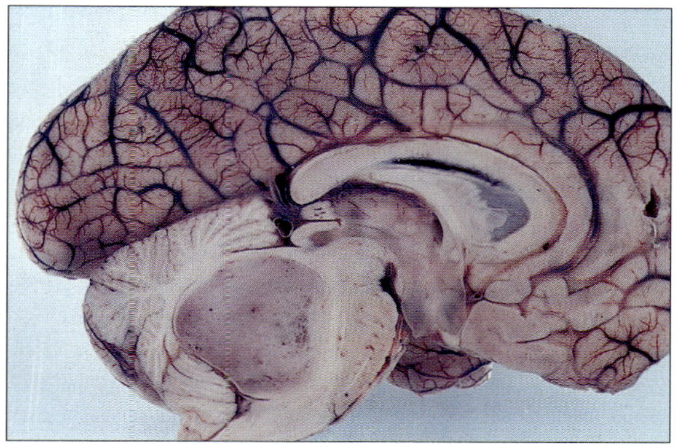

10.14 Male aged eight years with a brainstem astrocytoma. There is a predominantly exophytic growth pattern, filling the fourth ventricle and compressing the cerebellum. There is also invasion and expansion of the white matter in the pons and midbrain.

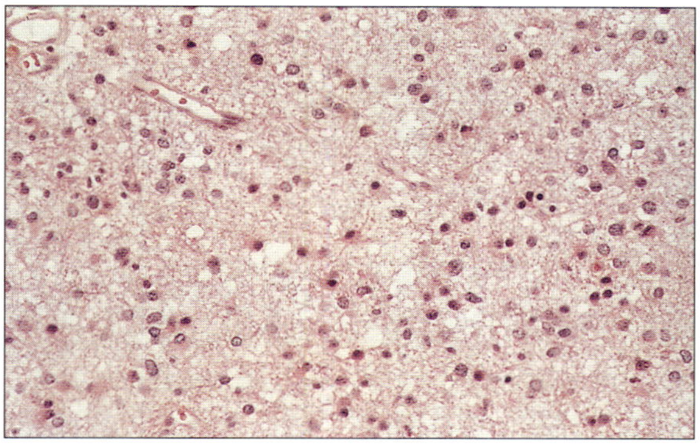

10.15 Histology of the tumour in **10.14** shows the appearances of a diffuse fibrillary astrocytoma. The tumour cells exhibit astrocytic differentiation and bear numerous cell processes (centre). There is no mitotic activity or necrosis and vascular endothelial hyperplasia is not a prominent feature.

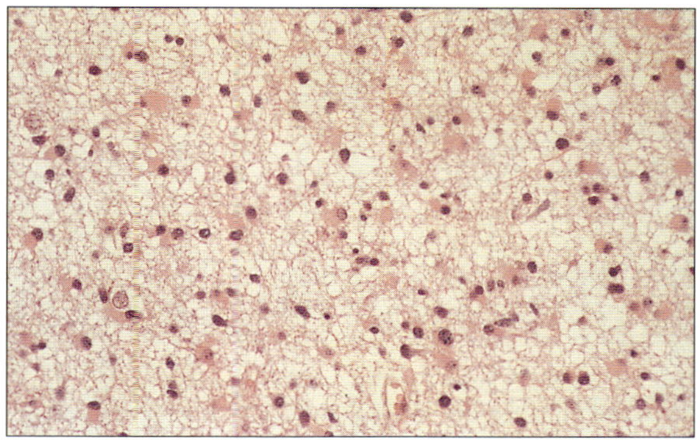

10.16 Histology of the tumour in **10.13** shows a protoplasmic astrocytoma, with small tumour cells containing a variable quantity of eosinophilic cytoplasm and relatively few cell processes, set in a loose microcystic matrix.

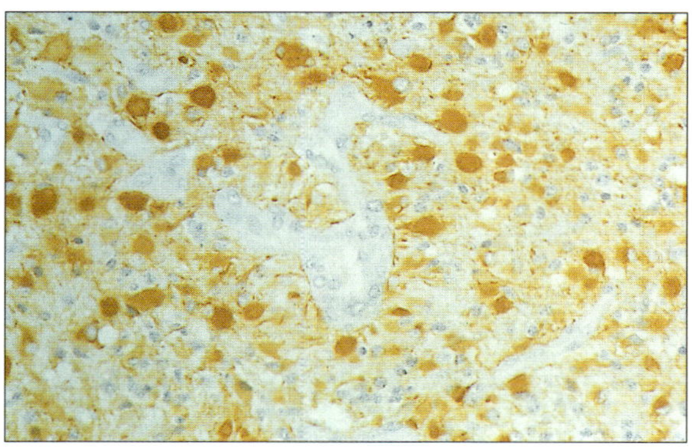

10.17 Gemistocytic astrocytoma. Immunocytochemistry for GFAP shows a strong positive reaction within the tumour cells which have numerous cellular processes. Vascular endothelium (centre) is unstained.

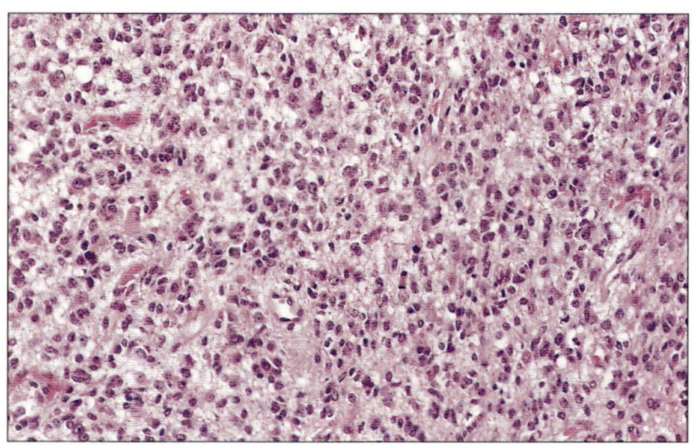

10.18 In contrast to well-differentiated astrocytomas, anaplastic astrocytomas have a higher cellular density, with less pronounced astrocytic differentiation. A moderate degree of nuclear pleomorphism and occasional mitotic figures (centre) are present.

tumours), with a peak incidence in the fifth to seventh decades of life.

Glioblastomas may arise *de novo* or as a consequence of dedifferentiation within a pre-existing astrocytoma. Most arise in the cerebral hemispheres, particularly in the frontotemporal region, but other sites including the brainstem, cerebellum and spinal cord may be involved (**10.20**). This tumour is characterised histologically by a markedly pleomorphic tumour cell population which includes multinucleate giant cells and small anaplastic cells (**10.21**). Mitotic activity is usually conspicuous and there is widespread vascular endothelial proliferation. Necrosis is present, often with a characteristic 'ribbon' pattern (**10.22**).

Vascular occlusion and haemorrhage are common in these tumours, which grow rapidly and extensively infiltrate the CNS; most patients die within one year of diagnosis. Variants of the glioblastoma include:

- the giant cell glioblastoma, in which bizarre multinucleate giant cells predominate;
- the gliosarcoma, in which a sarcomatous component exists alongside the neoplastic glial cell population, and which may resemble an angiosarcoma, fibrosarcoma, or malignant fibrous histiocytoma.

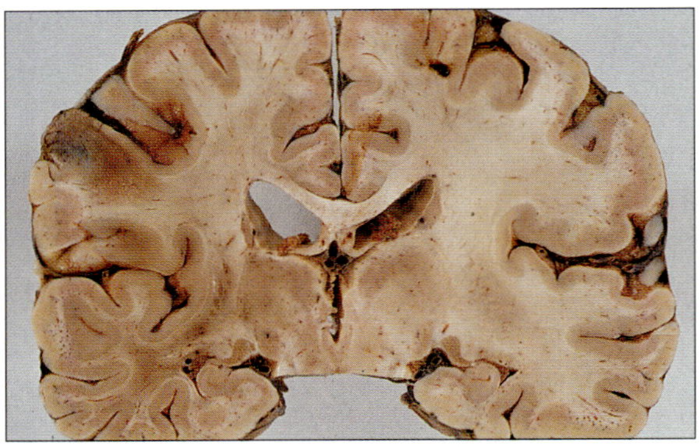

10.19 Male aged 42 years with an anaplastic astrocytoma in the left cerebral hemisphere, which is centred in the parietal lobe and accompanied by diffuse infiltration and discoloration of white matter.

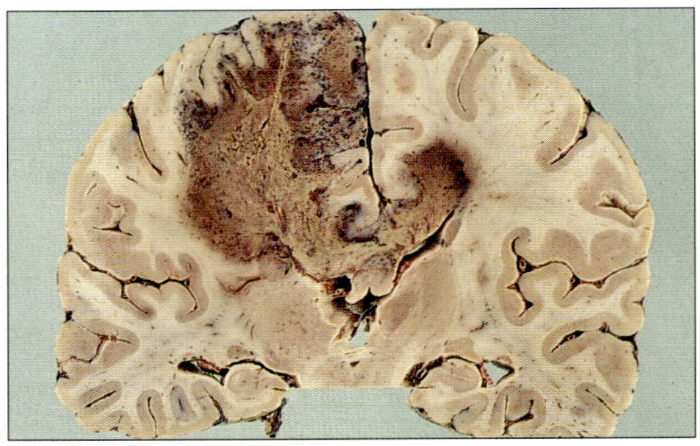

10.20 Male aged 62 years with a glioblastoma involving both hemispheres, with a predominant mass in the left parietal lobe and extensive spread through the corpus callosum into the right hemisphere. Extensive haemorrhage and multifocal necrosis are characteristic of this neoplasm (*see also* **10.5**).

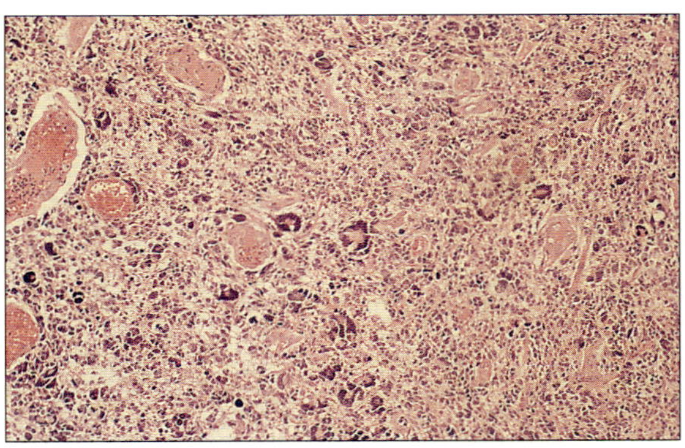

10.21 Histology of the tumour in **10.20** shows a characteristic pleomorphic cell population with numerous multinucleate giant cells and small anaplastic tumour cells. Vascular endothelial proliferation is a prominent feature (right) and numerous mitotic figures are scattered throughout the neoplasm.

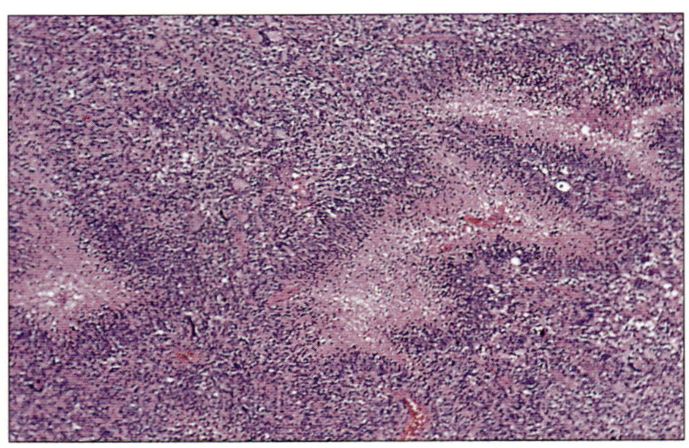

10.22 A low-power view of a glioblastoma shows a 'ribbon' pattern of necrosis with surrounding nuclear pseudopallisading. Multinucleate giant cells are evident throughout the tumour.

Astrocytoma variants

Pleomorphic xanthoastrocytoma

This usually occurs in a superficial location within the temporal lobe of children and young adults. Despite bizarre histological appearances, the neoplasm is usually well-demarcated and carries a favourable prognosis, although some have been demonstrated to progress to anaplastic astrocytoma or glioblastoma.

Subependymal giant cell astrocytoma

This is an extremely rare tumour which occurs in patients with tuberous sclerosis. It usually arises in a periventricular location, projecting into the lateral ventricles (**10.23**). These tumours grow slowly and are usually well-demarcated, being amenable to complete surgical resection.

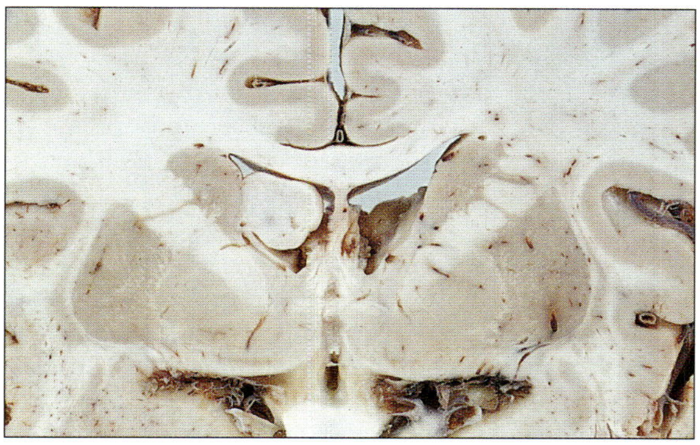

10.23 Male aged 10 years with tuberous sclerosis and a subependymal giant cell astrocytoma which projects into the lumen of the left lateral ventricle. This tumour has a nodular outline and is well demarcated from the caudate nucleus.

OLIGODENDROGLIAL TUMOURS

Oligodendroglioma

Oligodendrogliomas account for around 5% of all gliomas and occur most often in young adults. They are slow-growing lesions which arise in the cerebral white matter and basal ganglia, with extensive infiltration of surrounding tissues (**10.24**). Histologically, the tumours are characteristically composed of a uniform population of rounded cells that have small central nuclei and a clear perinuclear cytoplasmic halo with a well-defined cell membrane (**10.25**). A finely branching vascular network is usually present, and focal calcification is characteristic. Mitotic activity is usually inconspicuous. No specific immunocytochemical marker exists for oligodendrogliomas, but a proportion of cells in most of these tumours stain positively for GFAP, particularly if a tumour includes cells with a small quantity of eosinophilic cytoplasm.

Anaplastic oligodendroglioma

Malignant transformation in oligodendrogliomas can occur to produce an anaplastic oligodendroglioma, which is characterised histologically by nuclear pleomorphism and cellular atypia, mitotic activity and vascular endothelial proliferation with focal necrosis. Progression into a glioblastoma has been described occasionally.

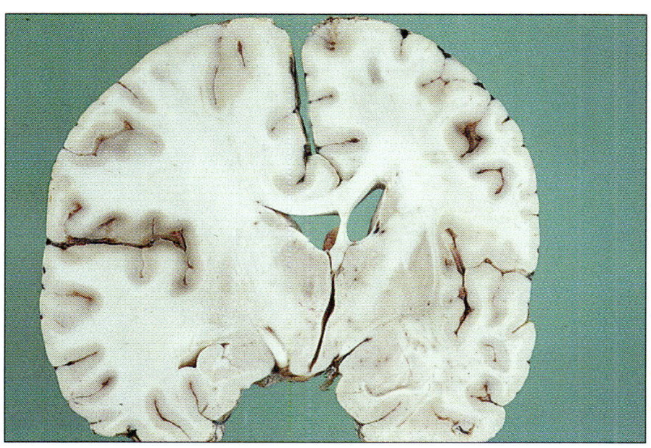

10.24 Female aged 25 years with a left hemispheric oligodendroglioma which diffusely infiltrates and expands the white matter, resulting in a midline shift and a subfalcine hernia.

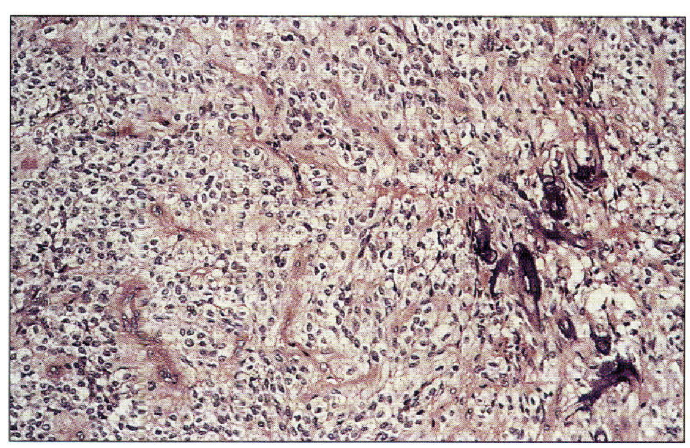

10.25 Histology of the tumour in **10.24** shows characteristic features of an oligodendroglioma, with a uniform tumour cell population characterised by well-demarcated cells containing a central rounded nucleus and clear cytoplasm. Finely branching blood vessels with focal calcification (right) are present.

MIXED GLIOMAS

It is recognised that intrinsic glial tumours composed of a mixture of cell types can occur, most often as an oligoastrocytoma. Anaplastic variants may also occur, in which the anaplastic component is usually astrocytic. These tumours occur most commonly in adults in the region of the white matter of the cerebral hemispheres.

EPENDYMAL TUMOURS

Ependymoma

Intracranial ependymomas characteristically occur in children, particularly in the region of the fourth ventricle, though other sites within the ventricular system may be involved, particularly in adults. In children, ependymomas are the third commonest group of intrinsic neoplasms. They tend to form a lobulated mass within the lumen of the fourth ventricle and may extend into the subarachnoid space and basal cisterns (**10.26**). The tumour growth is usually solid and well-demarcated with little invasion of surrounding structures.

Histologically, ependymomas can exhibit a variety of appearances, the most common of which is a perivascular pseudorosette arrangement of tumour cells around a hyalinised blood vessel (**10.27**). Ependymal rosettes and canaliculi are also characteristic, though less frequently encountered. Nuclear pleomorphism is variable, but mitotic activity and necrosis should raise the possibility of an anaplastic ependymoma. Occasional tumours exhibit a marked papillary growth pattern resembling a choroid plexus papilloma. Clear cell ependymomas may occasionally be confused with oligodendrogliomas.

Anaplastic ependymoma

Anaplastic ependymomas are uncommon, but may occur in both children and adults. In contrast to most ependymomas, there is extensive cellular atypia and nuclear pleomorphism, widespread mitotic activity, necrosis and vascular endothelial proliferation. Local invasion may occur and tumour seeding through the CSF pathway is a recognised complication.

Subependymoma

This uncommon tumour usually arises in the region of the fourth ventricle in adults. Subependymomas are nodular slow-growing lesions composed of small groups of ependymal cells in a dense fibrillary matrix, in which focal calcification is common. Some cases are asymptomatic and are found incidentally at autopsy. Larger lesions may compress the CSF pathway and cause hydrocephalus (**10.28**).

Myxopapillary ependymoma

This is an uncommon variant of ependymoma that occurs in the region of the cauda equina and lumbar spinal cord. The tumour cells are arranged in a striking perivascular papillary pattern around cores of hyalinised tissue, often within a mucinous matrix (**10.29**). Local infiltration into the conus medullaris is common, but myxopapillary ependymomas can frequently be surgically resected.

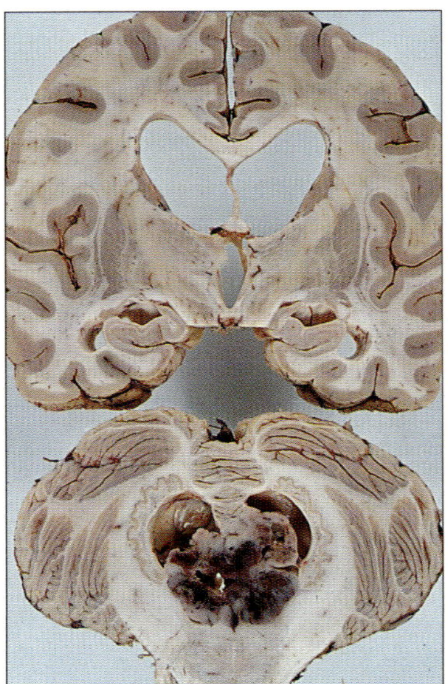

10.26 Female aged 14 years with a four-year history of ependymoma in the fourth ventricle which recurred following surgery. There is marked hydrocephalus involving all ventricles and the fourth ventricle is markedly distended by a lobulated partly haemorrhagic tumour.

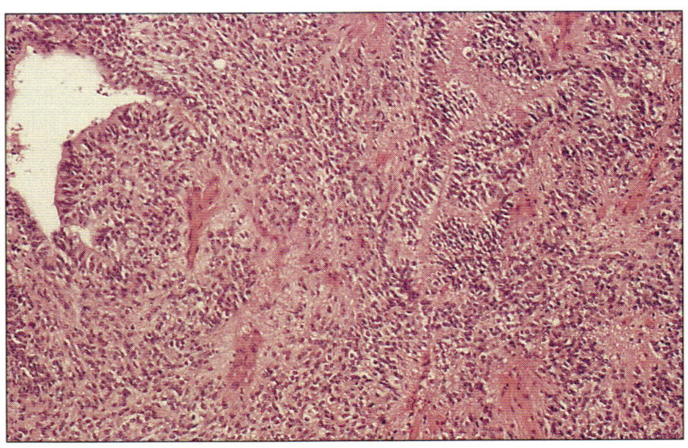

10.27 Histology of the tumour in **10.26** shows the appearances of an ependymoma, with numerous small blood vessels surrounded by eosinophilic cell processes, forming perivascular pseudorosettes. A canalicular structure lined by ependymal cells is present (top left).

CHOROID PLEXUS TUMOURS

There are two main groups of neoplasms which arise in the choroid plexus epithelium.

Choroid plexus papilloma

This is the commoner variety of choroid plexus tumours. Characteristically, they arise in the ventricular system in children or young adults. In children the fourth ventricle is predominantly affected, while in adults these tumours may arise in the lateral or third ventricles (**10.30**). Macroscopically, these tumours have a typical papilliform appearance, with finger-like fronds arising from a stalk attaching the tumour to the ventricular lining. On histology, the epithelium consists of an irregular layer of columnar cells, resting on a basement membrane overlying a fibrovascular core (**10.31**). A moderate degree of nuclear atypia is present in most cases, but invasion of the connective tissue stroma and adjacent structures is absent. Choroid plexus tumours may obstruct the CSF pathway, resulting in hydrocephalus.

Immunocytochemical investigations in choroid plexus papillomas show positive staining for epithelial markers, and immunoreactivity for transthyretin, carbonic anhydrase type II and cathepsin D is characteristic.

Choroid plexus carcinoma

This is a malignant tumour that characteristically occurs in children, and particularly involves the fourth ventricle (**10.6**). The macroscopic appearance is often

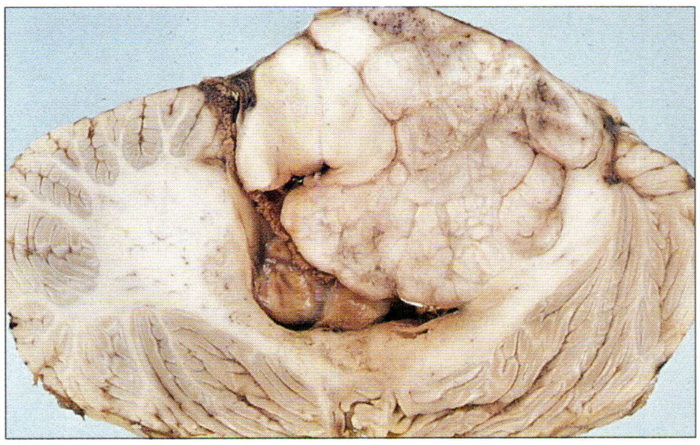

10.28 Male aged 47 years with a large subependymoma arising from the fourth ventricle, which forms a large nodular mass growing out of the exit foramina on the right. This caused hydrocephalus and displacement (but not invasion) of cerebellar and brainstem structures.

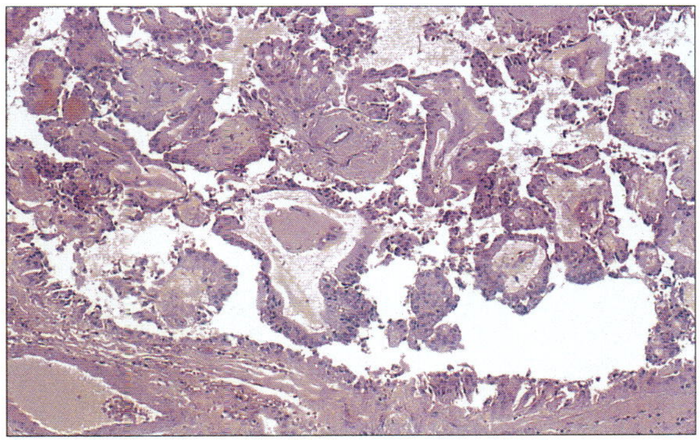

10.29 Histology of a myxopapillary ependymoma occurring at the L4 level in a female aged 24 years. There are numerous hyalinised blood vessels surrounded by ribbon-like groups of ependymal tumour cells.

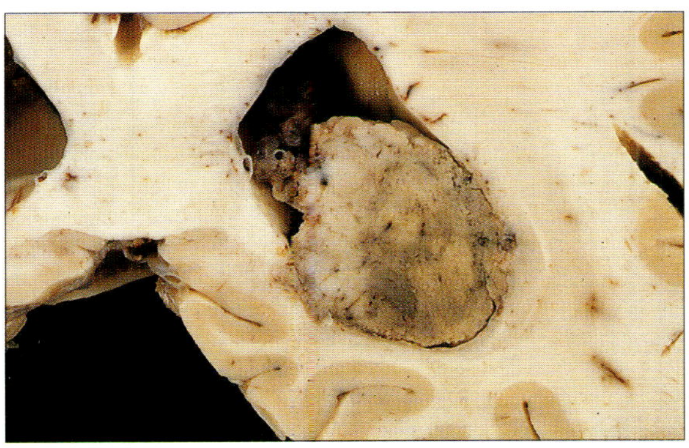

10.30 Female aged 33 years with a choroid plexus papilloma arising in the left lateral ventricle, filling most of the ventricle but not invading adjacent structures.

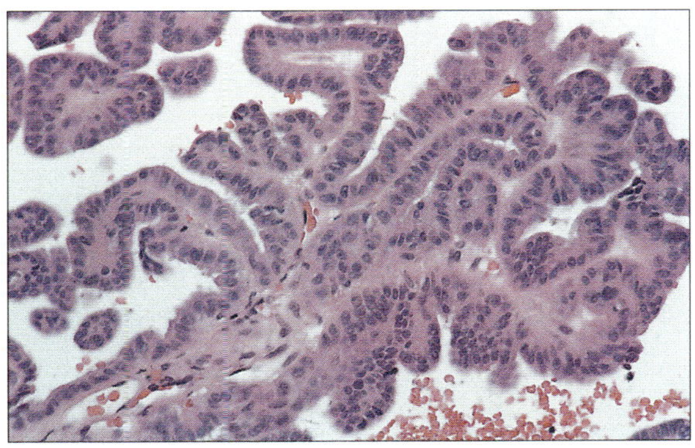

10.31 Histology of the tumour in **10.30** shows choroid plexus epithelial cells arranged in a single layer above a fibrovascular stroma. The tumour cells show a moderate degree of nuclear pleomorphism with occasional mitotic figures, but there is no evidence of stromal invasion.

similar to that of choroid plexus papilloma, but invasion of surrounding structures is much more common and the tumour often contains areas of haemorrhage and necrosis. These features are also identifiable on histology, which shows variable anaplasia with increased mitotic activity and a loss of the papillary pattern seen in benign tumours (**10.32**). Choroid plexus carcinomas can seed through the CSF pathway, resulting in distant CNS metastases. On immunocytochemistry, a similar pattern of reaction is observed to that for choroid plexus papilloma.

GLIAL TUMOURS OF UNCERTAIN ORIGIN

The WHO classification has recognised that certain very rare intrinsic CNS tumours have an uncertain histogenesis, while exhibiting characteristic and often striking histological appearances.

- Astroblastoma is a glial neoplasm in which perivascular radiating astrocytic cells predominate.
- Polar spongioblastoma usually occurs in young children. Histological examination shows elongated glial cells which exhibit striking nuclear pallisading.
- Gliomatosis cerebri describes diffuse infiltration of the brain by a glial neoplasm in which a primary tumour focus may be difficult to identify. Several lobes are characteristically involved and the cerebellum, spinal cord and brainstem are occasionally invaded (**10.33**).

NEURONAL AND MIXED NEURONAL–GLIAL TUMOURS

Neoplasms which contain a neuronal or ganglion cell component are uncommon. Several varieties occur, including the following.

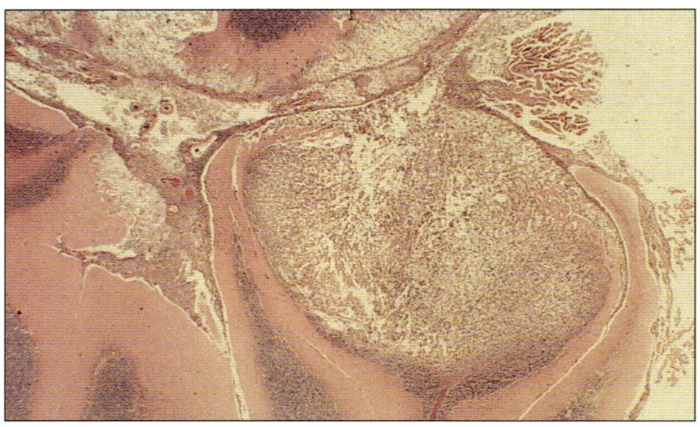

10.32 A low-power histological view of a choroid plexus carcinoma occurring in a four-year-old male. An anaplastic tumour is arising from the choroid plexus in the fourth ventricle and is invading adjacent cerebellum. It has spread extensively through the subarachnoid space (*see also* **10.6**).

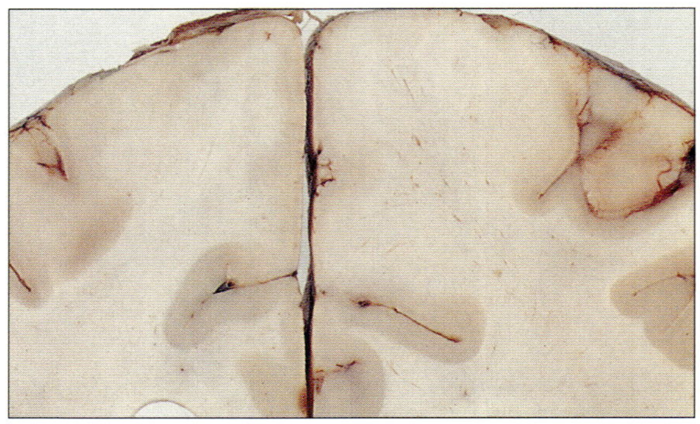

10.33 Male aged 39 years with gliomatosis cerebri. The boundary between the grey and white matter in the parietal parasagittal region is markedly blurred as a consequence of tumour infiltration.

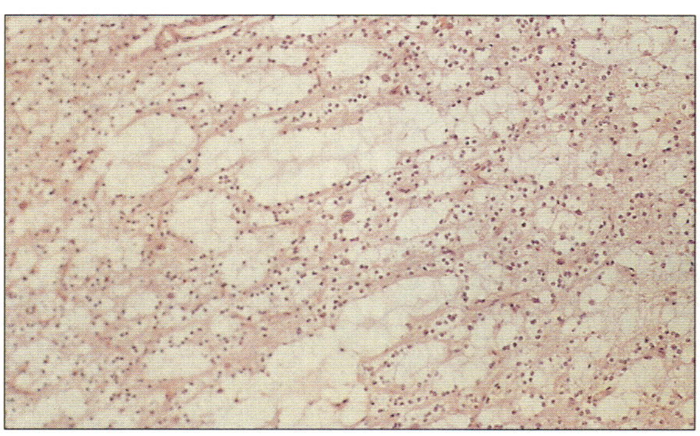

10.34 Male aged eight years with a dysembryoplastic neuroepithelial tumour characterised by numerous small oligodendrocyte-like cells surrounding cystic spaces, which contain larger neuronal cells (centre).

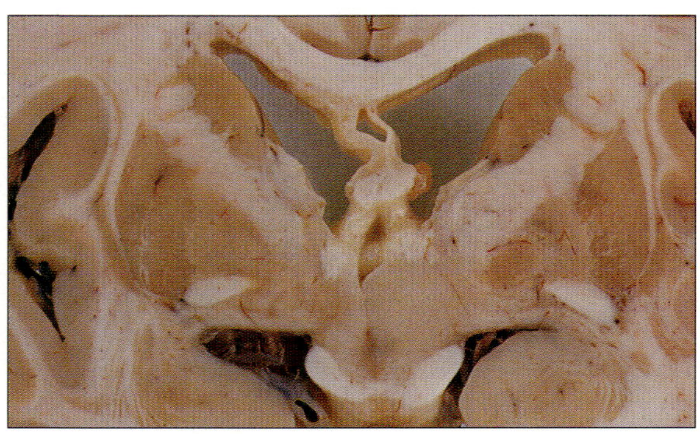

10.35 Male aged seven years with a gangliocytoma involving the hypothalamus, which is irregularly expanded on the right side with third ventricular compression and dilatation of the lateral ventricles, particularly on the right.

Dysembryoplastic neuroepithelial tumour

This is a relatively recently recognised lesion that usually occurs in children and young adults with a long history of partial complex seizures. The neoplasm is localised to the region of the cerebral cortex, often in the temporal lobe and comprises neoplastic oligodendrocytes, neurons and astrocytes. The tumour has a characteristic intracortical location with a nodular architecture in which cyst-like spaces can be identified (**10.34**). This tumour is curable by surgical resection.

Gangliocytoma

Gangliocytomas are slowly growing neoplasms that occur in children and young adults, particularly in the temporal lobe and hypothalamus (**10.35**). They are composed of mature neuronal cells and may be difficult to distinguish from neuronal heterotopias.

Ganglioglioma

This tumour has a similar incidence and distribution to the gangliocytoma, but the tumours are often cystic and contain a glial cell component, usually astrocytic. Vascular endothelial proliferation can be recognised and perivascular lymphocytic cuffing is characteristic (**10.36, 10.37**). The glial cell component in some tumours may exhibit anaplasia, corresponding to anaplastic astrocytoma, in which case a diagnosis of anaplastic ganglioglioma is appropriate.

Central neurocytoma

This is another recently recognised entity which characteristically occurs in young adults in the periventricular region, growing primarily within the cavity of lateral or third ventricles. The tumours are well-demarcated and comprise a uniform round cell population with clear cytoplasm reminiscent of oligodendroglioma (**10.38**). Fine fibrillar processes are present with a perivascular orientation. Immunocytochemistry confirms the neuronal nature of these cells with positive staining for synaptophysin and neuron-specific enolase (**10.39**).

Paraganglioma

This is an uncommon slowly growing neoplasm which arises from the filum terminale or lumbosacral

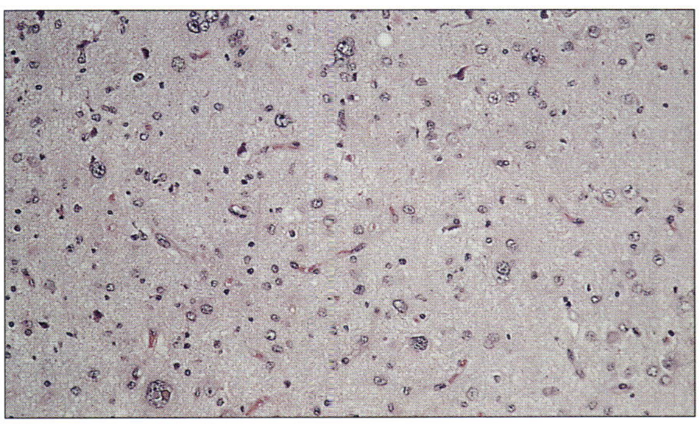

10.36 Histology of a ganglioglioma shows a non-homogenous tumour cell population forming a dense network. There are large bizarre neuronal cells with prominent nucleoli and smaller glial cells with numerous cellular processes.

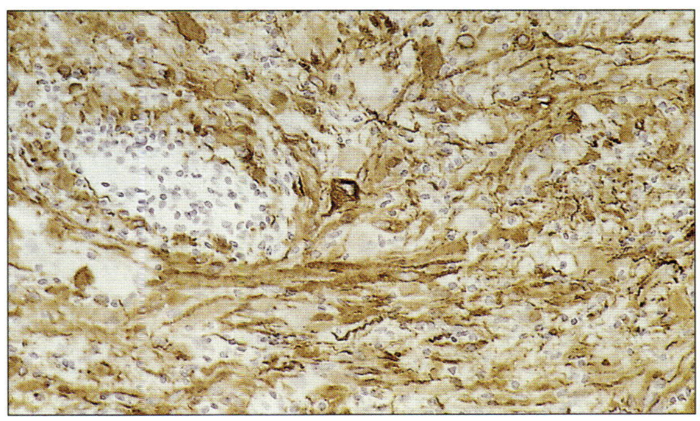

10.37 Immunocytochemistry for the 68kD neurofilament subunit in the tumour in **10.36** shows strong staining of the cytoplasm in the large neuronal cells and their processes, while the smaller glial cell component is unstained.

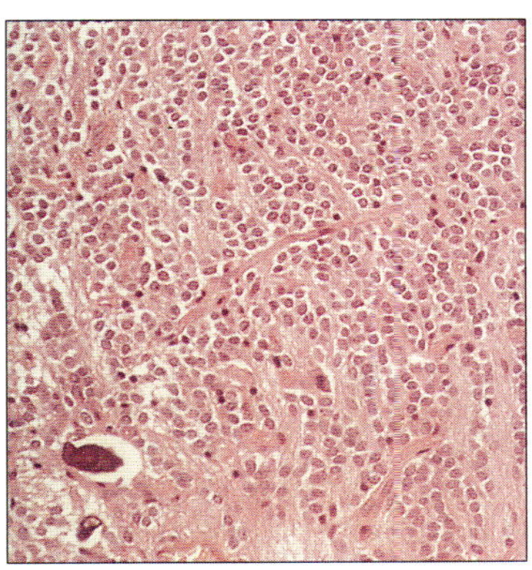

10.38 Histology of a central neurocytoma occurring in a 19-year-old male shows a small uniform tumour cell population set in a fibrillary matrix with finely branching blood vessels and focal calcification.

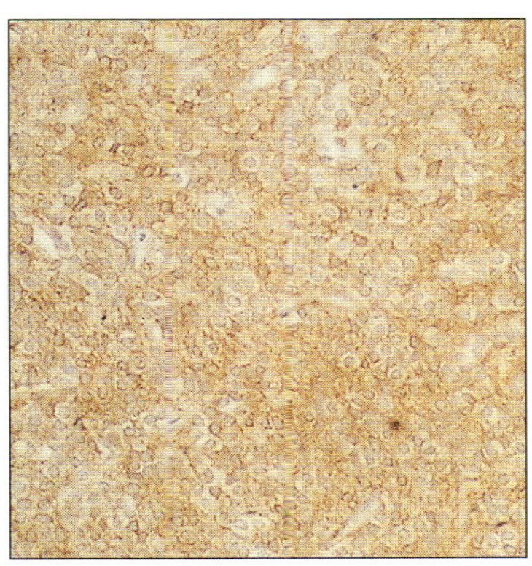

10.39 From the same case as **10.38**, immunocytochemistry for synaptophysin shows a strong positive reaction.

nerve roots in adults. These tumours are typically encapsulated (**10.40**) and show the characteristic histological appearances of a paraganglioma with polygonal pale-staining cells arranged in an alveolar pattern around delicately branching blood vessels (**10.41**). Immunocytochemistry shows a positive reaction for synaptophysin, chromogranin and neuron-specific enolase: the sustentacular cells of these tumours stain positively for S100 protein. Occasional tumours can contain mature ganglion cells and are referred to as gangliocytic paragangliomas. These tumours are curable by surgical excision.

Rarer neuronal tumours

These include the dysplastic gangliocytoma of the cerebellum, sometimes associated with other congenital malformations including megalencephaly, and the desmoplastic infantile ganglioglioma, a mixed neuronal–glial neoplasm occurring at a superficial location in the cerebral cortex in young children and infants. Despite the large size of these lesions, surgery is often curative. There is also the olfactory neuroblastoma, which arises in the vault of the nose in young adults. It is composed of immature neuronal cells which tend to infiltrate locally and may metastasise to regional lymph nodes.

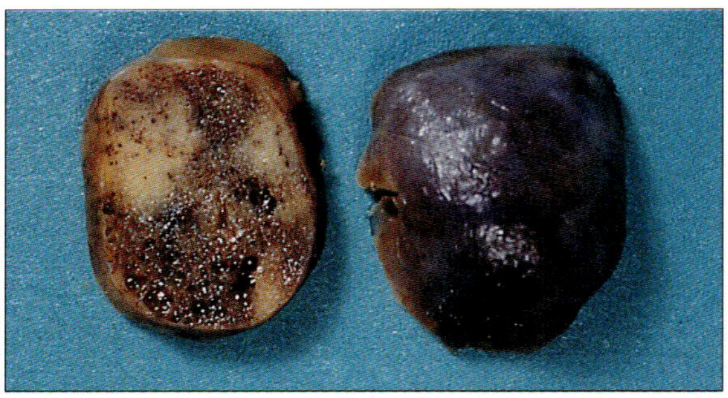

10.40 Macroscopic view of a resected paraganglioma arising in the filum terminale region in a 28-year-old female. The tumour is encapsulated and on cross-section contains numerous prominent vascular channels.

EMBRYONAL TUMOURS

Many pathologists use the term 'primitive neuroectodermal tumour' to denote the group of embryonal tumours occurring within the CNS, all of which are thought to have a common progenitor cell and have characteristic histological features. By far the commonest tumour of this type is the cerebellar medulloblastoma, but other rarer varieties are recognised; these are described below.

Medulloblastoma

This tumour is the second commonest CNS neoplasm in children, occurring characteristically in the cerebellar vermis (**10.42**). Medulloblastomas may also occur in young adults, when the cerebellar hemispheres are more often involved. These rapidly growing neoplasms often compress the CSF pathway, resulting in hydrocephalus, and invade adjacent structures including the brainstem. Meningeal invasion may also occur (**10.43**) and metastatic dissemination in the CSF pathway is common.

A wide range of histological features can occur, the commonest of which is a population of densely

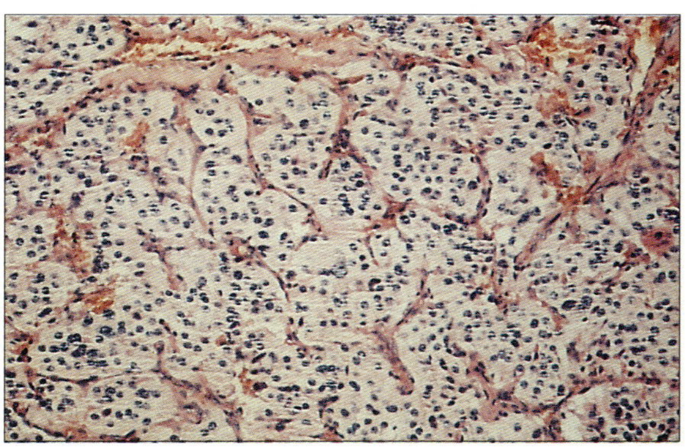

10.41 Histology of the paraganglioma in **10.39** shows a characteristic alveolar pattern of pale uniform tumour cells which are surrounded by a branching vascular network.

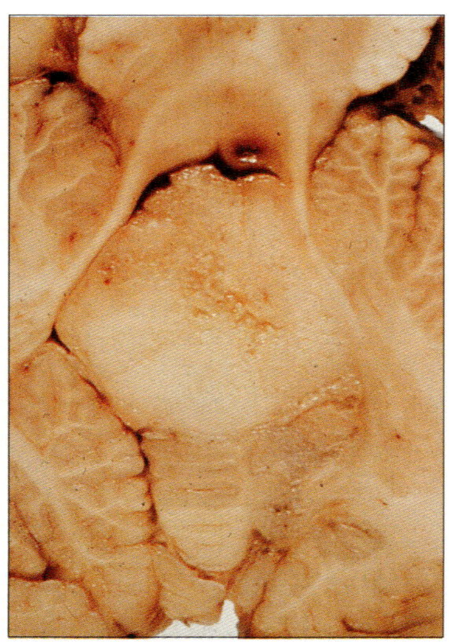

10.42 Male aged six years with a medulloblastoma arising in the cerebellar vermis, which fills the fourth ventricle. There is invasion of the vermis and right cerebellar hemisphere, and spinal metastases were found in the lumbar region at autopsy.

packed small elongated or round cells with oval or carrot-shaped nuclei and scanty cytoplasm (**10.44**). Mitotic activity is widespread and foci of necrosis may be identified. The tumour cells sometimes accumulate around blood vessels and neuroblastic rosettes can be identified in up to 40% of cases.

On immunocytochemistry, most medulloblastomas express neuronal proteins, though astrocytic differentiation (with GFAP positivity) is recognised. Some variants show extensive neuronal differentiation in larger pale-staining cells which occur in reticulin-free islands within the tumour. These are referred to as desmoplastic medulloblastomas (**10.45, 10.46**). A very rare variant, the medullomyoblastoma, includes a rhabdomyoblastic component; melanotic medulloblastomas contains foci of epithelial melanin-containing cells which may form glandular or papillary structures.

Cerebral primitive neuroectodermal tumour

This is also a tumour of childhood which usually occurs in the parietal or temporal lobes and may be multifocal. As with the medulloblastoma, CSF metastases occur and local spread can be extensive. Histologically, these tumours closely resemble medulloblastomas, though desmoplastic variants are extremely uncommon.

Other embryonal tumours

These are all rare lesions, which characteristically occur in children.

- Medulloepithelioma comprises glandular structures resembling the primitive medullary epithelium of the neural tube.
- Ependymoblastoma is characterised by the presence of numerous ependymoblastic rosettes with a central lumen (**10.47**).

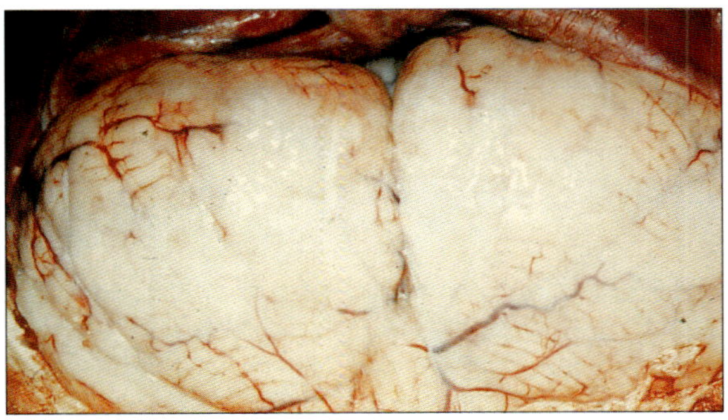

10.43 Female aged nine years with recurrent medulloblastoma which has spread extensively throughout the subarachnoid space, giving a pale coating over the cerebellar hemispheres.

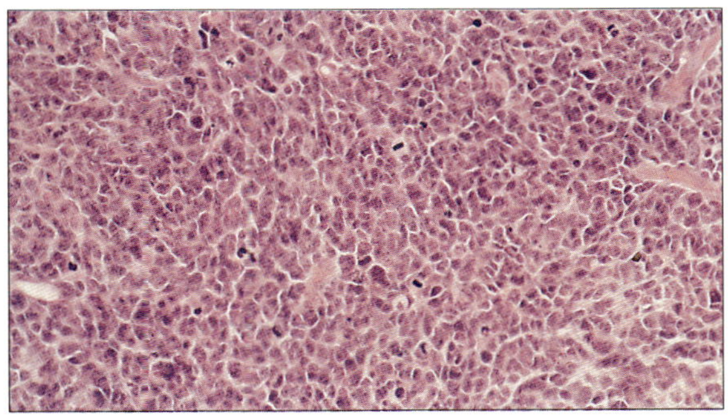

10.44 Histology of the tumour in **10.42** shows a densely cellular neoplasm composed of 'primitive' cells with elongated or carrot-shaped nuclei and scanty cytoplasm. Numerous mitotic figures are present throughout the neoplasm.

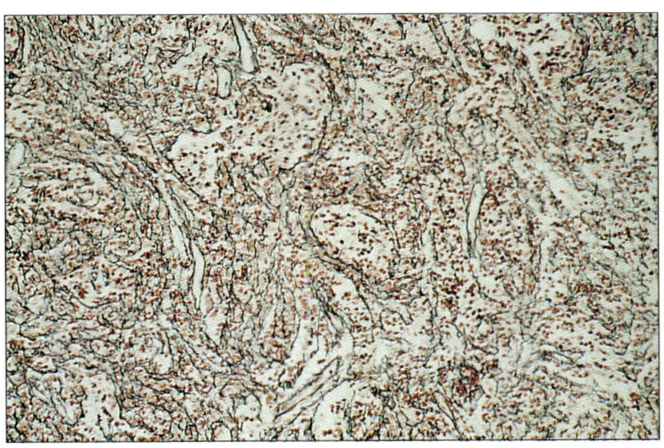

10.45 A reticulin stain in a desmoplastic medulloblastoma shows numerous reticulin-free pale islands of tumour cells.

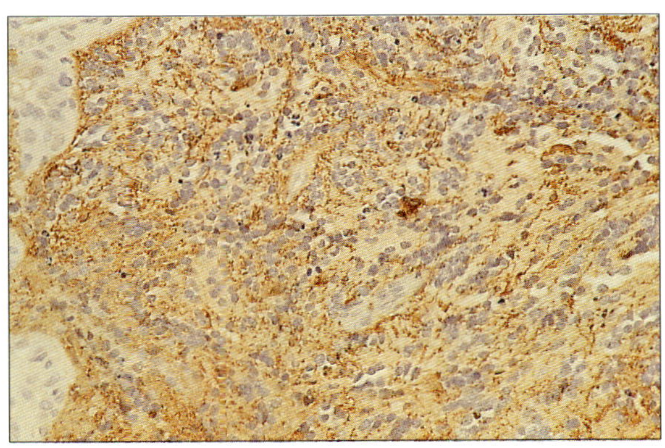

10.46 The islands of cells shown in **10.45** exhibit neuronal differentiation with a strong positive reaction for synaptophysin.

- Neuroblastoma characteristically occurs within the deeper regions of the cerebral hemispheres and may be apparently well-demarcated. Some varieties include mature ganglion cells, in which case the term ganglioneuroblastoma is appropriate.

All the above mentioned tumours can exhibit extensive local invasion and metastases within the CNS.

LYMPHOMAS

Although accounting for around 1–2% of all CNS neoplasms, the incidence of primary CNS lymphomas is increasing. These tumours occur at a markedly increased frequency in immunosuppressed individuals, particularly in those with AIDS. In immunosuppressed patients, the Epstein–Barr virus has been implicated in the pathogenesis of these tumours and viral RNA is demonstrable in many cases using *in situ* hybridisation (**10.48**).

CNS lymphomas may be multifocal and usually arise in the cerebral hemispheres particularly in the region of the deep white matter or basal ganglia (**10.49**). Larger tumours may be necrotic and CSF spread occurs in a few cases.

At the time of death, around 10% of cases may exhibit systemic spread, and ocular involvement may be noted. The diffusely infiltrating pattern of growth may resemble that of a glioblastoma, particularly if the corpus callosum is involved to give a 'butterfly' growth pattern.

Most lymphomas arising in the CNS are high-grade B cell non-Hodgkin's lymphomas with a diffuse growth pattern (**10.50**). A perivascular pattern of

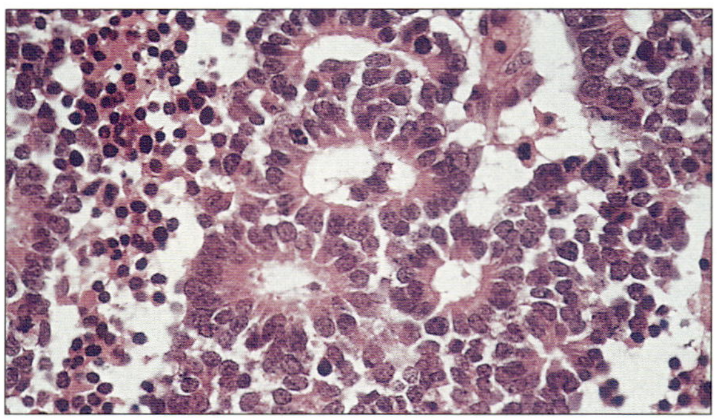

10.47 Male aged three years with an ependymoblastoma arising in the region of the third ventricle. This tumour shows evidence of ependymal differentiation with numerous small canalicular structures. Areas of necrosis are present (left) and mitotic activity is widespread.

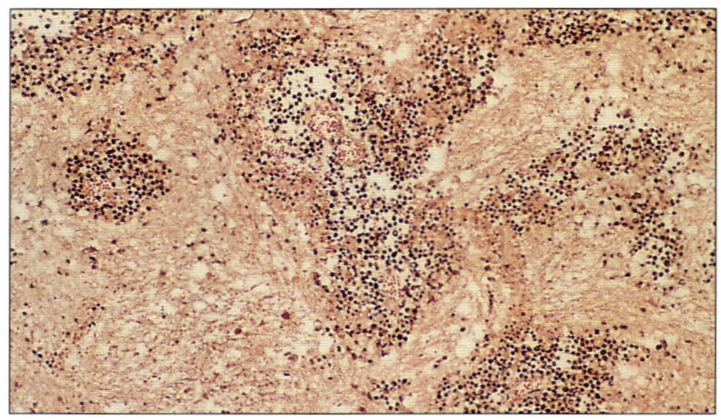

10.48 *In situ* hybridisation for Epstein–Barr virus RNA transcripts shows a positive dark reaction within the tumour cells of a CNS lymphoma in a 26-year-old male with AIDS.

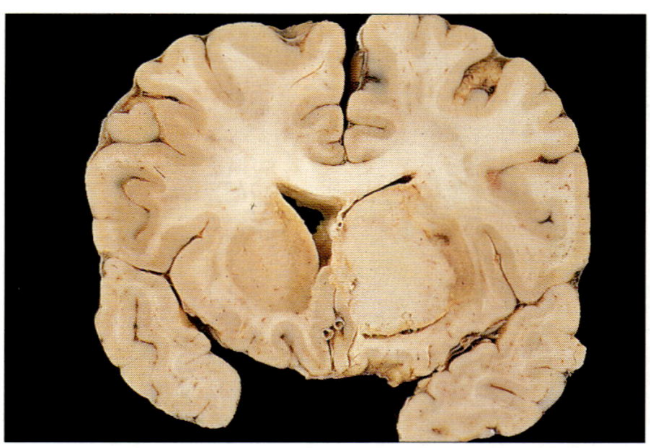

10.49 Male aged 37 years with AIDS and a large partly necrotic mass arising in the basal ganglia on the right side. This is a malignant lymphoma which extensively infiltrates the surrounding grey and white matter structures and contains small areas of haemorrhage.

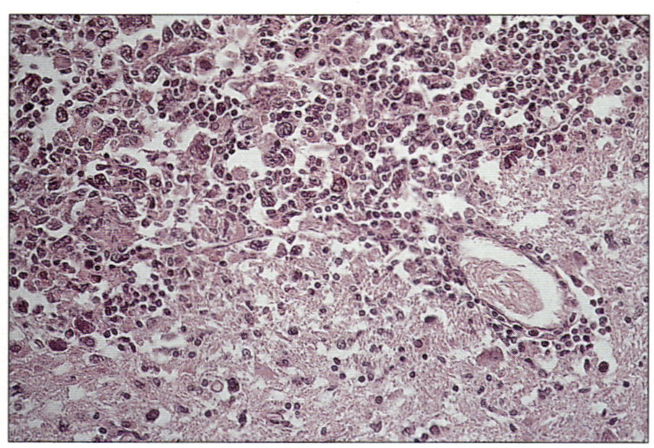

10.50 Histology of the tumour in **10.49** shows a pleomorphic tumour cell population composed predominantly of large malignant lymphoma cells, corresponding to immunoblasts and centroblasts. A smaller population of reactive T lymphocytes is present throughout the tumour and around adjacent blood vessels (right).

growth is characteristic with tumour cells present within the outer reticulin framework of small intracerebral vessels (**10.51, 10.52**).

GERM CELL TUMOURS

Most intrinsic CNS germ cell tumours occur in the midline region in, or around, the pineal gland and the suprasellar area (**10.53**). Most cases arise in children and young adults and males are affected more often than females.

Germinoma

The commonest germ cell tumour in the CNS is the germinoma, which usually arises in the region of the pineal gland and is a well-circumscribed slow-growing tumour. This is histologically identical to the testicular seminoma and is composed of uniform large cells with pale cytoplasm and a well-defined cell membrane (**10.54**). The prominent nucleus usually contains a large nucleolus and the cytoplasm is often PAS-positive. Immunocytochemistry shows a positive staining reaction for placental alkaline phosphatase (**10.55**), and occasional syncytiotrophoblastic giant

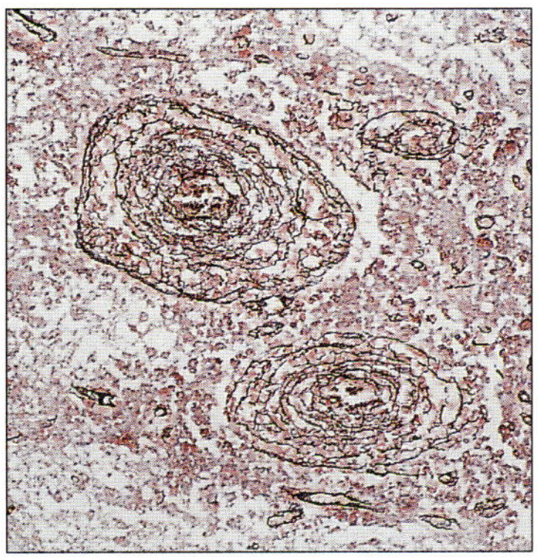

10.51 A reticulin stain in primary CNS lymphoma shows tumour cell invasion of vessel walls with separation of reticulin bands.

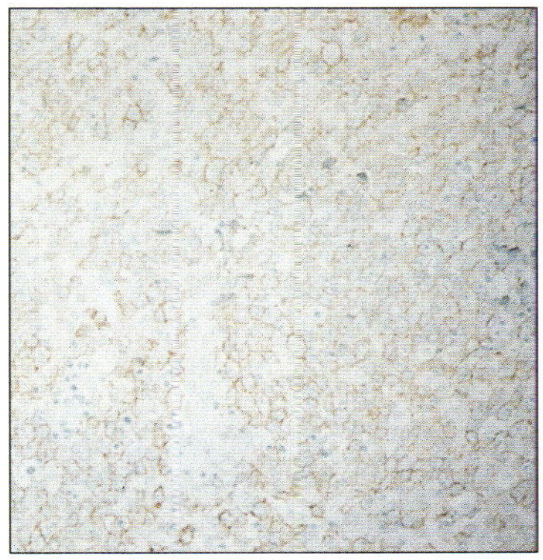

10.52 Immunocytochemistry on the tumour cell population shown in **10.51** shows a positive reaction for the B cell marker CD20.

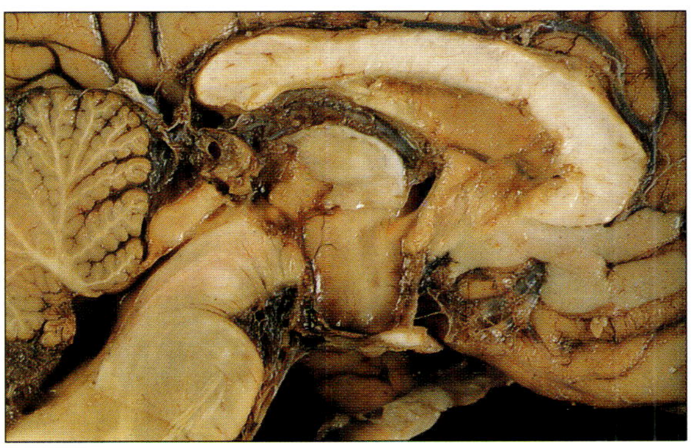

10.53 Male aged 13 years with a germinoma arising in the region of the pineal gland. The tumour is partly covered by thickened meninges and prominent blood vessels, and compresses the pulvinar region.

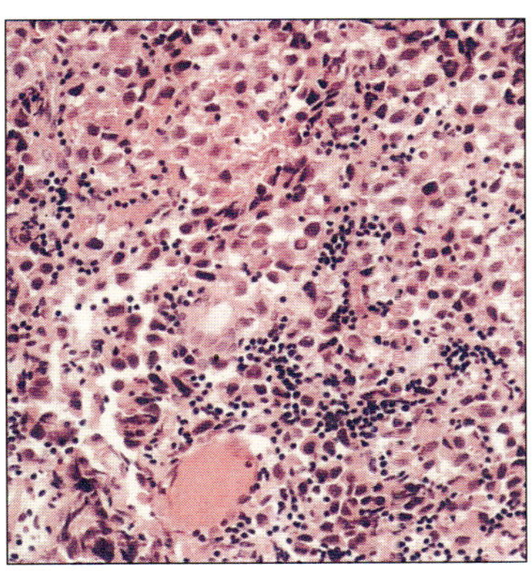

10.54 Histology of the tumour in **10.53** shows large tumour cells containing abundant eosinophilic cytoplasm arranged in solid sheets, with a prominent lymphocytic infiltrate.

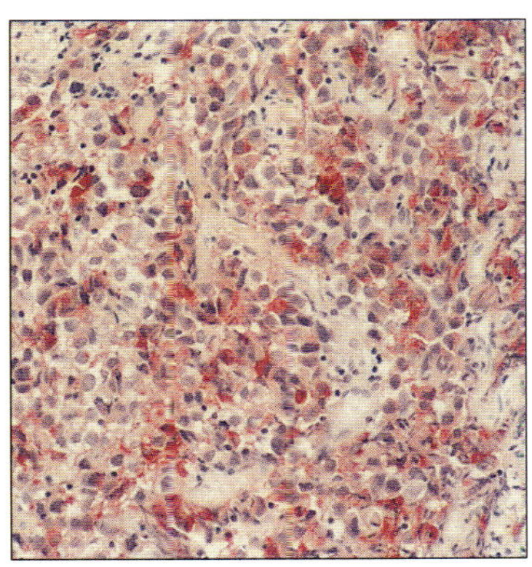

10.55 Immunocytochemistry for placental alkaline phosphatase gives a strong positive reaction (red) in the tumour cell population from the case in **10.53**.

cells may occur, which are positive for human chorionic gonadotrophin. Most tumours contain a multifocal lymphocytic infiltrate, which in some cases may be so conspicuous as to mask the underlying tumour cells. Germinomas may occur in a pure form or in combination with other germ cell tumours, particularly embryonal carcinoma or a yolk sac tumour. These tumours may be referred to as teratocarcinomas.

Other germ cell tumours

Other germ cell tumours include the following.

- Embryonal carcinoma, in which the tumour cells exhibit a primitive epithelial appearance, growing in solid sheets or poorly formed acini.
- Yolk sac tumour, a rapidly growing tumour composed of elongated cells growing in a tubular pattern. These cells have prominent cytoplasmic or stromal globules that are immunoreactive for alphafetoprotein.
- Choriocarcinoma, a highly malignant tumour composed of trophoblastic cells, is extremely uncommon as a primary lesion in the CNS, and exhibits positive staining for human chorionic gonadotrophin.
- Teratoma, which in the CNS is classified as mature (composed of fully differentiated tissues), immature (consisting of embryonic tissues with incomplete differentiation as in **10.56**), or teratoma with malignant transformation (in which mature epithelial tissue exhibits malignant change, e.g. squamous cell carcinoma or adenocarcinoma).

PINEAL NEOPLASMS

Intrinsic tumours of the pineal gland are uncommon, mostly occurring in children and young adults. They can be considered in two main categories.

Pineocytoma

This slow-growing neoplasm is well-demarcated from the surrounding brain. Compression of adjacent brain structures usually causes hydrocephalus, and infiltration of the surrounding CNS is uncommon (**10.57**). Histologically, most pineocytomas contain small

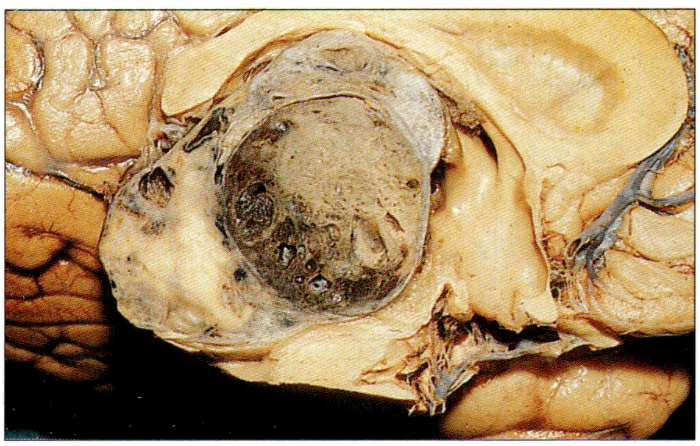

10.56 Male aged 10 years with an immature teratoma arising in the region of the pineal gland. This large neoplasm is compressing the adjacent brainstem and thalamus, with upward displacement of the corpus callosum.

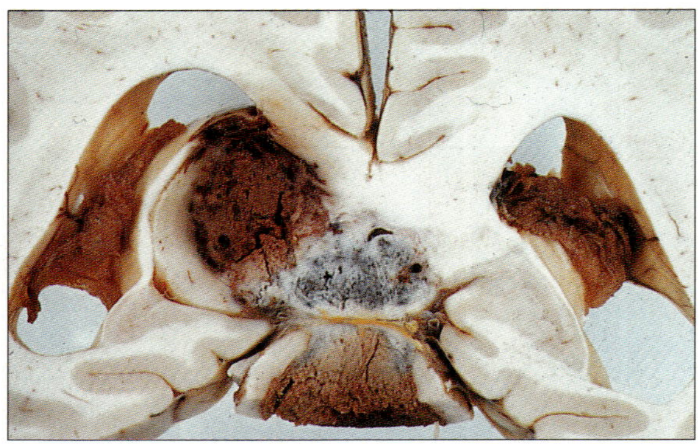

10.57 Female aged 19 years with a pineocytoma which has invaded the adjacent brainstem, left temporal lobe and thalamus with extensive haemorrhage.

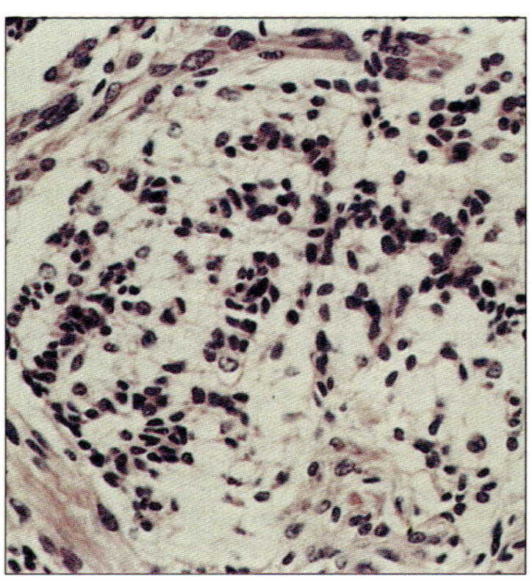

10.58 Histology of the tumour in **10.57** shows a population of small tumour cells set in a delicate fibrillary matrix.

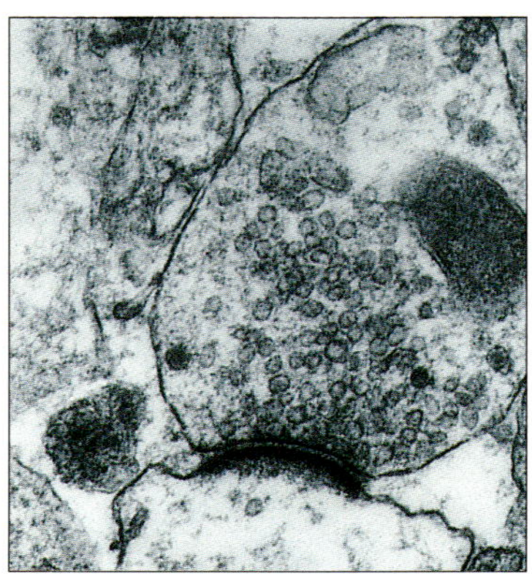

10.59 Electron microscopy of the tumour in **10.57** shows evidence of neuronal differentiation with synapse formation.

polygonal cells with a delicate connective tissue stroma (**10.58**). Pineocytic rosettes are common and immunocytochemistry shows reactivity to neuronal markers, e.g. synaptophysin, and some tumours show obvious neuronal differentiation with ganglion cells (**10.59**). Others may show retinal differentiation with fleurettes and immunopositivity for retinal S-antigen.

Pineoblastoma

This malignant tumour occurs most often in young children and has the histological features of a primitive neuroectodermal tumour. Neuroblastic rosettes are a common feature. Although neuronal and glial differentiation have been described, they are less common than in either cerebellar medulloblastomas or pineocytomas. These tumours invade locally and may metastasise via the CSF, as is characteristic of primitive neuroectodermal tumours.

TUMOURS OF UNCERTAIN HISTOGENESIS

Capillary haemangioblastoma

This tumour usually occurs in the region of the cerebellum in young adults. The lesions are well-demarcated and highly vascular, often with a prominent cyst (**10.60**). The lesion usually connects to the leptomeninges and multifocal cases have been described. These tumours are associated with von Hippel–Lindau disease, when multiple lesions are particularly common and involvement of other sites within the CNS, e.g. the medulla and spinal cord, may occur. Histologically, these are composed of an intricate vascular network composed of irregular, often dilated, capillaries and intervening stromal cells (**10.61**). The stromal cells are of variable histological appearance and range from small polygonal cells to larger cells with abundant foamy cytoplasm, occasionally exhibiting nuclear pleomorphism. Mitotic activity is uncommon.

The stromal cells can produce erythropoetin and extramedullary erythropoesis may be seen within the tumour. These cells also express vimentin and neuron-specific enolase, with a minority of cells also expressing GFAP. Immunostaining for epithelial markers (epithelial membrane antigen and CAM 5.2) is negative. This is helpful in establishing a differential diagnosis between haemangioblastomas and metastatic renal carcinoma, which may also occur in the von Hippel–Lindau syndrome.

EXTRINSIC TUMOURS

MENINGIOMAS

This group of tumours accounts for the vast majority of tumours arising in the coverings of the brain. Meningiomas account for around 18–20% of all intracranial CNS tumours in adults, but are extremely uncommon in children. Females are affected around twice as frequently as males. The tumours have a predilection for certain sites including:

- the parietal convexity;
- parasagittal region (**10.62**);
- sphenoid wing;
- olfactory groove;
- optic nerve (**10.63**);
- foramen magnum.

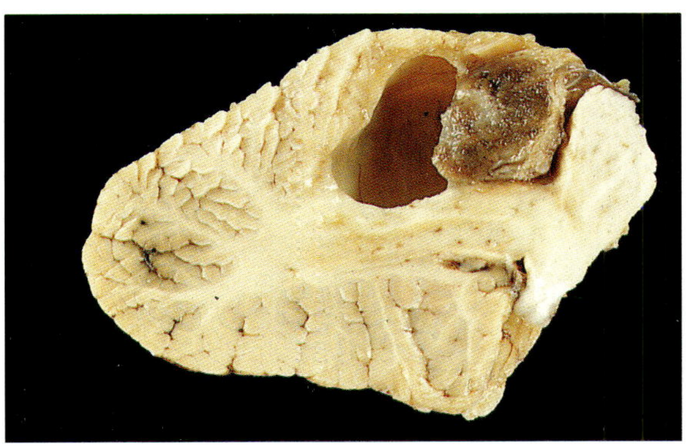

10.60 Male aged 52 years with Von Hippel–Lindau disease and a recurrent cerebellar haemangioblastoma. The tumour is associated with a large cyst and contains numerous areas of haemorrhage throughout the solid nodule.

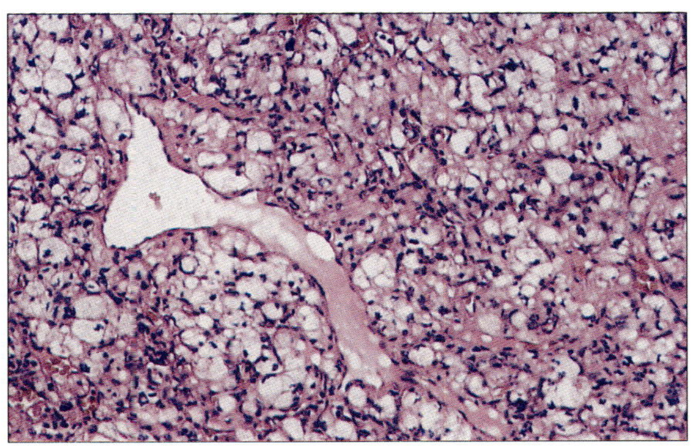

10.61 Histology of the tumour in **10.60** shows numerous vascular channels of varying calibre lined by a single endothelial layer, and surrounded by stromal cells which vary in appearance from large 'foamy' cells to polygonal cells with eosinophilic cytoplasm.

Spinal cord meningiomas account for around 5% of all meningiomas, and arise most often in the thoracic region (**10.64**). Meningiomas can occur within the ventricular system, usually in the lateral ventricle. Most meningiomas are attached to the dura and grow as solid lobulated masses which compress rather than invade the adjacent brain. At the base of the tumour, the dura and underlying skull bone may be extensively infiltrated; occasional meningiomas produce an osteoblastic reaction in the surrounding bone with secondary hyperostosis. A few tumours exhibit a diffuse pattern of infiltration, referred to as meningioma *en plaque* (**10.65**).

A wide variety of histological patterns is recognised, the commoner varieties of which are listed below. Immunohistochemistry for meningiomas shows a strong positive reaction for vimentin, desmoplakins and epithelial membrane antigen. Many tumours also exhibit focal positivity for cytokeratins and S100 protein.

On electron microscopy, meningiomas show a characteristic complex interdigitating network of cell processes, with hemidesmosomes as the predominant intercellular junction. The commonest varieties of histological patterns in meningiomas are described as follows.

Meningothelial pattern

In meningothelial meningiomas, there are well-demarcated solid lobules of polygonal cells with ill-defined

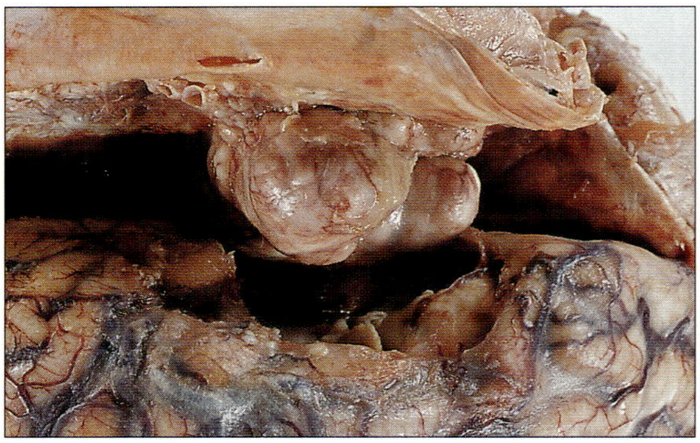

10.62 Female aged 52 years with a parietal convexity meningioma which is attached to the overlying dura and has extensively compressed the underlying cortex.

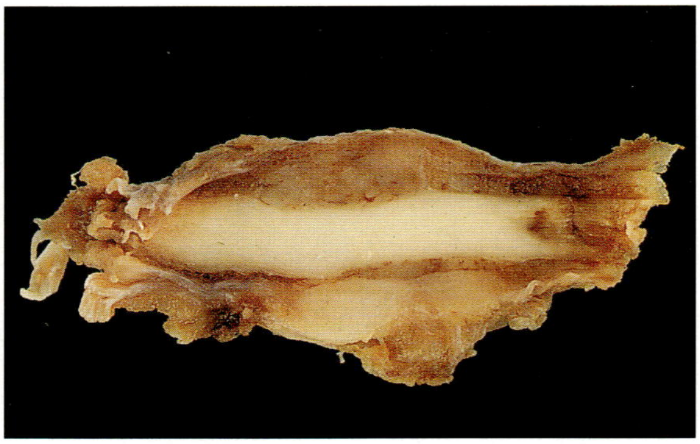

10.63 Female aged 35 years with a large optic nerve meningioma, which in resection surrounded the orbital portion of the nerve (centre) which is markedly compressed and distorted.

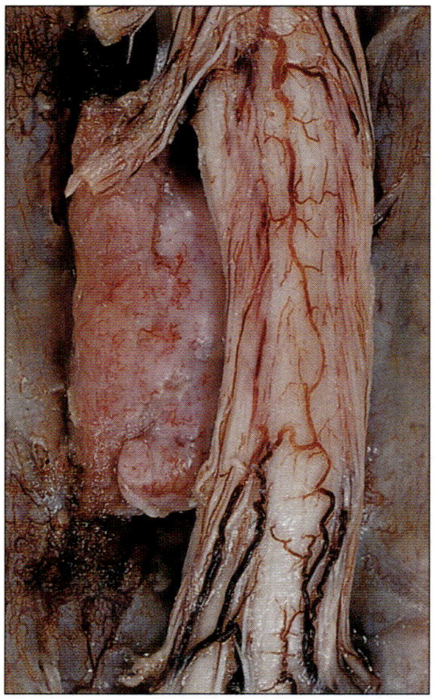

10.64 Female aged 45 years with a thoracic spinal cord meningioma arising on the posterior dura, displacing the spinal cord and adjacent nerve roots.

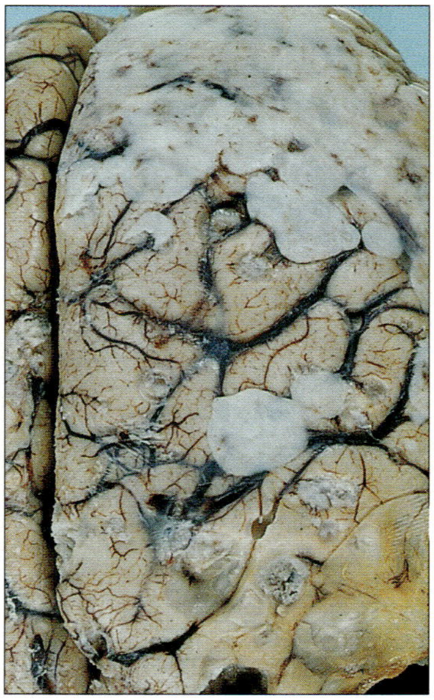

10.65 Male aged 61 years with meningioma *en plaque*. Numerous pale tumour nodules are present over the surface of the brain, forming a contiguous mass over the left occipital lobe.

cell membranes (**10.66**). Cytoplasmic invagination into the nucleus is common and can be recognised in smear preparations. Whorl formation is not particularly prominent, but calcification in the form of psammoma bodies may occur.

Fibrous (fibroblastic) pattern

In fibrous meningiomas, the tumour cells are spindle-shaped and elongated. They are arranged in a complex variety of bundles (**10.67**). Collagen and reticulin are present around the elongated cells, but whorl formation is uncommon.

Transitional pattern

In transitional meningiomas, the histological pattern is intermediate, combining features of meningothelial and fibrous tumours. Most show a number of concentric whorls, in which cells are arranged in a circular manner around a central capillary or psammoma body.

Psammomatous pattern

Psammoma body formation is pronounced and only a scanty number of meningothelial cells may be identified. These tumours occur particularly frequently in the spinal cord region and olfactory groove.

Rarer varieties

Rarer varieties of meningioma include:

- angiomatous, which contains numerous dilated blood vessels;
- microcystic;
- secretory, in which small glandular lumina may be formed;
- clear-cell;
- chordoid, which contains vacuolated cells resembling a chordoma;
- lymphoplasmacyte-rich, usually associated with polyclonal gammopathy;
- metaplastic, containing myxoid tissue, cartilaginous tissue, bone or fat.

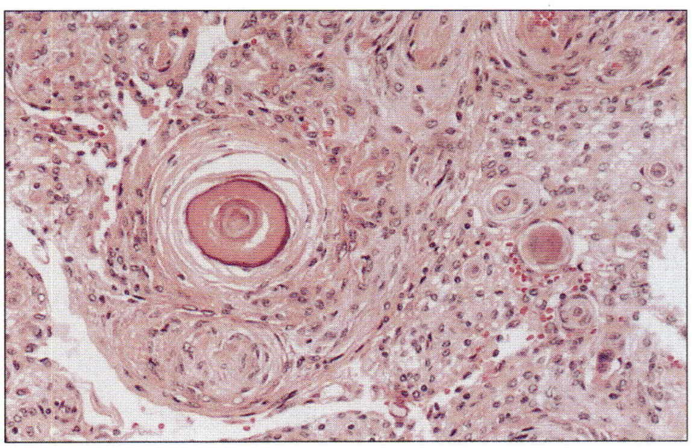

10.66 Histology of a meningothelial meningioma shows a population of polygonal cells arranged in whorls and solid sheets with several rounded calcified psammoma bodies.

ATYPICAL MENINGIOMAS

In this group of meningiomas, the tumour cells exhibit increased cellularity, often with mitotic figures, prominent nucleoli and multifocal necrosis (**10.68**). Necrosis in meningiomas may also result from therapeutic embolisation prior to surgery, resulting in multiple infarcts around blood vessels, which occasionally contain small fragments of embolic material. Superficial cortical infiltration may also be noted. These tumours have an increased tendency to recur following surgery when compared to the commoner varieties of meningioma.

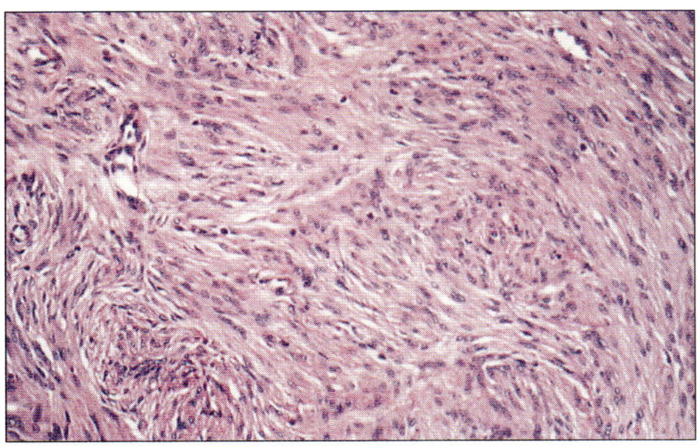

10.67 In a fibroblastic meningioma, the tumour cells are elongated and bipolar. They are arranged in parallel bundles with no evidence of whorl formation.

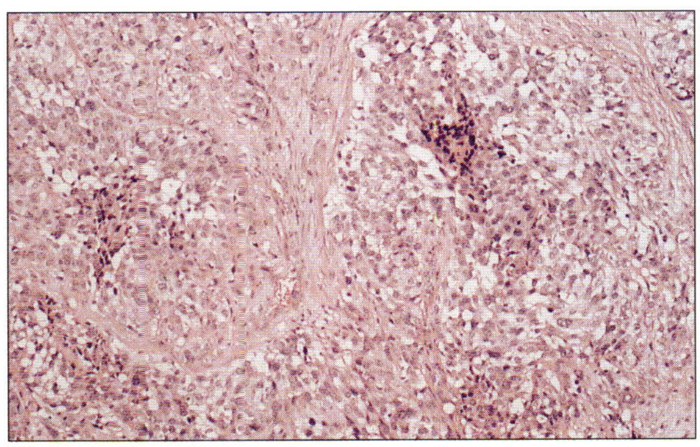

10.68 The atypical meningioma is characterised by multifocal necrosis, with a less well-ordered tumour cell architecture than its benign counterparts.

OTHER TYPES OF MENINGIOMA

Papillary meningioma

This rare variety of meningioma occurs most often in children and young adults. A prominent papillary pattern is present, but whorl and psammoma body formation is uncommon. Multiple foci of necrosis may be identified and mitotic figures are usually present. These tumours tend to invade the brain and may later metastasise to lung or bone.

Anaplastic (malignant) meningioma

The histological features of this tumour are those of a frankly malignant lesion, in which there is a greater degree of cellular atypia and nuclear pleomorphism than in the atypical meningioma. Cortical invasion is usually widespread and these lesions may metastasise systemically following surgery.

MESENCHYMAL TUMOURS

A wide range of mesenchymal tumours arise in the meninges, most of which correspond to soft tissue tumours arising elsewhere in the body. Benign tumours include the lipoma, fibrous histiocytoma, osteoma and chondroma.

Malignant tumours

A haemangiopericytoma is the commonest mesenchymal tumour arising within the cranial cavity. It may resemble a meningioma on radiology and at surgery, but tends to be highly vascular and may infiltrate surrounding brain and other tissues. Histologically, it is distinguished from a meningioma by its monotonous cell population, composed of polygonal cells with ovoid nuclei and ill-defined cytoplasm (**10.69, 10.70**), together with a prominent branching vascular network and a dense intercellular reticulin framework. Immunocytochemistry for epithelial membrane antigen and cytokeratin is negative; occasionally, a tumour exhibits immunoreactivity for desmin or smooth muscle actin. There is a strong tendency for these tumours to recur and they may metastasise systemically following surgery.

Other malignant tumours arising in the meninges include the chondrosarcoma, malignant fibrous histiocytoma, rhabdomyosarcoma and meningeal sarcomatosis (in which diffuse infiltration of meninges by a sarcoma has occurred). There are also the primary melanocytic lesions. These include:

- diffuse melanosis;
- melanocytoma;
- malignant melanoma.

In diffuse melanosis, there is diffuse proliferation of benign melanocytes within the leptomeninges sometimes extending into perivascular spaces in the CNS. A melanocytoma, however, is a nodular meningeal tumour usually well-demarcated from the surrounding brain. It often arises in the thoracic spinal region and in the basal region of the skull including Meckel's cave. Melanocytomas are abundantly pigmented and are composed histologically of uniform neoplastic melanocytes with characteristic fascicular nuclei. Malignant transformation is rare. Lastly, malignant melanoma is a rare primary tumour within the meninges, which can present diagnostic difficulty if an erroneous diagnosis of metastatic melanoma is made. These tumours closely resemble melanomas arising elsewhere in the body. Occasional diffuse infiltration of the meninges can occur by this tumour, resulting in meningeal melanomatosis.

NERVE SHEATH TUMOURS

Nerve sheath tumours may arise on cranial or spinal nerves, particularly sensory nerves, and in patients with neurofibromatosis multiple lesions may occur. The commonest categories are described below.

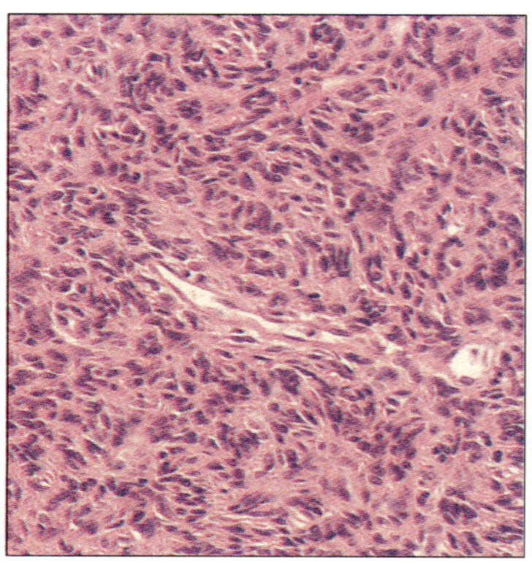

10.69 Histology of a meningeal haemangiopericytoma shows numerous thin-walled vascular channels surrounded by elongated 'twisted' tumour cells which are densely packed in a solid arrangement.

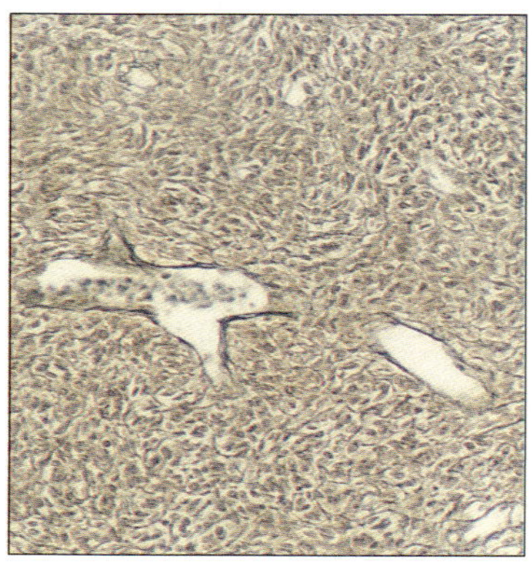

10.70 A dense reticulin framework is present around the tumour cells and blood vessels of the meningeal haemangiopericytoma shown in **10.69**.

Schwannoma (neurilemmoma)

These characteristically arise on the vestibular branch of the VIIIth cranial nerve (**10.71**) in the cerebellopontine angle (**10.72**), but can arise on other cranial and spinal sensory nerves. The lesions are usually located towards the edge of a nerve and are well-demarcated from surrounding tissues. Schwannomas are benign and usually slow-growing lesions. Bilateral VIIIth nerve tumours are a hallmark of type 2 neurofibromatosis. Histologically, two main patterns are seen (**10.73**).

- Antoni A tissue, in which there is a dense accumulation of elongated cells, often with nuclear pallisading.
- Antoni B tissue, where cells are less densely arranged in a loose myxoid matrix, within which xanthoma cells may also be present.

These tumours often contain hyalinised blood vessels and may show evidence of previous haemorrhage. Immunocytochemistry shows a strong positive reaction for S100 protein and Leu 7. Mitotic activity is uncommon in schwannomas, but nuclear pleomorphism is common and of no sinister prognostic significance. An abundant reticulin network is present around the tumour cells. On electron microscopy, tumour cells are surrounded by basement membrane.

Other variants of schwannoma include:

- the cellular schwannoma, in which Antoni A tissue predominates;
- the plexiform schwannoma, in which a worm-like arrangement of affected nerves is present, usually in the subcutaneous tissue;
- the melanotic schwannoma, which contains abundant melanin pigment.

Neurofibroma

This group of neoplasms characteristically occur on spinal sensory nerves. In contrast to schwannomas,

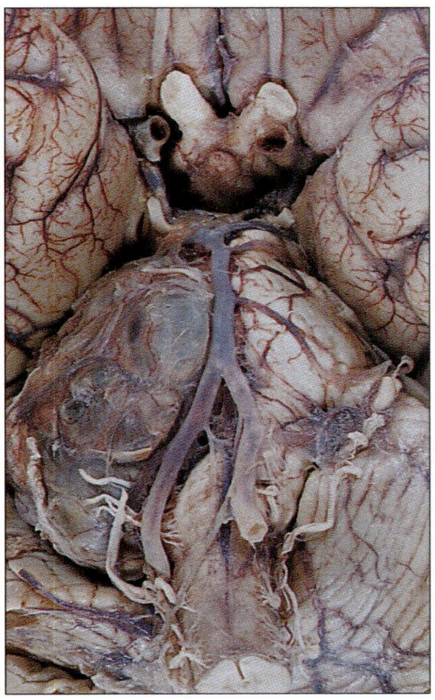

10.71 Female aged 58 years with a right-sided acoustic schwannoma. This well-defined neoplasm is sited in the cerebellopontine angle, with displacement of the brainstem and adjacent nerves and vascular structures.

The most common cerebellopontine angle tumours
Acoustic schwannoma
Meningioma
Epidermoid cyst
Choroid plexus papilloma
Metastatic carcinoma

10.72 The most common cerebellopontine angle tumours, arranged in ascending frequency.

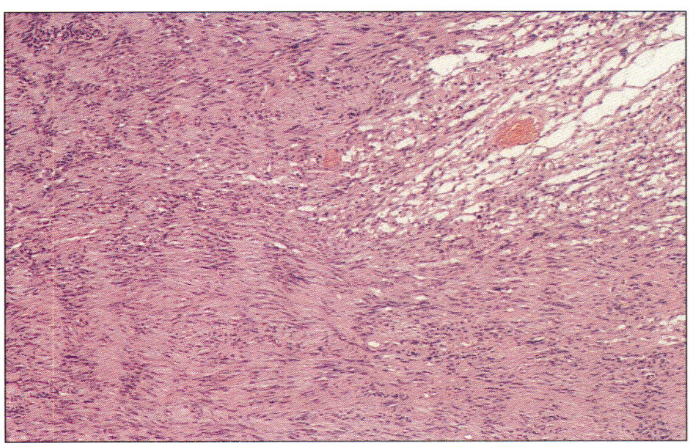

10.73 Histology of an acoustic schwannoma shows Antoni A tissue (bottom) which comprises elongated bipolar cells which are densely packed and exhibit nuclear pallisading. Antoni B tissue (top right) is also composed of elongated cells, but there is a looser arrangement often with a myxoid stroma and containing large hyalinised blood vessels.

they form diffuse tumours, within which nerve fibres are scattered. Multiple lesions are usually present in patients with type 1 and type 2 neurofibromatosis (**10.74**).

The histological pattern is variable, but characteristically contains wavy cells with elongated nuclei arranged in solid bundles (**10.75**). Focal pallisading or whorling may be found and mast cells are usually identifiable within the tumour. Nuclear pleomorphism may be observed, but is thought to be a degenerative feature of no sinister significance. Immunocytochemistry shows a positive reaction for S100 protein and Leu 7. Variants of neurofibroma include the circumscribed or globular neurofibroma, often unassociated with neurofibromatosis, and the plexiform neurofibroma which involves numerous branches of a nerve. A significant proportion of these lesions undergo malignant transformation with an increase in cellularity and mitotic activity, particularly in patients with neurofibromatosis type 1.

Malignant peripheral nerve sheath tumours

Malignant peripheral nerve sheath tumours generally correspond to malignant neurofibroma and occasionally arise from a pre-existing benign lesion, particularly in patients with neurofibromatosis type 1. These lesions are often composed of solid sheets of spindle cells, with little evidence of characteristic histological patterns in the corresponding benign tumours. Immunoreactivity for S100 protein is variable. These tumours are aggressively malignant and may metastasise. Variants of malignant peripheral nerve sheath tumours include the following.

- Malignant epithelioid schwannoma, in which plump eosinophilic cells may form a predominant part of the tumour cell population and may simulate carcinoma or malignant melanoma.
- Malignant nerve sheath tumours, with divergent differentiation, often into mesenchymal tissues, including malignant cartilage and bone or neuroendocrine or epithelial structures.
- Melanotic malignant nerve sheath tumours may also occur and can be confused on histology with malignant melanoma.

TUMOURS OF THE PITUITARY REGION

A wide range of tumours has been described arising in the region of the pituitary gland, either from the gland itself or from adjacent structures (**10.76**). Many of these lesions present with clinical symptoms

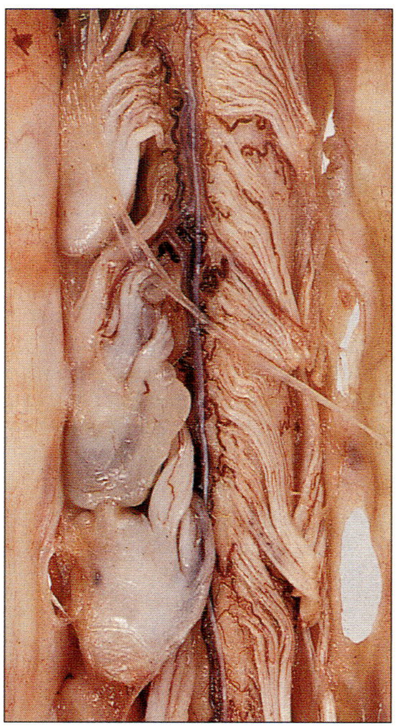

10.74 Female aged 38 years with neurofibromatosis type I. Multiple neurofibromas are present on sensory nerves in the cervical region. The tumours are attached to abnormally thickened spinal nerve roots; nerve fibres run throughout the neoplasm.

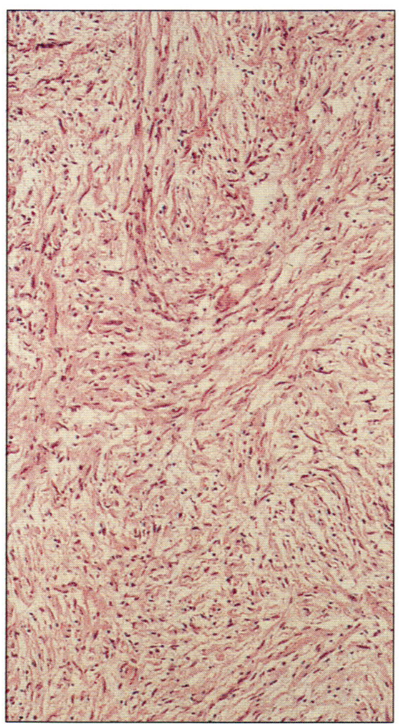

10.75 Histology of the tumour in **10.74** shows elongated tumour cells with 'wavy' nuclei arranged in irregular bundles within a loose myxoid stroma, characteristic of a neurofibroma.

relating to hypofunction as a consequence of pituitary gland compression, or hyperfunction due to an active endocrine secreting tumour. Visual impairment commonly occurs with large tumours due to compression or invasion of the optic chiasm. The commonest tumours to arise at this site are as follows.

Pituitary adenoma

These are common tumours, accounting for about 5–10% of neurosurgical tumour biopsies. The adenoma may be a microadenoma, which is less than 10mm in diameter and confined to the substance of the pituitary gland. However, larger macroadenomas may extend above the dural covering of the pituitary gland to compress adjacent structures (**10.77**). Some pituitary adenomas can grow to an extremely large size, particularly non-functional tumours in older patients. As well as their effects on adjacent local structures, pituitary adenomas can produce endocrine symptoms by the excess secretion of hormones. Hormone production in a pituitary adenoma can be detected immunocytochemically (**10.78, 10.79**); some pituitary adenomas produce only peptide subunits of the larger hormones. Pituitary adenomas are classified according to the predominant hormone produced, though many tumours are of null-cell type and do not produce active hormones. Evidence of hormone production can also be detected by electron microscopy, which reveals characteristic membrane-bound granules of varying size usually sited at the peripheral cytoplasm near the cell membranes (**10.80**).

Nowadays, the histological classification of pituitary tumours depends on the main cell type in relation to hormone production – conventional

Parasellar tumours and cysts	
Pituitary adenoma	Epidermoid cyst
Pituitary carcinoma	Dermoid cyst
Craniopharyngioma	Optic chiasm astrocytoma
Rathke's cleft cyst	Meningioma
Choristoma	Metastatic carcinoma
Chordoma	Sphenoid sinus carcinoma
Lymphoma	Nasopharyngeal carcinoma
Mucocoele	Olfactory neuroblastoma

10.76 Parasellar tumours and cysts.

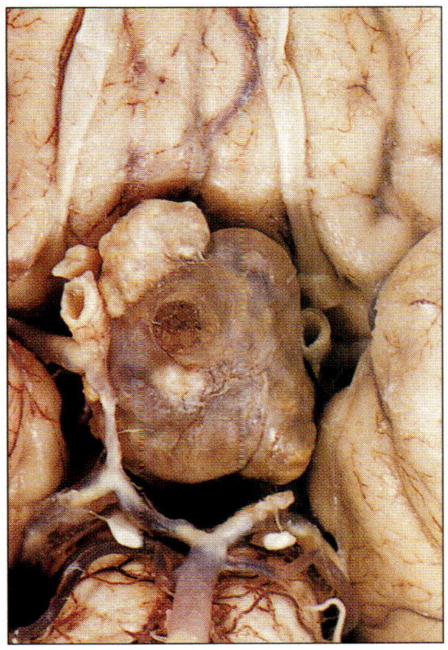

10.77 Female aged 49 years with acromegaly and a pituitary tumour. The tumour is displacing the adjacent internal carotid arteries and markedly compresses the optic chiasm. The small pale nodule on the upper left represents residual normal anterior pituitary tissue.

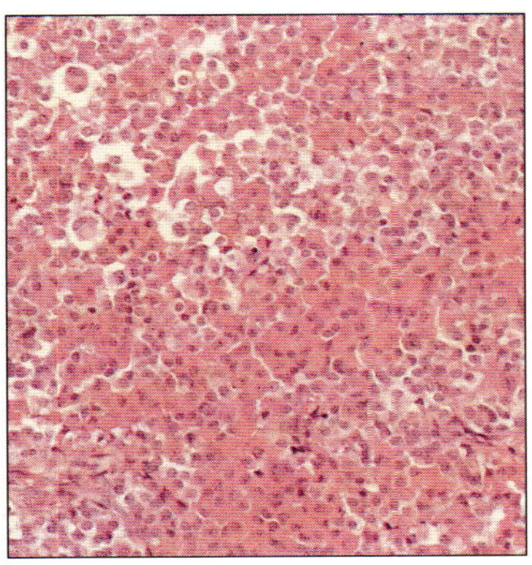

10.78 Histology of the tumour in **10.77** shows a pituitary adenoma composed of uniform polygonal cells containing eosinophilic cytoplasm.

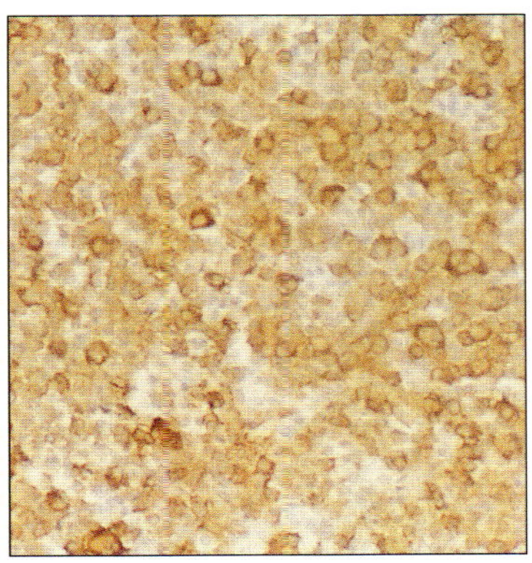

10.79 Immunocytochemistry for growth hormone shows a strong positive reaction in many of the tumour cells from the case in **10.77**.

classifications based on tinctorial stains are now less useful. Tumours which show no evidence of hormone production are referred to as null-cell adenomas. Some pituitary tumours are oncocytomas, and contain numerous mitochondria with relatively few neurosecretory granules. Large adenomas may undergo haemorrhagic infarction (which may result in a clinical episode of pituitary apoplexy) if the blood supply to the neoplasm is compromised. Although benign, pituitary adenomas may compress and occasionally infiltrate local structures, including soft tissue, blood vessels and bone, or cause signs and symptoms of raised intracranial pressure.

Pituitary carcinoma

This rare malignant tumour can be classified on the basis of hormone production; the majority are null cell carcinomas. These may resemble pituitary adenoma cytologically amd clinically, but exhibit mitotic activity and may invade the brain to metastasise both within the CSF pathway and to distant sites, including the lung and liver.

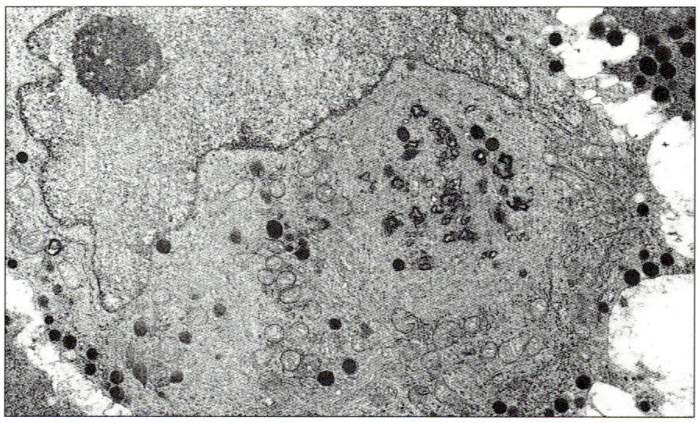

10.80 Electron microscopy of the tumour in **10.77** shows cells with numerous large dense secretory granules towards the peripheral cytoplasm. Many mitochondria are present within the cytoplasm and a fibrous body (right) composed of cytokeratin filaments and lysosome-like structures is present adjacent to the nucleus.

Craniopharyngioma

This benign tumour occurs in the region of the pituitary gland and third ventricle (**10.81**), and is thought to arise from the remnants of Rathke's cleft. Several distinct histological subtypes can be identified including:

- adamantinomatous craniopharyngioma;
- papillary craniopharyngioma.

Adamantinomatous craniopharyngiomas are cystic and contain keratin and cholesterol, often with focal calcification and extensive fibrosis with gliosis in the surrounding brain. Histologically, these tumours resemble the adamantinoma of the jaw, although some craniopharyngiomas show a closer resemblance to the calcifying odontogenic cyst of the jaw (**10.82**). The tumours characteristically occur in children and young adults, and are slow-growing benign neoplasms.

Papillary craniopharyngioma is a rare variant of craniopharyngioma. It comprises a cystic lesion containing well-differentiated squamous epithelium with a pseudopapillary pattern. It is uncommon in children, tends to involve the third ventricular region and has a better prognosis than other craniopharyngiomas.

Other tumours in the pituitary region (10.76)

These include the Rathke cleft cyst. This comprises a thin-walled cyst lined by ciliated cuboidal or columnar epithelium. It resembles the small Rathke pouch remnants occasionally found at the junction between the anterior and posterior parts of the pituitary gland. There is also the rare granular cell

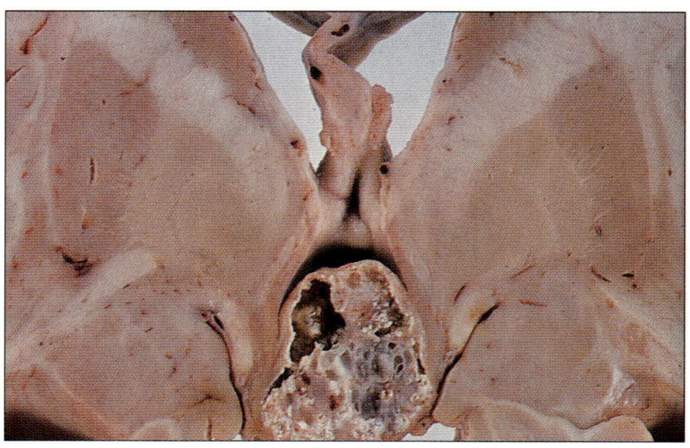

10.81 Male aged 15 years with a craniopharyngioma which shows extensive cystic change and has grown upwards to fill most of the third ventricle, resulting in obstructive hydrocephalus.

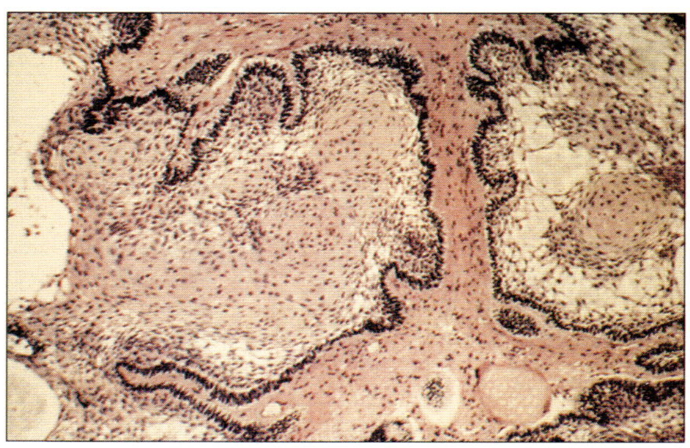

10.82 Histology of the tumour in **10.81** shows typical adamantinomatous appearances of a craniopharyngioma, with cystic change and evidence of keratin production.

tumour or pituicytoma, which arises in the posterior lobe of the pituitary gland. It comprises neoplastic glial cells with abundant granular cytoplasm.

CYSTS AND TUMOUR-LIKE STRUCTURES

A variety of cysts and tumour-like structures can occur within the CNS. They present with features similar to those of either intrinsic or extrinsic neoplasms.

CYSTIC LESIONS

Colloid cyst of the third ventricle

This cystic lesion occurs in children and young adults in the anterior region of the third ventricle near the foramen of Monro (**10.83**). It is lined by cuboidal or columnar epithelium which is occasionally ciliated. These lesions can move within the CNS pathway to obstruct the foramen of Monro, and thus may result in sudden death.

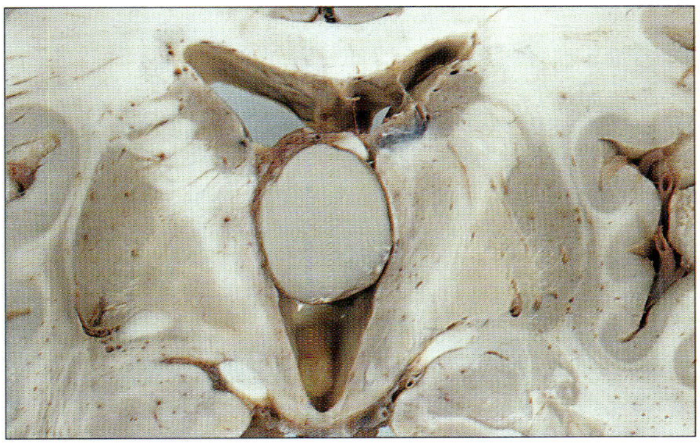

10.83 Female aged 32 years who died suddenly as a consequence of ventricular obstruction by a colloid cyst arising in the region of the foramen of Monro and obstructing the third ventricle.

Epidermoid cyst

These lesions tend to occur in children and young adults, usually in the midline structures of the brain (**10.84**), or adjacent to the spinal cord. Occasionally, spinal cord epidermoid cysts arise from the implantation of epidermal tissues following trauma, repeated lumbar puncture, or previous surgery. These cysts are lined by a keratinising stratified squamous epithelium, within which the contents can break down into cholesterol. Leakage of cholesterol can result in a foreign-body giant-cell reaction in the surrounding tissues. Malignant change within the squamous epithelium has been described, resulting in squamous cell carcinoma.

Dermoid cyst

This cyst is also lined by squamous epithelium but contains adnexal structures within the cyst wall, including hair follicles and sweat glands. The contents of dermoid cysts (**10.85**) can include hair and sebaceous debris which, if liberated, result in a foreign-body giant-cell reaction. Malignant change is rare.

Other rarer cystic lesions

These include enterogenous cysts, which characteristically occur in the upper region of the spinal cord, and are lined by ciliated cuboidal or columnar epithelium resembling that of the respiratory and upper gastrointestinal tracts. They are usually associated with a malformation involving the vertebral bodies. There is also the neuroglial cyst. This is lined

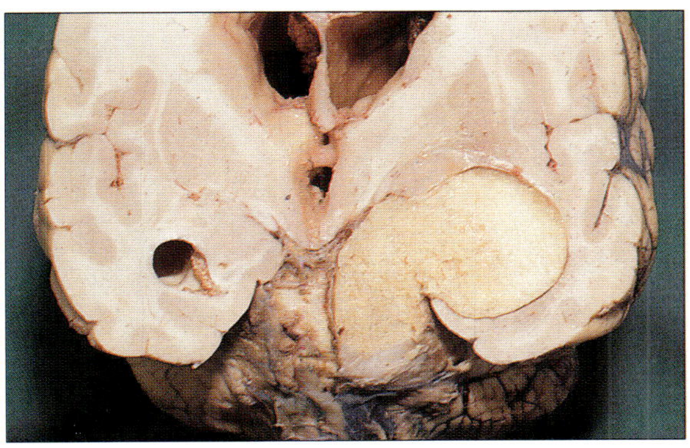

10.84 Male aged 27 years with a large epidermoid cyst arising at the base of the brain, which contains abundant yellow-white keratin. The cyst has displaced the temporal lobe, basal ganglia and adjacent structures on the left.

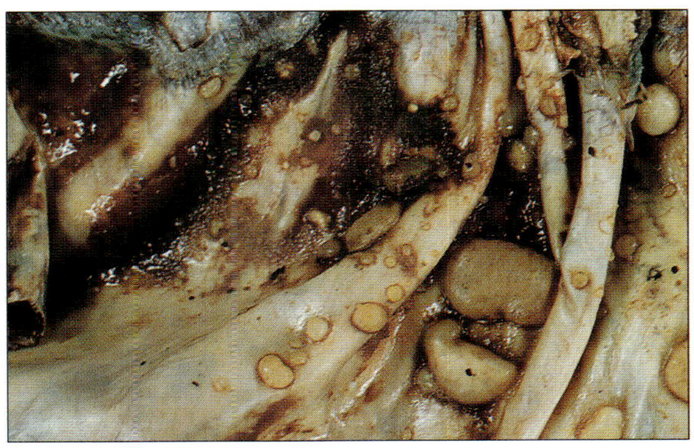

10.85 Male aged 62 years with a recurrent dermoid cyst, which ruptured into the subdural space, seeding cyst contents, and throughout the dura, which is studded by numerous small keratinous deposits.

by ependyma and may occur in the periventricular regions.

OTHER TUMOUR-LIKE STRUCTURES

Hypothalamic neural hamartoma

This non-neoplastic mass is composed of irregularly clustered neurons within a fibrillary glial stroma. Most of these lesions occur at the base of the brain and are attached to the floor of the third ventricle. In some cases, these lesions are associated with hypothalamic disturbances and endocrine imbalance. They tend to present in young children, occasionally causing precocious puberty.

Nasal glial heterotopia

This is a congenitally displaced mass of neural glial tissue in the paranasal regions. Sometimes, these lesions communicate with the brain through a defect in the skull base and represent an encephalocele.

LOCAL EXTENSIONS FROM REGIONAL TUMOURS

The brain and spinal cord may be directly invaded by a large number of tumours arising from surrounding structures. The commoner varieties include paraganglioma (chemodectoma), a neuroendocrine tumour arising in the middle ear or in the glomus jugulare. A chordoma is an uncommon bone tumour of notochordal origin usually presents in middle age. The commonest sites for chordomas are at the lower sacral region, compressing the spinal cord and cauda equina and in the region of the clivus, and leading to brainstem compression and cranial nerve palsies as the skull base is infiltrated. This is a lobulated tumour composed of vacuolated (physaliphorous) cells (**10.86**). On immunocytochemistry, these tumours give a positive reaction with antibodies to cytokeratins, epithelial membrane antigen, vimentin and S100 protein. These characteristic staining reactions and morphology usually allow a clear definition from a chondroma or chondrosarcoma, which may also arise in the skull or vertebral column.

Neoplasms arising from adjacent structures, e.g. the paranasal sinuses, orbit, and skeletal muscle, may secondarily invade and compress the CNS. Common examples of these lesions include the nasopharyngeal carcinoma, the adenoid cystic carcinoma (which exhibits perineural extension) and myelomas, plasmacytoma and lymphomas arising in the extradural tissues of the spinal cord.

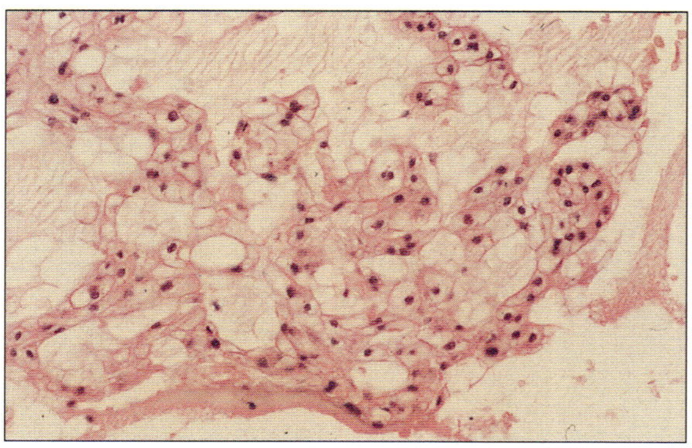

10.86 Histology of a chordoma arising at the skull base shows a population of physaliphorous tumour cells with extensive cytoplasmic vacuolation set in a loose myxoid stroma.

METASTATIC TUMOURS

Metastatic tumours to the CNS are common, and over the age of 65 years represent the commonest variety of intracerebral neoplasms. Metastases in children are uncommon, but the CNS is a well-recognised site

Incident cases of metastatic tumour diagnosed between January 1989 and December 1990 in southeast Scotland, UK

Primary site	Number of patients	Percentage (%)
Lung	135	54.2
Unknown	35	14
Breast	32	12.9
Melanoma	16	6.4
Gastrointestinal	10	4.1
Renal	6	2.4
Ovary, uterus, cervix	6	2.4
Bladder	4	1.6
Others	5	2

10.87 Incident cases of metastatic tumour diagnosed between January 1989 and December 1990 in southeast Scotland, UK.

for the relapse of acute lymphoblastic leukaemia. Most neoplasms metastasise to the CNS by the haematogenous route, though perineural spread and direct extension from adjacent tumours may also occur. The commonest tumours to metastasise to the CNS are listed in **10.87**. Many malignant tumours may spread to involve the CNS, including a wide range of carcinomas, leukaemias, lymphomas, sarcomas and malignant germ cell tumours.

Mestastases within the substance of the brain usually form multiple, irregularly rounded deposits, often at the junction between the grey and white matter in the cerebral hemispheres and deep grey matter structures (**10.88**). Central necrosis within these lesions is common, and there is often oedema and lymphocytosis in the surrounding grey and white matter (**10.89**). Secondary haemorrhage may occur within the metastases, particularly in cases of metastatic malignant melanoma (**10.90**). Metastases within the substance of the spinal cord are less common than intracerebral metastases.

Neoplastic cells may also invade the CSF pathway rather than producing a solid lesion within the substance of the brain or spinal cord. This results in a malignant meningitis (**10.91**), which is often associated with multiple cranial nerve palsies. Neoplastic cells may be identified on lumbar puncture and sometimes repeated punctures are required to yield a satisfactory population of well-preserved tumour cells (**10.92**). In the investigation of metastatic

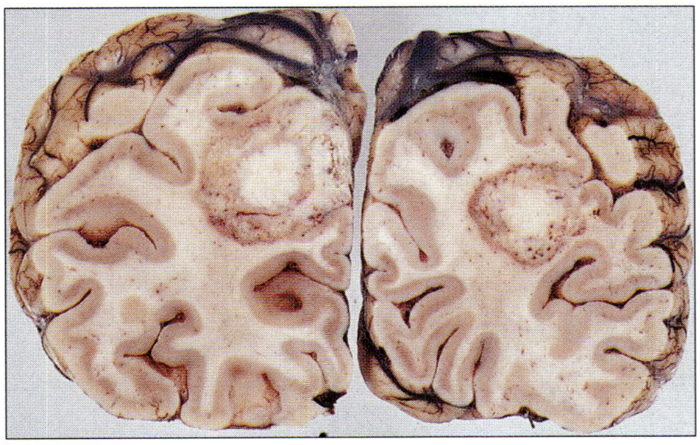

10.88 Male aged 78 years with a right bronchial carcinoma and cerebral metastases. The metastatic deposits are present bilaterally in the occipital lobes and show extensive central necrosis.

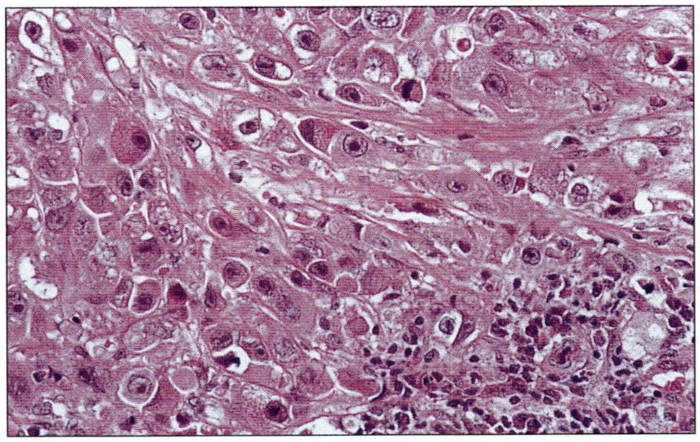

10.89 Histology of the metastatic tumours in **10.88** shows the appearances of a large-cell anaplastic carcinoma, containing mitotic figures and a chronic inflammatory cell infiltrate (top left).

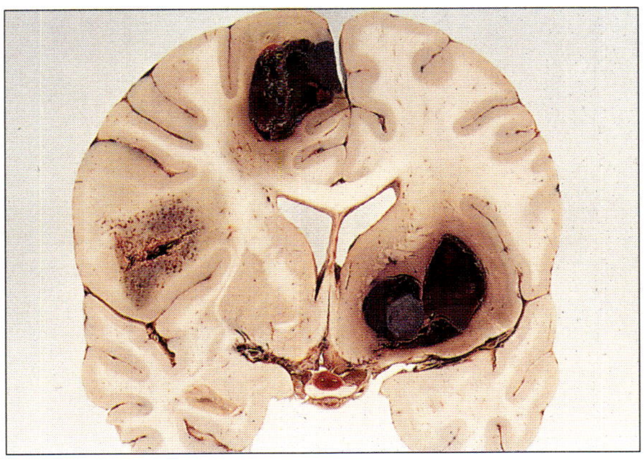

10.90 Female aged 52 years with multiple pigmented metastatic deposits from a malignant melanoma which are markedly haemorrhagic.

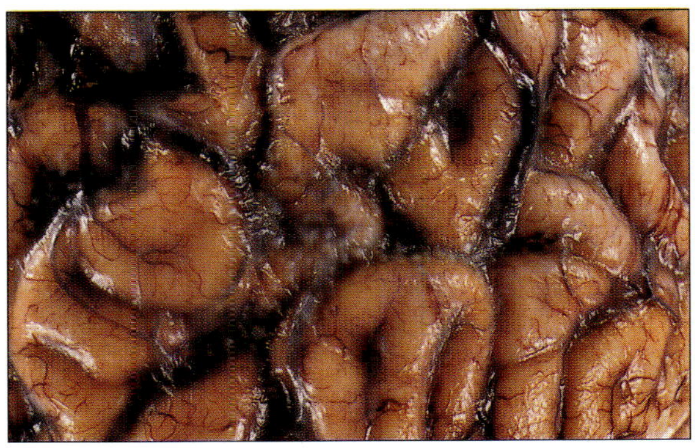

10.91 Female aged 52 years with metastatic breast carcinoma and carcinomatous meningitis. Numerous pale nodular aggregates of tumour cells are present in the subarachnoid space, with linear deposits outlining the smaller blood vessels.

carcinomas within the CSF, immunocytochemistry for epithelial markers including cytokeratins and epithelial membrane antigen is helpful in establishing a diagnosis (**10.93**). Systemic lymphomas and leukaemias may also invove the CSF pathway. Spinal cord compression may result from metastatic tumour deposits in the spinal epidural space (**10.94**) or bone (**10.95**). Solid spinal intradural metastases are uncommon. The prognosis for patients with either intraparenchymal or CSF metastases is very poor, and most patients die within six months of diagnosis. Occasional large solitary metastases can be surgically resected, resulting in symptomatic relief and often prolonging survival for several months.

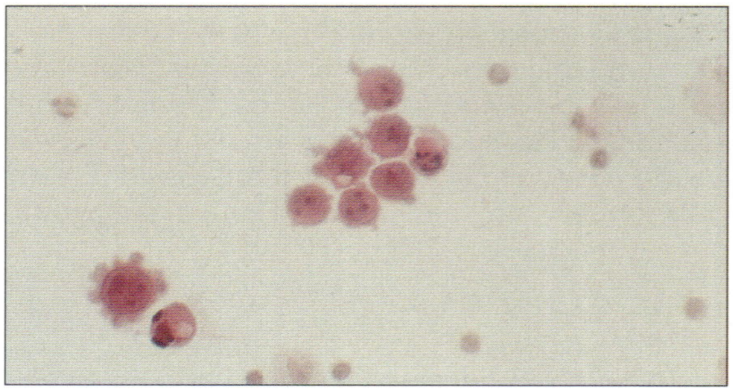

10.92 CSF cytology from the case illustrated in **10.91** shows numerous large malignant cells containing eosinophilic cytoplasm, occasional cytoplasmic vacuoles, and large irregular nuclei with multiple nucleoli. These appearances are characteristic of carcinomatous meningitis.

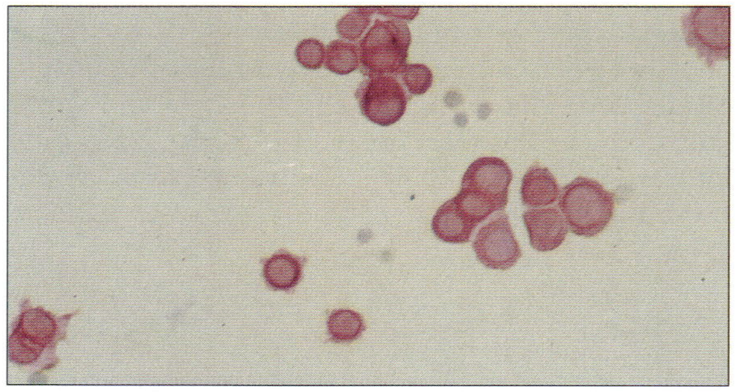

10.93 Immunocytochemistry for cytokeratins (CAM5.2) on CSF cytology from the case illustrated in **10.92** shows a brown positive reaction with the neoplastic cells, confirming the diagnosis of carcinomatous meningitis. Small lymphocytes are unstained.

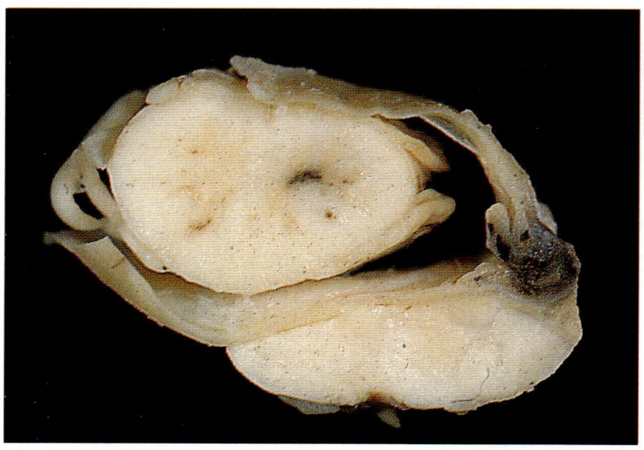

10.94 Male aged 52 years with spinal cord compression from an epidural myeloma.

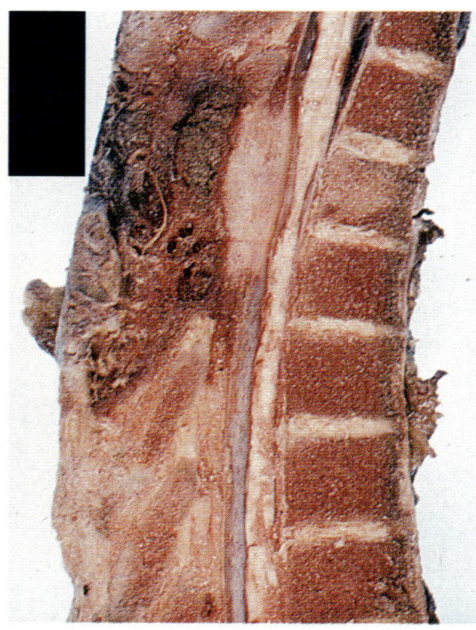

10.95 Male aged 69 years with spinal cord compression from vertebral collapse, as a result of multiple metastatic deposits from a transitional cell carcinoma in the bladder.

FURTHER READING

Burger PC, Scheithauer BW. AFIP *Atlas of Tumor Pathology. Central Nervous System. Series III.* Washington, Armed Forces Institute of Pathology, 1994.

Burger PC, Scheithauer BW, Vogel S. *Surgical Pathology of the Nervous System and its Coverings.* 3rd edn. New York, Churchill–Livingstone, 1991.

Daumas–Duport C, Scheithauer B, O'Fallon J, Kelly P. Grading of astrocytomas. A simple and reproducible method. *Cancer* 1988; **62**: 2152–2165.

Kleihues P, Burger PC, Scheithauer BW. *Histological Typing of Tumours of the Central Nervous System.* WHO Series. 2nd edn. Berlin, Springer-Verlag, 1993.

Russell DS, Rubinstein LJ. *Pathology of Tumours of the Nervous System.* 5th edn. London, Edward Arnold, 1989.

Weller RO. Tumours of the Nervous System. In: Weller, RO (ed). *Nervous System, Muscle and Eyes: Systemic Pathology.* 3rd edn. Vol. 4. Edinburgh, Churchill–Livingstone, 1990, pp 427–503.

INDEX

Numbers in bold print refer to captions and illustrations.